FOURTH EDITION

Therapeutic Modalities for Musculoskeletal Injuries

Craig R. Denegar, PhD, ATC, PT

Ethan Saliba, PhD, ATC, PT

Susan Saliba, PhD, ATC, PT

WITH

Michael Joseph, PhD, PT

AND

Kavin Tsang, PhD, ATC

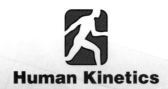

Human Kinetics

Library of Congress Cataloging-in-Publication Data

Denegar, Craig R., author.

Therapeutic modalities for musculoskeletal injuries / Craig R. Denegar, Ethan Saliba, Susan Saliba. -- Fourth edition.

   p. ; cm.

"With Michael Joseph and Kavin Tsang."

Includes bibliographical references and index.

I. Saliba, Ethan, 1956- , author. II. Saliba, Susan Foreman, 1963- , author. III. Title.

[DNLM: 1. Athletic Injuries--therapy. 2. Musculoskeletal System--injuries. 3. Pain--prevention & control. 4. Physical Therapy Modalities. 5. Rehabilitation--methods. QT 261]

RD97

617.1'027--dc23

2014041127

ISBN: 978-1-4504-6901-2 (print)

The web addresses cited in this text were current as of July 2015, unless otherwise noted.

Acquisitions Editor: Joshua J. Stone; **Developmental Editor:** Melissa J. Zavala; **Managing Editor:** Carly S. O'Connor; **Copyeditor:** Kevin Campbell; **Indexer:** Nancy Ball; **Permissions Manager:** Dalene Reeder; **Graphic Designer:** Fred Starbird; **Cover Designer:** Keith Blomberg; **Photograph (cover):** © Human Kinetics; **Photographer (interior):** Neil Bernstein, unless otherwise noted; **Photographs (interior):** © Human Kinetics, unless otherwise noted; **Visual Production Assistant:** Joyce Brumfield; **Photo Asset Manager:** Laura Fitch; **Photo Production Manager:** Jason Allen; **Art Manager:** Kelly Hendren; **Associate Art Manager:** Alan L. Wilborn; **Illustrations:** © Human Kinetics, unless otherwise noted; **Printer:** Walsworth

We thank the University of Virginia in Charlottesville, Virginia, for assistance in providing the location for the photo shoot for this book.

The video contents of this product are licensed for private home use and traditional, face-to-face classroom instruction only. For public performance licensing, please contact a sales representative at **www.HumanKinetics.com/SalesRepresentatives**.

Human Kinetics
1607 N. Market Street
Champaign, IL 61820
USA

United States and International
Website: **US.HumanKinetics.com**
Email: info@hkusa.com
Phone: 1-800-747-4457

Canada
Website: **Canada.HumanKinetics.com**
Email: info@hkcanada.com

Tell us what you think!
Human Kinetics would love to hear what we can do to improve the customer experience. Use this QR code to take our brief survey.

E6167

Contents

Part I
Principles of Therapeutic Modalities and Rehabilitation
1

Part II
Physiology of Pain and Injury
55

Part III
Electrical Modalities and Nerve Stimulation
123

Part VI
Mechanobiology, Exercise, and Manual Therapies
273

Part VII
Putting it All Together
325

Preface

The paradigm of evidence-based medicine has influenced the delivery of health care for more than 20 years. Central to this paradigm is the integration of the best available evidence in the care of each patient, from diagnosis to the documentation of the outcomes of treatment. In reality, the best available evidence is often insufficient to confidently identify the best diagnostic, evaluative, and treatment procedures or develop a prognosis. Moreover, critically appraising and comparing evidence from an increasingly deep volume of research can be a daunting task. The fourth edition of *Therapeutic Modalities for Musculoskeletal Injuries* provides updated basic and clinical research to guide informed management of common musculoskeletal conditions and build a foundation for lifelong learning.

As in previous editions, this revised text begins with an introduction to the application of therapeutic modalities in the context of evidence-based clinical practice (Part I: Principles of Therapeutic Modalities and Rehabilitation) followed by a strong foundation in injury, inflammation, repair, pain, and pain modulation (Part II: Physiology of Pain and Injury). The chapters that follow address the theory and application of common modalities. Part III (Electrical Modalities and Nerve Stimulation) examines the use of TENS for pain control, provides an extensive discussion of arthrogenic muscle inhibition, and then addresses neuromuscular electrical nerve stimulation.

The next two parts (IV and V) are devoted to a critical evaluation of the principles and applications of cold, superficial heat, ultrasound, electromagnetic fields and low-power laser. These chapters present the underlying theory and technologies and then go beyond addressing the laboratory studies of their effects to focus on the evidence for their effectiveness in clinical practice.

New to this edition is a chapter in mechanobiology, exercise, and mechanical loading as repair stimuli. The emerging field of mechanobiology offers us a new understanding of the effects of movement and activity on cell function and gene expression. Increasingly, mechanical stimuli are being recognized for their role in tissue homeostasis, tissue repair, and even pain sensation and percep-

tion. Understanding how cells receive and respond to external stimuli is essential to understanding and advancing recovery from musculoskeletal injury.

These new chapters, found in Part VI: Mechanobiology, Exercise, and Manual Therapies, take readers beyond the conventional view of exercise as a means of restoring function and enhancing performance into an understanding of how and why exercise is an essential component in the musculoskeletal tissue repair process.

Lastly, a new chapter of case reviews has been added to encourage you to integrate the basic science, clinical research, and clinical reasoning you will need to provide high-quality, cost-effective care in an increasingly complex health care system in which information technology plays an important role.

There are many additional features in this edition to help you understand and retain the content. Each chapter opens with objectives, and a scenario provides the context for the subject. Throughout the chapters, many terms are set apart as key terms, and definitions are provided in the glossary. Sidebars illustrate the applications of concepts in clinical practice. Each chapter concludes with a summary of the content and a Key Concepts and Review section that shows how each objective was supported by the chapter's content. A thorough set of references is provided.

For instructors, the test package, instructor guide, and image bank will help you present the topics covered in this book. The test package includes hundreds of true-or-false, multiple-choice, and fill-in-the-blank questions that you can use to build or supplement tests and quizzes. The instructor guide includes a sample syllabus as well as chapter summaries, chapter objectives, lecture outlines, and activities. The PowerPoint includes more than 380 slides. The image bank contains most of the figures, tables, and content photos, which you can then use to build lecture notes, PowerPoint presentations, or other lecture and learning materials. You can

eBook
available at
your campus bookstore
or HumanKinetics.com

find these ancillaries at www.HumanKinetics.com/ TherapeuticModalitiesforMusculoskeletalInjuries.

New to this edition is an online video with 21 clips demonstrating practical applications of various treatment modalities so that students may learn how to appropriately and accurately apply modalities for therapy. Exercises included in the online video are highlighted by this icon:

Information on accessing the online video is on page xi.

Each author has experienced enormous changes in practice resulting from advances in basic science and the integration of high-quality research into clinical practice. This edition reflects our ongoing pursuit of knowledge that improves the care provided to our patients. We hope that your journey as a health care professional is as long and fascinating as ours has been and that our text sets you on the path to success.

Accessing the Online Video

New to this edition is high-definition online streaming video. The video clips demonstrate the application of 21 various treatment modalities discussed throughout the book. The online video can be accessed by visiting www.HumanKinetics .com/TherapeuticModalitiesforMusculoskeletal Injuries. If you purchased a new print book, follow the directions included on the orange-framed page at the front of your book. That page includes access steps and the unique key code that you'll need the first time you visit the *Therapeutic Modalities for Musculoskeletal Injuries* website. If you purchased an e-book from HumanKinetics.com, follow the access instructions that were e-mailed to you following your purchase.

Once at the *Therapeutic Modalities for Musculoskeletal Injuries* website, select Online Video in the ancillary items box in the upper left corner of the screen. You'll then see an Online Video page with a description about the video. Select the link to open the online video.

You will now be taken to a web page with three buttons for the seven chapters that feature video. Select the button for the chapter you want. Once you select a chapter button, you'll see a video player. The video numbers along the right side of the player correspond with video number cross-references in the book, and the title under the player corresponds with the exercise title in the book. Scroll through the list of clips until you find the video you want to watch. Select that clip and the full video will play.

Here are the therapeutic modalities supported by online video:

Chapter 8

Video 8.1   Setup of a multi-modality device

Video 8.2   Demonstration of motor TENS

Video 8.3   Using a TENS device at home

Video 8.4   Application of interferential current

Chapter 9

Video 9.1   Progression of NMES with volitional effort

Video 9.2   Demonstration of NMES stimulation protocol for the quadriceps using the Russian stimulator

Chapter 11

Video 11.1   Demonstration of cryokinetics for an ankle sprain

Video 11.2   Demonstration of the clinical application of a hydrocollator pack

Video 11.3   Demonstration of proper home application of a heating pad

Chapter 13

Video 13.1   Use of ultrasound on an anterior elbow

Video 13.2   Use of ultrasound on an ankle

Chapter 15

Video 15.1   Application of a laser treatment to the Achilles tendon

Video 15.2   Application of laser for treatment of carpal tunnel symptoms

Chapter 17

Video 17.1   Demonstration of eccentric loading on the Achilles tendon

Video 17.2   Demonstration of eccentric loading for patellar tendinopathy

Chapter 18

Video 18.1   Demonstration of cross-friction massage

Video 18.2   Demonstration of myofascial release

Video 18.3   Demonstration of strain–counterstrain technique

Video 18.4   Demonstration of joint mobilization

Video 18.5   Demonstration of the muscle energy technique on the sacroiliac joint

Video 18.6   Demonstration of manual cervical traction

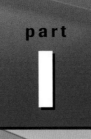
Principles of Therapeutic Modalities and Rehabilitation

Part I provides an overview of the use of therapeutic modalities in the context of a comprehensive plan of care for musculoskeletal injuries. Key steps in a progression from injury to return to play and work are identified, and regulations related to modality application are reviewed. Injury and illness are not simply physical ailments. The patient's psychological responses must be considered in order to individualize care and optimize outcomes. Strategies are identified to maximize compliance with a plan of care and to remove barriers to success.

An ever-growing body of research is available to help clinicians and patients to make sound plan-of-care decisions and guide optimal treatment applications. Part I introduces the skills needed for locating and critically appraising research so that decisions and techniques are based on the best available information. The paradigm of evidence-based care is no longer novel, nor is it static. The delivery of efficient, patient-centered care requires clinicians to learn the patients' preferences and goals, tap their clinical experiences to individualize care, and use the best available research in practice. Part I spans these critical components in the context of the use of therapeutic modalities in clinical practice.

Fundamentals of Therapeutic Modalities

OBJECTIVES

After reading this chapter, you will be able to

1. discuss how an evidence-based approach to health care affects the use of therapeutic modalities;

2. discuss how regulation of health care may influence the use of therapeutic modalities in the care of physically active individuals;

3. identify the varying groups of therapeutic modalities and their purposes;

4. describe the principles of physics that affect energy transfer and how they affect the application of therapeutic modalities;

5. identify the hierarchy of components in a progressive rehabilitation plan; and

6. discuss guidelines for guiding an athlete through a comprehensive plan of care.

It is your first day working as a certified athletic trainer for a sports medicine clinic. Your position primarily involves service to a local high school but also involves a few hours in the clinic each morning. A varsity football player for the high school sprained his ankle on the first day of practice yesterday. The team physician has evaluated the injury and referred the athlete to the clinic for treatment.

Questions arise, and the answers lead to more questions. What will be the plan of care for this injured athlete (i.e., short- and long-term treatment goals)? Can therapeutic modalities be used to achieve any of these goals? You identify pain control, restoration of range of motion, and return to full weight bearing as goals to be achieved within 7 to 10 days, and you choose therapeutic modalities that include cold and transcutaneous electrical nerve stimulation (TENS). Can you, as a certified athletic trainer, administer these modalities to this athlete in the sports medicine clinic? Who has the answers?

Chapter 1 introduces a progressive rehabilitation paradigm from which treatment goals can be developed. The chapter also discusses basic legal issues, including negligence and the regulation of practice, that affect the use of therapeutic modalities by athletic trainers and physical therapists.

The use of therapeutic modalities or physical agents in the treatment of human ailments is not new. Massage, "cupping" (applying heated shells over painful areas), and the use of electric eels are mentioned in the archives of early Greek and Roman cultures. However, there was little scientific evidence to support those early treatments. Today, the use of therapeutic modalities in patient care is primarily undertaken by providers whose professional origins date back less than 100 years, physical therapists and athletic trainers (figure 1.1). Although other medical and allied medical care providers, such as physicians, chiropractors, podiatrists, and dentists, may apply therapeutic modalities, this happens to a lesser degree. Experts in athletic training and physical therapy have significantly contributed to the collective knowledge of therapeutic modalities through writing and research.

Therapeutic modality literally means a device or apparatus that has curative powers. Heat, cold, massage, ultrasound, and **diathermy** have been used by health care practitioners for many years. Perhaps these treatments are better classified as **physical agents**, that is, treatments that cause some change to the body. The scientific basis for their use has grown stronger over time, giving us a better understanding of how modality applications may help injured patients achieve treatment goals and return to normal activity, including sport and work.

A CONTEMPORARY VIEW

Sackett (Sackett et al. 2000, p. 1) described an evidence-based approach to clinical practice as the "integration of best research evidence with clinical expertise and patient values." The use of therapeutic modalities in patient health care should follow the same principles. However, there is often little evidence that the application of a therapeutic modality improves treatment outcomes or hastens the return to active function. Complicating the matter are those clinicians who adhere to "menu-driven" protocols or adopt practices based on the rationale of "that's how it has always been done." These hurdles should not discourage the use of therapeutic modalities but rather highlight the importance of clinicians' being

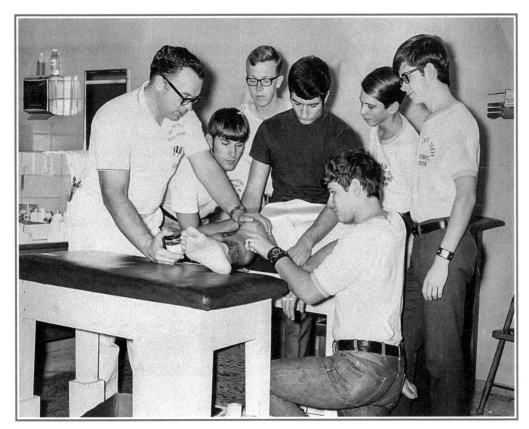

Figure 1.1   An early athletic training room.

Photo courtesy of Minnesota State University Mankato.

well educated and up to date on current research, approaching patients and their condition individually, and setting goals for the use of modalities.

The health care system is ever changing, and all providers are under increasing scrutiny to demonstrate improved patient outcomes and cost-effectiveness. To effectively use therapeutic modalities to treat physically active individuals and other patients, health care providers must stay current and follow evidence-based practices. Our collective understanding of the physics of therapeutic modalities, the physiological responses to therapeutic modalities, and the clinical benefits of these modalities is continually evolving. Researchers are exploring how to best use therapeutic modalities. As we learn more, clinical practices change, which benefits health care professionals and patients alike.

The theoretical basis for the application of therapeutic modalities after musculoskeletal injuries continues to evolve, but the rationale for clinical use has often been based on "logical argument" or empirical value. In the last two decades, however, a model of evidence-based practice in health care has emerged. Databases have been developed to provide clinicians rapid access to reports of clinical trials,

including the application of therapeutic modalities for the treatment of several musculoskeletal disorders. Information gathered from new research on the evolution of **evidence-based health care** is integrated into this text. This topic is discussed in greater detail in chapter 3.

Much has been learned about how therapeutic modalities affect the body; over the last 70 years, cold agents, therapeutic ultrasound, diathermy, and the

Challenges for Certified Athletic Trainers

The practice of athletic training is recognized through state credentialing and the establishment of **practice acts**. Although practice acts define what is within a scope of practice, these documents do not define when an intervention is appropriate. It is critical that educators, as well as practicing clinicians, value and use the best available science to safely and effectively integrate therapeutic modalities with patient care.

therapeutic use of electricity have been developed. The efficacy of many therapeutic modalities has been supported through research on physiological responses to various physical agents. Current research efforts are focused on examining the clinical outcomes of integrating therapeutic modalities into the plan of care. Until more is discovered through research, health care providers must integrate sound theory, clinical observations, and research evidence to guide their use of therapeutic modalities in clinical practice.

Deciding to Use Modalities

The selection of any health intervention, including those related to the use of therapeutic modalities, should be purposeful and goal directed; this theme will resonate throughout this text. In recommending a plan of care, the clinician must evaluate the efficacy and benefits while also weighing the risks of each intervention under consideration. The first and only hard rule is "do no harm." Clinical research, when available, and clinician experiences and expertise will influence judgments about one treatment versus another. Specific indications for each modality are identified in the chapter on that modality.

Of equal importance in choosing a treatment are the patient's beliefs, preferences, and values. The patient's perspective is important for several reasons. Patients who have had positive experiences with certain treatments may seek interventions in which they have confidence, and they may wish to avoid those they perceive as having no benefit. As discussed in chapter 2, confidence in the clinician and belief in the effectiveness of a treatment will affect the patient's cognitive appraisal, emotional response, and adherence to rehabilitation. Without doubt, placebo (literally meaning "to please") plays a role in treatment responses. Time, cost, and risk of adverse responses, along with evidence of treatment effectiveness, are weighed in making clinical recommendations. However, if a placebo fosters perceptions of benefit and ultimately a positive outcome of care, so be it. Conversely, a belief that a treatment is not beneficial may become a self-fulfilling prophecy.

Patients may choose not to comply with instructions for medication use, therapeutic exercise, and other types of self-care. Adherence to treatment recommendations is a concern across health care; in chapter 2 we identify strategies designed to improve adherence to rehabilitation. Adherence can be improved when patients are involved in program design (e.g., establishing goals) and when they understand the nature of their problem, the reasons for each element in a plan of care, and their role in the treatment and recovery process. When a clinician proposes the use of a therapeutic modality, the patient deserves to know what the clinician believes will be achieved through the treatment. The patient should also be informed of what to expect during and after the treatment and should appreciate the possible consequences of refusing the treatment or choosing a different intervention. This can best be accomplished by establishing a positive rapport by recognizing the whole patient rather than just the injury that is being treated.

Concerns When Using Modalities

Although therapeutic modalities are applied to make injured individuals more comfortable and speed rehabilitation, these treatments can also cause harm. Before applying any therapeutic agent, be sure that the equipment is in proper working order. Make sure that any electrical equipment such as a whirlpool is powered by a circuit served by a ground fault interrupter, and identify known contraindications or conditions that warrant special caution. Specific contraindications and cautions for each modality are identified in its respective chapter.

Types of Modalities

Therapeutic modalities can be classified or grouped based on the form of energy used: thermal, electrical, acoustical, electromagnetic, or mechanical. Exchange of *thermal energy* occurs with ice packs, cold or warm water immersion, and moist heat packs. *Electrical energy* that stimulates biological tissues is used in various waveforms of TENS, high-volt, or interferential currents. Effects of *sound energy* (based on the acoustical spectrum) are achieved with ultrasound and extracorporeal shockwave therapy. *Electromagnetic energy* is used with shortwave diathermy, low-level lasers, infrared lamps, and ultraviolet lights. *Mechanical energy* is applied through intermittent compression devices, traction units, and manual massage.

Depending on the form of energy, different physiological actions may be achieved. Cold removes heat or thermal energy from the body, while diathermy adds to it. Electrical energy is most commonly used to stimulate or depolarize neurological tissue. Some forms of energy can also create different effects based on their application parameters. For instance, sound energy can be adjusted to achieve thermal or nonthermal effects. Improper energy exchange may harm the patient (e.g., pain from stimulation of nociceptive fibers or scalding the skin). Therefore, the clinician must have a sound understanding of the type of energy used by the modality as well as the parameters for operating it.

- Thermal energy is used to increase or decrease tissue temperature. Thermotherapy adds energy to tissue and increases its temperature while **cryotherapy** removes energy from tissue and decreases its temperature. Cold and superficial heat modalities are discussed in chapters 10 and 11.

- Electrical energy is used to depolarize neural tissue to modulate pain or produce muscle contractions, to produce local chemical changes by eliciting ion movement, or to facilitate tissue and bone healing. Electrical stimulation modalities are discussed in chapters 7-9.

- Mechanical energy is generally used to create motion in a body segment or area. This can be achieved by mechanical or manual means. Manual and mechanical therapies are discussed in chapters 16-18.

- Acoustical energy is most commonly used to increase tissue temperature, but nonthermal effects may also be attained. Therapeutic ultrasound is discussed in chapters 12 and 13.

- Electromagnetic energy is generally used to increase tissue temperature. Although some applications of electromagnetic energy are for the purpose of damaging tissue (such as sterilization with UV light), this is beyond the scope of most therapeutic applications. Diathermy and low-level laser therapy are discussed in chapters 12, 13, 14, and 15.

Principles of Energy Exchange

Therapeutic modalities create physiological change by means of an exchange of energy to or from the body. Energy exchange is guided by varying the following:

- *How much.* The *Arndt-Schultz principle* states no reactions or changes will occur in body tissues if the amount of energy is insufficient to stimulate the target structure and too much energy will actually be detrimental to the tissues. In addition, the *law of Grotthus-Draper* describes the inverse relationship between energy absorption and penetration; energy that is absorbed by superficial tissues is not available to be transmitted to deeper layers. Conversely, energy that is not reflected or absorbed at superficial levels will be transmitted to deeper tissues. Mechanisms of energy exchange are subject to various principles of physics, which determine if energy is reflected, transmitted, refracted, or absorbed.

- *The distance between.* The *inverse-square law* implies that the amount of energy transfer varies inversely with the square of the distance between the two objects, the modality and the body (figure 1.2); the greater the distance, the lower the amount of energy transfer. For example, if a lamp were lowered from 60 cm above the skin to 30 cm, the distance would be reduced by 1/2. The inverse of 1/2 is 2, and the square of 2 is 4. Thus, the heating effect is

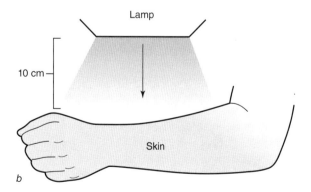

Figure 1.2 The inverse-square law: *(a)* Heating effect equals x. *(b)* When the distance between the lamp and the skin is reduced by half, the heating effect is increased to $4x$ (the inverse of 1/2 equals 2, and 2^2 equals 4).

increased fourfold when the height of the lamp is reduced by 1/2.

• *The angle between.* The *cosine law* states that energy exchange varies with the cosine of the angle formed between the beam of energy and the perpendicular (figure 1.3); the greater the angle, the less the amount of energy transfer. This relationship assumes that the energy strikes the skin perpendicularly; if the energy strikes the skin at an angle, some is reflected, reducing the overall effect. For example, if ultrasound waves form a 30° angle with the perpendicular, the reduction in acoustical effects is calculated by multiplying the cosine of 30°, which is 0.86. Thus, only 86% as much effect occurs when sound waves strike a surface at an angle 30° from perpendicular as when they strike perpendicular to the surface. In other words, the effect is reduced 14%.

• *The difference between.* A gradient is established by the difference in energy possessed by the two sources, the body and the modality. The gradient describes the direction as well as the rate of energy exchange. Energy will move from the higher source to the lower source; hence energy transfer occurs from the therapeutic modality to the body, except in the case of cold modalities, where the body has a higher source of energy than the modality. The magnitude of difference between the two sources will affect the rate of energy transfer; the larger the difference, the greater the rate of exchange. For example, the body will exchange energy more quickly with a whirlpool circulating water that is 30° lower than body temperature than with one that is only 5° lower. In addition, the latter would result in a smaller amount of change in tissue temperature.

• *How long.* The duration of application is more a treatment parameter than a principle, but it can affect the amount of energy transfer based on the previously identified principles. In general, the longer the application period, the more energy transfer will occur. The amount of time for modality application should be adjusted (usually increased) to accommodate applications, as they vary based on the inverse-square law or cosine square law. For example, performing ultrasound through a bladder will result in a decreased amount of energy transfer (as compared to direct contact with the skin); therefore the treatment time should be extended. While there is no exact correlation or algorithm between time adjustment and differences in each principle, the general concept should be considered when applying therapeutic modalities.

LEGAL ASPECTS OF THERAPEUTIC MODALITY APPLICATION: PRACTICE ACTS AND NEGLIGENT TREATMENT

Recognition of the profession and higher educational standards influence the practice of athletic training. Athletic training has been recognized as a distinct allied medical profession in most states through the development of practice acts and state credentialing. As recognition and regulation varies, it is prudent

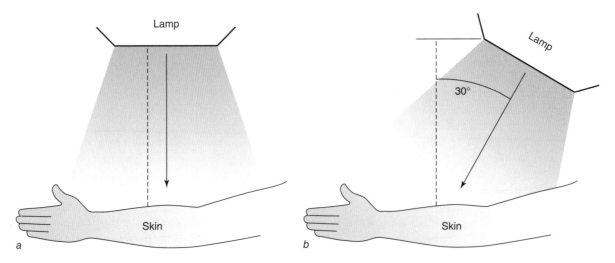

Figure 1.3 The cosine law: *(a)* The heating effect equals *x*. The angle of the light does not deviate (= 0°) from the vertical. The cosine of 0 equals 1; thus, the heating effect equals 1*x*. *(b)* The light strikes the skin at a 30° angle. The cosine of 30° is 0.86. Thus, the heating effect is only 86% of the effect of light beaming straight down.

for athletic trainers to be cognizant of the standards established in the state in which they practice.

Changes in athletic training regulation and the education of athletic trainers also have elevated the standard of care expected from certified athletic trainers. Before the days of certification by the National Athletic Trainers' Association (NATA), there was no standard by which to judge athletic trainers' actions. Today, certification by the Board of Certification, Inc. (BOC) for athletic trainers, recognition of athletic training as a profession by individual states through licensure or certification, and higher educational standards have defined the standards of athletic training and elevated levels of practice. Failure to practice according to these standards, including causing injury by improper application of therapeutic modalities, may constitute negligence.

Athletic trainer certification by the BOC is determined by an examination that tests the applicant's knowledge and skills in preventing, recognizing, treating, and rehabilitating athletic injuries as well as performing administrative aspects of athletic training. A standard of preparation for the certified athletic trainer has been established through the examination.

Therapeutic modalities are addressed in a subsection of *Athletic Training Education Competencies, Fifth Edition* (NATA 2011). Through education and supervised clinical experience, the athletic trainer learns how and when to apply therapeutic modalities and then demonstrates the associated knowledge and skills during the certification examination. The certified athletic trainer has met established standards to practice athletic training and to use therapeutic modalities. One might then assume that a certified athletic trainer's practice is governed by the National Athletic Trainers' Association's *Code of Ethics* (NATA 2005), the *Role Delineation Study/Practice Analysis, Sixth Edition* (BOC 2010), and the *Athletic Training Education Competencies, Fifth Edition* (NATA 2011); however, this assumption is incorrect.

Practice acts and state credentialing regulate the utilization of therapeutic modalities with patient health care. Health care providers must comply with regulations set forth by the state in which they practice, including regulations that affect which therapeutic modalities may be applied, to whom the treatment can be administered, and the setting in which the treatment may be rendered. The various agencies responsible for regulating health care practice can provide or direct the clinician to the relevant practice act. These materials may also be available through the health care provider's state associations or societies.

Other medical and legal considerations relate in general to the use of therapeutic modalities. This text is not intended to cover all legal and administrative aspects of health care, but two issues closely related to the application of therapeutic modalities are covered, informed consent and liability in tort.

Challenges for Athletic Trainers

The Commission for Accreditation of Athletic Training Education (CAATE) has established criteria for accreditation of educational programs that include preparation in the knowledge and use of therapeutic modalities. The examination administered by the BOC assesses this preparation. The BOC further requires evidence of continuing education to maintain certification. Although an athletic trainer may be well qualified to use a specific therapeutic modality or administer a particular treatment, individual state laws specify what the athletic trainer may legally do. Moreover, in states that do not regulate the practice of athletic training, the application of a modality may infringe upon the practice of other disciplines as defined in that state. The athletic trainer must understand and practice within the boundaries of the state's practice act. Failure to do so may lead to revocation of a state license or certification and loss of practice privileges or charges of practicing another discipline without proper credentials.

A review of regulations of all states is beyond the scope of this text. In addition, regulations may change. This text and the instruction provided are intended to develop knowledge and skills related to the clinical competencies established by the profession. It is the responsibility of athletic trainers to learn the laws of the state they practice in and how these laws affect what they can do and who they can treat.

Informed Consent

Informed consent refers to the right of patients to receive information about their diagnosis and treatment options and to grant consent to receive treatment. In some settings, there are no formal policies about informed consent for modality application or participation in therapeutic exercises. Informed consent is often viewed simply as forms that have to be completed before treatment or a formality. Nothing could be further from the truth. Often parental consent to provide immediate treatment of injuries (used by schools and sport programs) is misconstrued as informed consent. Furthermore, although people who enter a clinic routinely sign forms giving health care providers permission to treat them, these forms often do not include informed consent for specific treatments.

The components of informed consent as described by Scott (1990) are presented in the next paragraph. Items 2 through 5 are directly related to the application of therapeutic modalities. This text describes the physical and physiological principles of modality application, the mechanisms by which the therapeutic benefits of modalities are achieved, and the contraindications and precautions for

modality use. With this information, the clinician can in turn provide patients with information they need to make informed decisions about their health care. We believe that clinicians can establish a positive rapport with their patients by adopting a policy of discussing expectations during each treatment session. This practice will fulfill the requirements of informed consent, but just as important, it will affect the patient's cognitive appraisal and contribute to better adherence to the rehabilitation program.

Components of Informed Consent

The injured physically active person should be informed of the following:

1. The diagnosis or findings of a physical examination
2. The recommended treatment procedures and rehabilitation plan
3. The prognosis if the recommended treatment is administered or rehabilitation plan completed
4. The risks and benefits of the recommended treatment and rehabilitation plan

Challenges for Athletic Trainers

Often a bond of trust exists between the physically active individual and the athletic trainer, whereby the individual believes that the athletic trainer will provide the best possible care. Additionally, the injured person may have observed treatments administered to others and may know what to expect. Failure to receive consent prior to treatment does not routinely lead to litigation against an athletic trainer. However, the athletic trainer should not ignore this issue. Make it a habit to explain any proposed treatment to the injured person and provide an opportunity for questions. This facilitates communication in the sports medicine clinic, where the injured person is encountering an unfamiliar health care facility and providers. It is also good practice in the athletic training room, where explaining the rehabilitation plan and proposed treatments engages the injured individual and allows the athletic trainer to review his or her responsibilities in the rehabilitation plan (figure 1.4).

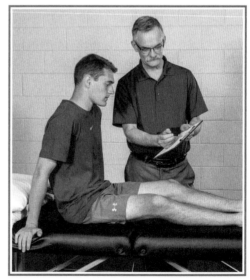

Figure 1.4 Explaining the rehabilitation plan and proposed treatments allows the clinician to review his or her own responsibilities as well as inform the injured individual.

5. Reasonable alternatives to the proposed treatment and rehabilitation plan, with the potential risks, benefits, and prognosis

6. The prognosis if no treatment is administered or rehabilitation completed

This article was published in *Professional ethics: A guide for rehabilitation professions*, R.W. Scott, pgs. 60, Copyright 1998, with permission from Elsevier.

Liability in Tort for Negligent Treatment and Professional Negligence

A **tort** is a private, civil legal action brought by an injured party (in this case, the patient), or the party's representative, to redress an injury caused by another person (in this case, the care provider). **Negligence** entails doing something that an ordinary person under like circumstances would not have done (a negligent act or an act of commission), or failing to do something that an ordinary, reasonable, prudent person would have done under similar circumstances (a negligent action or an act of omission). This general definition can be more clearly focused if *ordinary person* is replaced with *health care provider*. The professional standards established through national certification, the *Code of Ethics* and Standards of Practice, and state regulation have created a level of expectation for health care services.

When a health care provider fails to act appropriately or acts inappropriately in providing services and injures someone, the clinician may be found negligent in tort. In relation to the application of therapeutic modalities, negligence in tort is likely to involve a negligent act. The clinician is responsible for ensuring that the equipment used to apply modalities is properly maintained and calibrated and is in good working order, and that the modalities are applied in a manner that does not harm the patient. Negligent acts include burns caused by a moist heat pack with too little toweling for insulation, cold-induced nerve injury caused by inadequate instructions for applying ice packs at home, and electrical shock caused by faulty wiring on a poorly maintained transcutaneous electrical nerve stimulator. The health care provider must recognize when the application of a modality is contraindicated, must know how to apply a modality safely, and must instruct the individual properly if he or she is to self-administer a modality. Failure to do any of these things may constitute negligence if harm occurs with the use of a therapeutic modality.

REHABILITATION PLAN OF CARE

The treatment of physically active patients requires a team approach because no single health care provider has all of the skills and resources needed for guiding the patient through rehabilitation. The rehabilitation plan of care is founded on the medical diagnosis provided by the physician and the physical examination of the injured patient by the clinician. The medical diagnosis is critical to determining whether surgery is necessary, to determining whether medications are indicated, and to estimating the rate of progression that the healing tissues will tolerate.

In establishing a plan of care for recovery, the physician, clinician, and patient must identify specific short-term goals. A medical diagnosis may be a grade II lateral ankle sprain. However, the rehabilitation plan of care addresses not the lateral ankle sprain but the pain, loss of motion, loss of strength, decreased **neuromuscular control**, and inability to fully bear weight, walk, run, jump, cut, or play basketball—in other words, the **signs**, **symptoms**, **impairments**, disabilities, and handicaps resulting from the injury. Clinicians must also identify factors that may limit adherence to rehabilitation, including the patient's psychological-emotional response to the injury. Finally, the short-term goals that are established to address specific needs such as pain control or improved neuromuscular control must be tied to the individual's achievement of long-term goals. Thus, the medical diagnosis is only part of determining the best approach to rehabilitation.

Developing a rehabilitation plan of care may sound difficult; however, some basic concepts make the process much easier. First, a basic rehabilitation model should be used as the framework for the plan of care. Second, the plan of care must address the problems identified in the physical examination; thus, a plan of care is *individualized*. Third, the plan of care should be progressive, with clearly identified performance or time-specified criteria for progression to more complex and challenging activities.

Clinicians generally agree on the order of priorities in a progressive rehabilitation plan of care. The model presented in figure 1.5 provides a guide to progression of a rehabilitation plan of care. After a complete clinical examination, the first priority in all health care is to do no harm. It is necessary to protect injured tissues from further damage and to allow for healing and the restoration of tissue

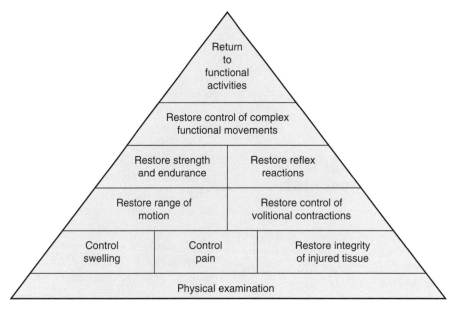

Figure 1.5   A progressive model for rehabilitation of physically active individuals.

Reprinted, by permission, from J. Hertel and C.R. Denegar, 1998, "A rehabilitation paradigm for restoring neuromuscular control following athletics injury," *Athletic therapy today* September 3(5): 13.

integrity. The control of pain and swelling is also a high priority early in the rehabilitation process. Pain is one of the worst of human experiences; it makes us miserable, affects sleep, and alters neuromuscular control and function. Once a diagnosis is established, pain has served its purpose (warning the person that something is wrong) and should be alleviated to the greatest degree possible.

Injury and inflammation result in swelling, muscle guarding, and loss of motion. Once the certified athletic trainer is assured that damaged tissues have been properly protected and pain and swelling have been addressed, attention is given to restoring range of motion about the involved joints. Functional recovery usually requires normal amounts of joint range of motion.

In addition to working to restore motion lost due to injury, the clinician must work to restore neuromuscular control and muscular endurance (neuromuscular control is discussed in greater detail in chapters 7, 9, and 10). Pain, swelling, and joint instability change the way the nervous system coordinates muscle contractions. Neuromuscular control and muscular endurance must be reestablished so the patient can perform the low-resistance, high-repetition activities that are the foundation of muscular power and strength training.

As the injured athlete recovers, the rehabilitation plan progresses to address losses of strength and power and muscular endurance. *Strength* is the ability

to do work, whereas *power* is a measure of the rate at which the work is done. Success in physical activity including sports requires muscular strength and power. Generally, strength is addressed first with slow, controlled exercises. Power training is then added through plyometric exercises, sprinting, and other rapid movement training. In most sports, repeated or sustained muscular activity is required. Thus, *endurance*, or the ability to repeat and sustain activity, must also be retrained.

Finally, the activity-specific needs of the patient must be met. The functional requirements, much like the endurance requirements, differ among activities, sports, positions, and events. A basketball player who can run, jump, and cut may not be ready to return to the game because of an inability to backpedal, a football player may not be ready to return to the offensive line because of poor footwork, or the loading dock employee may not be able to return to work because he cannot climb in and out of the forklift. Each activity and sport places unique demands on the body. As a rehabilitation plan of care progresses, it should become more specific to the demands of the individual's activities.

Therapeutic modalities are most commonly used to alleviate pain and allow patients to initiate therapeutic exercises to improve range of motion and regain neuromuscular control. The clinician should understand how the modality affects the body and the rationale for each modality application. Modality application is not an all-inclusive treatment or cure, but a passive intervention that enables patients to meet specific, short-term rehabilitation goals.

In addition to working toward specific goals related to the injury, the health care team must also strive to maintain the patient's overall fitness level. Exercise to maintain cardiovascular fitness and strength should be incorporated into the rehabilitation plan as soon as it is safe to do so. Stationary cycling, stair climbing, aquatic exercising, and circuit training can be used to maintain fitness while protecting healing tissues, and they can provide some variety in the injured person's routine. Physically active individuals also experience a withdrawal phenomenon when their regular physical exercise routine is disrupted by injury. Including safe aerobic exercise and weight training in the rehabilitation plan helps individuals cope with this disruption. Figure 1.6 provides an example of an individualized plan of care.

Monitoring Progress

Progress implies change. A team physician we once worked with was fond of saying, "If things do not stay the same they will get better or worse." There are many potential pitfalls in evaluating and rehabilitating injured persons. Incomplete diagnoses, poor adherence to the plan of care, and excessive activity

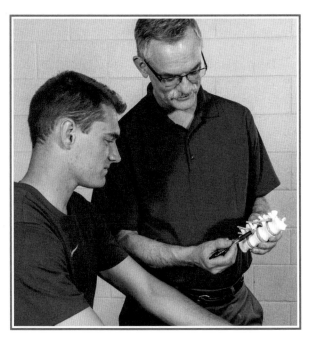

Figure 1.6 A plan of care is individualized with clear criteria to check progress toward more complex and challenging activities and recovery.

can slow or prevent recovery from injury and return to full activity. The health care team must monitor an individual's progress during rehabilitation, discouraging excessive or inappropriate activities and adding challenging activities when appropriate.

Two factors guide progression. The first is tissue healing. In some cases, such as fractures and anterior cruciate ligament reconstruction, the time the body needs to repair the tissues is relatively well established. Although pain is often a reasonable guide for exercise progression, the physician may specify a time frame of restricted activity to allow for substantial tissue repair. The second factor is successful completion of short-term goals related to the earlier stages of rehabilitation. If healing tissues are adequately protected, the initial short-term goals will be based on the first three rehabilitation priorities. For example, after a lateral ankle sprain there may be a considerable amount of pain. Appropriate short-term goals may include reducing pain to a rating of 2 (on a scale of 0 = *no pain*, 10 = *worst pain imaginable*) at rest in 2 days and a rating of 2 in full weight bearing in 1 week. If range of motion is lost, restoring full ankle range of motion in 10 days is a reasonable short-term goal.

Progression should be performance based. For example, a physically active person may ask how long she must remain on crutches after spraining her lateral ankle ligaments. These ligaments are not stressed by walking, only by extreme ankle inversion. Thus, a good guide for return to full weight bearing is a normal, pain-free walking gait. The person may adopt a limp while walking; the limp is an altered neuromuscular pattern to avoid pain. If walking is painful, the first goal of rehabilitation has not been fully achieved. Thus, for this physically active person, progression is simple and performance oriented.

Communication is essential to monitoring the injured person's progress through rehabilitation. Each person will respond differently, and feedback from the patient is vital. Some must be cautioned repeatedly about being too aggressive, whereas others must be encouraged to do more. Much of the individual response hinges on a person's response to pain. Some people approach therapeutic exercise with a "no pain, no gain" mentality. The health care team must help these people to interpret their pain sensations in order to protect healing tissues. Other people will stop exercise at the first sensation of pain, even though some discomfort is expected at various stages of most rehabilitation programs. Those who know what to expect will be better able

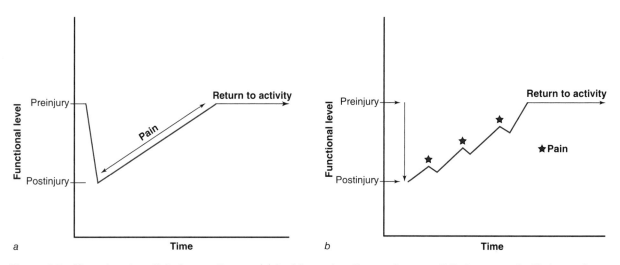

Figure 1.7   The return to activity is a continuum: *(a)* Avoiding pain with exercise as activity increases facilitates early functional recovery. *(b)* Recovery of function is delayed when the threshold of healing tissue is exceeded and pain occurs.
Adapted from Gieck and Saliba 1988.

to interpret their pain and make progress with their rehabilitation. Figure 1.7 shows theoretical and realistic return-to-activity models.

The final stage in recovery from injury is the return to unrestricted activity, such as work, training, practice, or competition. Clearance to return to full activity is a team decision. The patient must feel physically and psychologically ready. The physician and clinicians must consider whether the injured tissues can withstand the stresses of the activity and whether the person's overall level of fitness is sufficient for him or her to participate effectively without undue risk of injury. Others, including coaches and parents, can provide valuable insight into the physical capabilities and psychological motivation of physically active individuals. Most importantly, clearance to return to activity must be based on performance assessment as well as physical examination. The person evaluated solely in a physician's office or health care clinic may appear capable of returning to activity, yet field or work site evaluation may reveal significant losses of activity-specific agility, power, or endurance. Ideally, the clinician should evaluate the individual's functional performance and gain physician approval before giving final clearance for unrestricted activity.

Documenting Progress

Paperwork is the bane of health care providers. Preparing and maintaining good records is often challenging, but it is essential work. This subject is given considerable attention in *Management Strategies in Athletic Training, Fourth Edition* (Ray 2011). However,

it would be remiss not to mention documentation in this chapter.

Good records are needed to assess the benefits of treatment and rehabilitation. There is a growing demand in the managed care environment for health care providers to demonstrate that they do make a difference in patient care. The use of patient self-reports (figure 1.8) can facilitate communication between the patient and the clinician. These forms allow the patient to document improving or worsening symptoms. Patient self-reports can also improve our understanding of which interventions are most beneficial in the treatment of the injured person.

Good records also are essential in a defense against a charge of negligence. Malpractice cases often take years to reach the courtroom, and a good memory will never prevail over good documentation. Figure 1.9 provides an example of an individual injury evaluation and treatment record.

Without a complete record of the case, specific details of the individual's problem and treatments will not be available. Develop good record-keeping skills and make a habit of documenting the modalities and specific parameters you select in treating each person. Perhaps an integration of technology into the traditional therapy environment may alleviate the stresses of documentation. Modern computer hardware (smartphones, tablets) and software (apps) can expedite the process of recording treatment. Physicians (surgeons) have long used dictation services to record their work; today, voice-activated software is readily available to perform the same task.

Patient Pain and Activity Inventory

Name _____ Date _____

1. Date of injury or date of onset of symptoms: _____

2. New injury: ☐ Yes ☐ No   Reinjury: ☐ Yes ☐ No

3. Please rate your general health (circle one):

   Excellent   Good   Fair   Poor

4. Please rate your pain with 0 being no pain and 10 being pain as bad as it can be since injury or in the last four weeks.

Now	0	1	2	3	4	5	6	7	8	9	10
Best	0	1	2	3	4	5	6	7	8	9	10
Worst	0	1	2	3	4	5	6	7	8	9	10
With activity	0	1	2	3	4	5	6	7	8	9	10

5. Please choose the best word or words that describe your pain (circle as many as apply):

   Sharp   Dull   Ache   Burning   Tingling   Numbness

6. How long does the pain last? _____ hours/day   _____ hours/week

7. Please mark location of your pain with an "X."

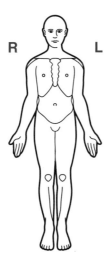 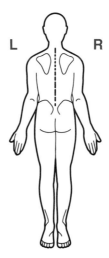

8. Please list three (3) important activities that you are unable to do or that you are having difficulty doing as a result of your problem with 0 being unable to perform the activity and 10 being able to perform activity at preinjury level.

Activities												
1.	0	1	2	3	4	5	6	7	8	9	10
2.	0	1	2	3	4	5	6	7	8	9	10
3.	0	1	2	3	4	5	6	7	8	9	10

Figure 1.8   A sample patient self-report.

Reprinted, by permission, from P.A. Houglum, 2005, *Therapeutic exercises for musculoskeletal injuries*, 2nd ed. (Champaign, IL: Human Kinetics), 168.

Individual Injury Evaluation and Treatment Record

Name: *Jones, Mike*   Sport: *Basketball*   Body part: *R-Ankle*

Date injury occurred: *2/5/12*   Date injury reported: *2/6/12*

Primary complaint: *R-ankle pain*   Secondary complaint: *None*

Subjective data: *Pt. inverted R-ankle while playing basketball. Reports "a loud snap." No previous hx. of ankle injury. Otherwise normal medical hx. Pain w/walking is 5/10. Pain at rest is 3/10. Pain to palpation over the ant. talofibular ligament. No other bony or soft tissue tenderness noted.*

Objective data: *Moderate swelling over lateral malleolus. No discoloration or deformity. Ankle is warm to touch. Lacks 5 deg dorsiflexion and 10 deg plantar flexion in both AROM and PROM compared to L-ankle. Strength is 4+/5 for DF, PF, Inv. & Ev. compared to 5/5 for L-ankle. Anterior drawer test is remarkably positive w/ mushy end point. Talar tilt test equivocal due to swelling. Neg. Klieger's test. Pt. walks w/a noticeable limp and cannot bear wt. on the R-foot w/out assistance. Applied RICE for 20 minutes. Issued compression sleeve and ankle brace. Fitted crutches and provided instruction in crutch walking. Educated pt. on RICE techniques for home program. Provided pt. w/ ankle home care brochure. Pt. indicated he understood instructions.*

Assessment: *Probable 3° ATF sprain.*

Plan: *Will refer to Dr. Smith. Appt. arranged for 3:00 pm today. Applied RICE for 20 minutes. Issued compression sleeve and ankle brace. Fitted crutches and provided instruction in crutch walking. Educated pt. on RICE techniques for home program. Provided pt. w/ankle home care brochure. Pt. indicated he understood instructions.*

Evaluator's signature: *David Black*

Date	Treatments and progress
2/6/12	*RICE × 20 min. Instructions for home care program. Crutches w/instructions. Compression sleeve and ankle brace. Pt. tolerated tx. well. Pain at rest 2/10. Swelling reduced.* **DB**

Figure 1.9 A sample form used to record the evaluation and treatment of an injured athlete.

Reprinted, by permission, from R.R. Ray, 2011, *Management strategies in athletic training,* 4th ed. (Champaign, IL: Human Kinetics), 194.

SUMMARY

This chapter addresses several concepts related to the application of therapeutic modalities in contemporary practice, including types of modalities, principles of energy transfer, state regulation, consent to treatment, liability, and the development of a progressive plan of care. Providers should know and practice within the limits of the regulations established in the state where they work. Patients should understand the treatments that are recommended, including potential benefits as well as potential risks and alternative interventions. The failure to administer treatments safely and receive consent to treat may constitute negligence. All applications of therapeutic modalities should be part of a comprehensive plan of care leading to a return to activity and competition.

1. *Discuss how an evidence-based approach affects the use of therapeutic modalities.*

An evidence-based approach to the use of therapeutic modalities requires the clinician to seek out and evaluate the best evidence available demonstrating effectiveness and efficacy. This practice adds to and supplements the expertise of the clinician. In addition, treatment decisions should be individualized as the clinician attends to the needs and values of each patient.

2. *Discuss how regulation of health care may influence the use of therapeutic modalities in the care of physically active individuals.*

Athletic training is regulated in many states through state practice acts. The state practice act defines what an athletic trainer may do, whom the athletic trainer may treat, and where treatments can be administered. Although the certified athletic trainer may be educated and trained to use therapeutic modalities to treat musculoskeletal injuries, state regulations may restrict modality application depending on the setting, amateur or professional status of the individual being treated, or modality used.

3. *Identify the varying groups of therapeutic modalities and their purposes.*

Therapeutic modalities are grouped based on energy form: *thermal, electrical, acoustical, electromagnetic,* or *mechanical.* Each form of energy will exert an effect on the patient that is physiological, psychological, or both. Common effects include changes in tissue temperature, pain modulation, changes in cellular membrane permeability, or muscle contraction.

4. *Describe the principles of physics that affect energy transfer as related to therapeutic modalities.*

Energy is transferred to or from the body through the application of different modalities. The amount and rate of energy transfer are affected by the established gradient, the distance between the modality and the tissues, and the angle of the energy source from the perpendicular. These factors are unique to each application, and the clinician should account for them along with consideration for the duration of application.

5. *Identify the hierarchy of components in a progressive rehabilitation plan.*

A progressive rehabilitation plan consists of six stages: (1) a complete clinical examination; (2) controlling pain and swelling and protecting damaged tissues; (3) restoring range of motion and volitional neuromuscular control; (4) restoring reflexive neuromuscular control, strength, and muscular endurance; (5) restoring power and control over complex functional movement; and (6) resuming sport-specific training.

6. *Discuss guidelines for guiding an athlete through a comprehensive plan of care.*

Progression through a comprehensive rehabilitation plan of care is based on protecting healing tissues and achieving short-term goals. If healing tissues are adequately protected, pain during and after activity is the primary guide to progression. Active exercise should be pain free, and the individual should be able to do tomorrow what was done today.

Psychological Aspects of Injury and Rehabilitation

OBJECTIVES

After reading this chapter, you will be able to

❶ compare and contrast the contemporary stage model and the biopsychosocial model of psychological response to injury;

❷ discuss the impact that cognitive appraisal can have on the physically active patient's psychological and emotional responses to injury;

❸ identify influences on one's ability to cope with a musculoskeletal injury;

❹ identify factors that improve an athlete's adherence to a rehabilitation plan;

❺ identify common barriers to successful completion of rehabilitation; and

❻ discuss the assessment of treatment outcomes in the context of natural history, placebo, and "true" treatment effect.

A retired man who is an avid golfer enters a sports medicine clinic for treatment of his shoulder, which was injured when he tripped while carrying his golf bag. He complains of stiffness and a loss of motion in the shoulder. However, his primary concern is that the injury is preventing him from playing golf and that this **disability** might be permanent. Physical examination reveals an extensive contusion to the right shoulder; however, the joint appears to be stable and the rotator cuff intact. He responds well to transcutaneous electrical nerve stimulation (TENS) and moist heat, prescribed to reduce pain and spasm, and active assistance and active range of motion exercise during his initial treatment. Swinging a short iron is included in the initial therapy session. The patient is far less anxious on leaving the clinic than when he entered.

He complies well with his home care program and requires just four additional treatments in the clinic. He gradually progresses his golfing activities, beginning on the driving range, then playing 9 holes, and after four weeks of recovery playing 18 holes.

Musculoskeletal injury is usually an unexpected and undesired consequence of participation in competitive athletics, physically demanding work, and recreational physical activities. It is estimated that 3–17 million sport and recreational injuries occur annually in the United States to children and adults. Effective treatment and rehabilitation require a comprehensive plan of care with specific, progressive goals that are appropriate to the needs and status of each patient. Using evidence-based practices in selecting and applying therapeutic modalities will allow you to achieve the treatment and rehabilitation goals. Two important concepts were introduced in chapter 1: (1) the rehabilitation plan of care is based on medical diagnosis and evaluation of the injured person's needs, and (2) each person will respond uniquely to injury, requiring you to individualize the plan of care to treat the person, not just the injury. An additional concept introduced in this chapter is the deliberate involvement of patients during the development of their treatment and rehabilitation programs.

We have an abundance of information about the physiological dimensions of injury, such as etiology, epidemiology, outcome measures, diagnosis, tissue healing processes, and the effectiveness of interventions. Yet, once injury occurs, the patient

will experience cognitive, emotional, and behavioral responses that are linked to the paleocortical pain tract that is discussed in chapter 5. The abundance of interneurons in the emotional centers of the brain can trigger various responses that can affect recovery. Our knowledge about the psychological dimensions of injury has been limited until recently, as athletic trainers, psychologists, and other members of the sports medicine community have become increasingly aware of the vital role psychosocial factors play in recovery. Varying models—conceptual, theoretical, or integrative in nature—have been proposed in an effort to establish a framework for investigating and describing the psychological response to injury and rehabilitation.

Recognizing and appreciating the mind–body connection is perhaps the most important concept in treating individuals with musculoskeletal injuries. The relationships between physical injury and psychological response and between psychological dysfunction and somatic pain are complex. The anatomical connection is obvious and not a new concept, yet the appreciation of patient psyche is often overlooked or ignored. The situation described at the beginning of this chapter is an example of attending to both areas: the patient's program included swinging a golf club, a sport-specific exercise (physical) that alleviated much of the individual's anxiety (psychological) about playing golf again. Before applying a therapeutic modality, the clinician should appreciate the psychological aspects of injury and rehabilitation just as much as the physical aspects of injury and tissue healing.

While psychological factors do affect the likelihood that an injury will occur (Andersen and Williams 1999), this topic is beyond the scope of this text. The focus of this section is on the role psychological factors play in patients' responses to injury and their adherence to rehabilitation. Key attributes affecting outcomes are characteristics of the injury, situational factors, interactions with health care providers, differences in personalities, and individual cognitive appraisal. How the person assimilates these factors will affect his or her emotional responses (e.g., fear, tension, anger) and behavioral responses (e.g., adherence to rehabilitation) (Walker, Thatcher, and Lavallee 2007). Positive appraisal will lead to supportive emotional and behavioral responses and will move the patient toward full recovery. You should remember that not all outcomes are positive, especially if the clinician does not monitor the reciprocal relationship between appraisal and responses.

Successful return to competition or daily activity is contingent not only on the clinician's development of a rehabilitation program that uses evidence-based techniques but, just as importantly, on the patient's adherence to the program. Psychosocial barriers caused by factors other than the injury can have a negative impact on adherence to rehabilitation. A holistic focus on treating the entire patient and not just the physical injury raises awareness of the patient's psychological responses, thereby offering the chance to address adverse responses that could disrupt rehabilitation. Behavioral economists and social psychologists say that implementing holistic strategies will lead to better patient compliance and adherence to treatment plans and ultimately to better outcomes.

Much has been learned about the psychological response to musculoskeletal injuries through the study of sport-related injuries. Certified athletic trainers work closely with individuals before and after injury; the understanding, personal attention, and caring attitude that athletic trainers provide can strongly influence a person's psychological and physical recovery and response to treatment with therapeutic modalities. Other members of the sports medicine team may not have as close a working relationship with the athlete-patient as the trainer does,

but they have an impact on all aspects of recovery. Regardless of the role a clinician plays on the health care team, establishing a positive rapport and earning the trust of the patients who seek advice and assistance are essential to their successful recovery.

PSYCHOLOGICAL RESPONSE TO INJURY

It is important that all clinicians understand their scope of practice and their role on the health care team. All providers should be aware of the potential psychological responses to injury and should be able to recognize behaviors and actions that might be harmful or disruptive. Organizations should have appropriate patient mental health programs in place that include management protocols, educational materials, and professional resources for referral. The clinician should not demean a patient's concerns; most important, the clinician must be able to recognize when an appropriate referral should be made. A few common models describing the individual's psychological response to injury include Grief and Stage, Biopsychosocial, and Cognitive Appraisal.

Grief and Stage Models

Early on, scholars adopted the grief model (as observed in those suffering loss or bereavement, illness, and disability) in describing the psychological response to musculoskeletal injury. Kübler-Ross (1969) described a five-stage psychological response to terminal illness (death and dying): denial and isolation, anger, bargaining, depression, and acceptance. In the 1980s and early '90s, sport psychologists adopted this paradigm with musculoskeletal injury, suggesting the injured person first *denies* the severity of the injury and then expresses *anger*. A *bargaining* stage might include statements such as "If the ligament isn't torn, I will train in the weight room every day." Unrealistic bargaining was thought to give way to *depression*, followed by *acceptance* of the injury and the consequences.

More recent work has emphasized that physically active people such as athletes may experience some of these responses after musculoskeletal injury but do not progress through all of the stages. For example, a high school soccer player may be angry (at the opponent) when he sustains a displaced fracture to his tibia, but he cannot deny the injury exists and therefore will not progress through the remaining stages. These individuals may express anger at the time of the injury, or when they become bored with the routine and slow progression of rehabilitation. In addition, experts have found that most injured athletes do not experience depression following musculoskeletal injury (Leddy, Lambert, and Ogles 1994, Brewer, Linder, and Phelps 1995). Others have proposed that athletes do not deny the existence of an injury but are more likely to be trying to make sense of it and determine its severity. Thus, the paradigm described by Kübler-Ross does not adequately describe the typical psychological response to musculoskeletal injury.

Within the current literature, opinion about the grief and stage model in defining psychological responses to injury appears equivocal; some researchers suggest that grief stages might only occur in response to severe or traumatic injuries (season or career ending) (Smith et al. 1990, Heil 1993), while other researchers offer minimal support for the denial stage and no support for the bargaining stage (Udry 1997). Evans and Hardy (1995) suggest that the more recent conceptualization of the grief model represents a less stage-like and more dynamic model than earlier versions and is therefore worthy of further attention. Currently, the consensus is that emotions consistent with the various stage models are observed in athletic injury research (e.g., depression, anger, frustration), but a common sequence of discrete responses or stages of responding to athletic injury is not supported. Recognizing the limitations and applicability of grief response models, such as their lack of accommodation for individual differences, researchers have challenged and over time replaced the grief response models.

Biopsychosocial Models

Several biopsychosocial models have been used to describe psychological responses to musculoskeletal injury. The International Classification of Functioning, Disability, and Health (ICF) (World Health Organization 2002) is a model that incorporates a disorder or disease, structure and bodily function, activity and participation, and how these are affected by environmental and personal factors. Nagi (1965) described a model with four components of injury and response: (1) disease, (2) impairment, (3) **functional limitation**, and (4) disability. If *musculoskeletal injury* replaces *disease*, this model is easily applied to injured physically active people (figure 2.1).

For example, consider a volleyball player who injured her knee. The injury was diagnosed as a grade II tibial collateral ligament sprain. The sprain to the ligament was the *musculoskeletal injury*. The player had pain, loss of motion, and loss of strength following the injury. These *impairments* resulted in *functional limitations*, among them the inability to walk without assistance or perform physical tasks, including sport-specific activities such as running and jumping. This volleyball player could not play her sport, work part-time as a waitress on the weekends, participate in physical education, or go hiking with her family. These limitations on performance in sport, school, employment, and family activities represent her *disabilities*.

In biopsychosocial models, injury is more than tissue damage; attention is focused on the person's entire response to the injury. These models present an enlightening concept: To understand the physically active person's psychological response to an injury, one must appreciate the impact of the injury on the person's life, not just the pathology. The ICF model also acknowledges that personal and environmental factors influence the response and ability to cope with injury and illness. The clinician should discuss the impact of the injury with the patient and try not to assume he or she knows the patient's goals. For example, a retiring football player may not want to return to a highly competitive program but instead may choose to exercise at a recreational level after a significant injury. The clinician should help motivate and encourage the patient in a manner consistent with the patient's values.

Cognitive Appraisal Models

In response to the inadequacies of grief and stage models such as the death-and-dying paradigm, cognitive-based appraisal models were identified

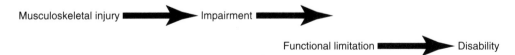

Figure 2.1   Nagi model of the process of disablement in the context of musculoskeletal injury in physically active people.

as a framework for understanding the psychological response to injury. Cognitive appraisal models suggest that personal (attributes of the individual) and situational (social and physical environment) factors mediate how people appraise and respond to their injuries (Brewer 2001). The appraisals affect emotional responses and subsequently influence behavioral responses (e.g., adherence to rehabilitation). Wiese-Bjornstal, Smith, and LaMott (1995) proposed that cognitive appraisal and grief process models are not mutually exclusive, and they developed a broader integrated stress process model that describes the psychological response to injury as well as rehabilitation. Therefore cognitive appraisal occurs not just once (upon occurrence of injury) but also as the individual progresses through the healing/rehabilitation process.

Cognitive appraisal models are established from the roots of stress and coping theories and are predicated on the uniqueness of individual responses to a physical injury and the recognition that many factors influence how individuals cope and how well they adhere to a plan of care after injury. Weiss and Troxel (1986) identified the importance of examining personal and situational factors for their effect on responses to injury. Grove (1993) identified personality as a factor that influences the thoughts, feelings, and behaviors of patients during rehabilitation. Therefore, injury can be viewed as a stressor prompting cognitive appraisal by the individual, which influences her emotional responses and in turn affects her behavioral responses. This response process applies both to the injury itself and to rehabilitation. The integrated model proposed by Wiese-Bjornstal et al. (1995, 1998) describes the influences of the social environment on response to injury. The common feature in these models is that an individual's psychological and emotional responses to injury depend on his or her appraisal or understanding of the injury and the stressors present in the context of the injury and rehabilitation.

Cognitive appraisals are processes through which a potentially stressful situation is assessed as being stressful and the individual's evaluation of the extent of that stress. Appraisals influence the way in which an individual copes with a stressful situation. Lazarus (1991) defined coping as an individual's ever-changing efforts to manage circumstances that are appraised as stressful. The injured patient is said to experience two forms of appraisals, primary and secondary (Lazarus 1991). Primary appraisal is an assessment of what is at stake with respect to challenge, benefit, threat, and harm or loss. Secondary appraisal is similar to the primary appraisal but involves assessment of the coping options available to the individual. Therefore, coping varies within individuals and is dependent upon the circumstances (their environment), individual differences, and the individual's cognitive appraisals. Recall the case study of the golfer presented at the beginning of this chapter. His response to injury changed dramatically after he understood the nature of his injury and the limitations it was likely to place on his life. He did not progress through stages of response to the injury, but rather his psychological and emotional responses were altered by his cognitive appraisal of his injury, what was at stake, and what coping options were available.

Cognitive appraisal models are distinguished from the stage models in three important ways. The first distinction is that some or most of the labeled stages may be absent in the cognitive appraisal models. For example, most injured athletes do not become depressed (Wegener 1998/1999). Depression can be a significant barrier to recovery and must be recognized and treated when it occurs, but its occurrence is the exception rather than the rule. The second distinction is that the psychological and emotional responses to injury do not progress in a structured order in the cognitive appraisal models (Wegener 1998/1999; Yukelson and Heil 1998). Injured persons may express little anger and frustration after an injury, accept their situation and cope, and then become angry and confrontational after a setback in rehabilitation. Such a response may also be associated with individuals' perceptions that their progress is slower than expected. This response seems to be associated with programs that vary little from day to day and week to week. The third distinction is that cognitive appraisal models imply that the individual's psychological and emotional responses to injury are affected by his or her understanding of the injury and the psychosocial environment (figure 2.2). Thus, whether a physically active person adapts and copes after injury or demonstrates **maladaptive behaviors** can be influenced by members of the health care team as well as the patient's peers, friends, family, and coaches.

Again, recall the golfer described at the beginning of this chapter. Understanding the patient's perception of the injury and our natural fear of the unknown is crucial. Had attention been focused solely on the injured shoulder and not on the person, the golfer's primary concern and goal may have been

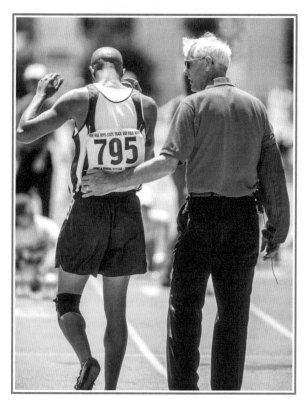

Figure 2.2 A strong support network can help people cope and adapt following injury.

overlooked. More important, however, the certified athletic trainer would have lost the opportunity to affect the psychological response to the injury. Swinging a golf club is not standard in shoulder rehabilitation programs. However, including this activity assured the athlete that his season was not over.

Critical components of the model relate to the mediating role of the characteristics of the injury, the sport-specific situational factors, interactions with care providers, individual differences, and the resultant cognitive appraisals. Knowledge and understanding (cognition) alter the psychological-emotional response to injury (Wegener 1998/1999). Providing the type and amount of information that injured people need takes experience and practice. Some individuals ask a lot of questions and want detailed information. For others, the information needs to be more general and less detailed. Finding the right level is important and quite subjective, and success is often achieved through trial and error by the clinician. Avoid "talking down" or being overly simplistic, but also do not try to impress and overwhelm the patient with your knowledge. If an injured person wants more information than he has been

provided, he may lose confidence in the care provider and become less compliant with the plan of care. However, someone who feels overwhelmed by information will be confused and anxious, resulting in the same negative outcomes. Clinicians must listen and observe; the initial evaluation is a critical time to promote effective coping after injury. Similarly, it is important to continually monitor the patient for changes throughout the rehabilitation process.

Personality and Environmental Influences

One's ability to cope after injury is influenced by many factors that can produce varying emotional and behavioral responses. Some people are natural worriers, tending to overreact to life's frustrations, whereas others seem to manage the ups and downs effectively. Someone's ability to cope also depends on his or her current situation and life stressors. An athlete who coped effectively with an off-season injury in high school may maladapt to a similar in-season injury in college because the college environment, the pressure to return to competition, and decreased daily support from family, teammates, and coaches make for different stressors and coping resources (Wegener 1998/1999). In addition, an important component of the treatment plan is an objective assessment of the patient's response to injury.

Emotional Responses

The ways in which people appraise their injuries influence their emotional responses (Walker, Thatcher, and Lavallee 2007). Musculoskeletal injuries generally produce negative emotions. Tension, anger, depression, frustration, and boredom are common. It is important to remember that emotions are in constant flux and are influenced by a variety of internal and external factors such as personality, situation, and available support resources. These emotions occur at the onset of injury and usually are temporary as the person copes and begins the rehabilitative process. Wiese-Bjornstal et al. (1995, 1998) propose that if emotions are appropriately controlled and focused, they may have a positive effect on coping. McDonald and Hardy (1990) discussed the importance of athletes' accepting the reality of the injury and of experiencing and expressing their fluctuating emotions so that they can eventually progress toward concentrating their energy on recovery.

Although we have said that most injured athletes do not experience depression after sustaining an injury, several studies have pointed out that a minority of injured athletes do experience extreme responses, such as depression and suicidal tendencies, at levels that call for clinical referral (Smith et al. 1990). Recent data indicate a growing prevalence in the percentage, types, and severity of mental illnesses in young adults, thus prompting efforts to develop plans for the recognition and referral of psychological concerns in collegiate student-athletes (Neal et al. 2013). This point reminds the clinician that the psychological response to injury is a complex and dynamic process, not a standard condition that can be applied to all individuals. Experts (Grove 1993; Brewer 2001; and Wiese-Bjornstal 1998) have suggested that personal factors (e.g., self-esteem, self-worth, self-confidence, self-efficacy) continually exert their effects on the individual's psychological response to the injury throughout rehabilitation.

Emotional responses to injury are influenced by various components of self-perception: self-worth, self-confidence, and self-efficacy. These components of self-perception have been examined in the sport injury literature and have been found to influence emotional and behavioral response to sport injury. How we view ourselves does not prevent us from experiencing negative emotions when we are injured, but it determines the degree and severity of those emotions and how long it takes us to cope and progress toward positive emotions and behaviors. The reciprocal relationship is easily understood—high self-perception tends to produce quicker coping and transition to rehabilitation (McDonald and Hardy 1990; Bianco, Malo, and Orlick 1999; Brewer, Linder, and Phelps 1995). The initial negative emotions are often accompanied with thoughts of "what-ifs" and self-doubts that lead to internally directed anger, but those with strong self-perception quickly summon their resolve and focus their energy on working diligently during recovery.

Although not extensively examined in the research, positive emotional responses to injury have been purported to occur. For example, athletes may express relief, as injury removes the external pressures imposed by parents, coaches, and teammates or the internal pressures created by their own perfectionism or commitment. An example of this was presented by Wiese-Bjornstal et al. (1998) in a case report when an adolescent female star basketball player initially expressed disappointment that her second major knee injury in two years was not diagnosed as an ACL tear. When a subsequent diagnosis revealed it was a torn ACL and would require surgery, she expressed relief, a "positive" emotion. She was tired of being the star player and saw injury as her way out of an unbearable situation.

It is also possible for high levels of self-perception and self-worth to be detrimental and lead to negative emotions and an inability to cope. People may base their self-perception primarily on how much they contribute to or gain status from their given environment. They may find it difficult to identify coping strategies when their self-perception is threatened, leading them to act out their frustration through negative behaviors. For instance, a collegiate athlete may feel like an important member of the team based on her role as a starter and her successful performances, and she may gain little of her self-worth from her efforts in the classroom. When an injury removes her from participation on the team, she may appraise her situation with despair and become negative and reclusive. The elimination of sport participation can pose difficulty for participants because such an important part of their lives is temporarily taken away (Gould et al. 1997a; McDonald and Hardy 1990; Udry et al. 1997). Tracey (2003) identified the choice to continue attending practices while injured as an emotionally difficult experience that influenced the athlete's affective states.

Experts have discussed the concepts of invulnerability and "athletic masculine identity" as factors that establish the identity of the individual and contribute significantly to emotional responses (Messner 1992; Young, White, and McTeer 1994). They suggest that many athletes, especially those with high self-perception, may possess these characteristics, which contribute to their self-confidence and sense of self-worth. An injury can take a profound emotional toll because the athlete normally considers himself strong and invincible. Loss of fitness, independence, and status on the team results in difficult emotions for the athlete and threatens his perception of invulnerability and identity.

The clinical care team cannot influence all of the factors that promote a maladaptive response. However, a holistic approach to care for physically active people will improve your understanding of their situation. It is essential for athletic trainers and clinicians to foster an environment that promotes attention to the individual's needs. Crowded, noisy facilities can leave the injured person asking, "Does anybody care?" Such an environment also diminishes the likelihood of identifying maladaptive behaviors, intervening within the limits of one's training and ability, and making appropriate referrals (Fisher and Hoisington 1998; Fisher et al. 1993).

An injury will force the patient to adapt. Whether that adaptation is functional or dysfunctional depends on many factors. Certainly the severity of the injury, timing of the injury, and the athlete's coping resources strongly influence the response. The psychological and emotional responses do not proceed through a common sequence of stages—they can differ significantly from person to person and within the same person under different circumstances. The care provider must create an atmosphere conducive to compliance with rehabilitation, must respect the unique nature of each person's response, and must identify barriers to treatment compliance and recovery.

Behavioral Responses

As we have indicated, behavioral responses to athletic injury are predicated upon the athletes' appraisal of their situation and their subsequent emotional responses. The direction and nature of behavioral responses that will affect their adherence to rehabilitation (Duda, Smart, and Tappe 1989; Fisher et al. 1993; Fisher and Hoisington 1998) include the use of psychological skills (Rotella and Heyman 1993; Ievleva and Orlick 1991), the use of social networks (Pearson and Jones 1992), and risk taking (Rose and Jevne 1993). Experts, including Wiese-Bjornstal et al., have found that athletes who adhere to rehabilitation, use psychological skills, effectively use available social support, reduce risk taking, and pursue rehabilitation goals with maximum effort and intensity return to previous athletic levels more quickly than those who do not. Research also indicates a positive correlation between successful rehabilitation and the most consistently linked factor to adherence, self-motivation.

The benefit of integrating psychological skills is well documented in the injury rehabilitation literature. Skills such as goal setting, imagery, and positive self-talk are associated with rapid recovery of function in athletes with ankle or knee injuries (Ievleva and Orlick 1991). Others have indicated that relaxation can positively affect sport injury rehabilitation outcomes. Brewer et al. (2000) and other experts (Laubach et al. 1996, Murphy et al. 1999) suggest athletes who use psychological techniques during recovery believe they can influence the outcome of rehabilitation. Thus, these athletes are more likely to take action to exert control and follow their injury rehabilitation program more completely.

Social support is an important component in dealing emotionally with being injured as well as during recovery (Gould 1997a and 1997b; Gyurscik 1995; Rose and Jevne 1993; Udry 1997). Social support is considered a buffering factor that mediates the stress-injury relationship. Not only does social support help the person cope with the stress of injury, it also provides a feeling of attachment to others. Athletes have identified the lack of social support as a stumbling block in recovering from an injury. For athletes, the most common sources of social support are family, friends, athletic trainers, sport psychologists and researchers, teammates, coaches, and other health care clinicians. A key part of providing support to injured athletes is to avoid erroneously assuming that you understand their subjective experience. While the clinician may have an extensive history and background in treating a particular type of injury, it is very likely to be the patient's first experience with it. Clinicians should take steps to enhance their insight and establish clear communications with the patient to gain a complete picture of the injury and the athlete's emotional state.

Tracey (2003) identified the medical staff—that is, the athletic trainer—as an important source of support for injured participants, who may rely on the trainer's input for information upon which they base their emotional responses. Some athletes have reported consciously suspending their emotional response until they have communicated with the athletic training staff. Therefore, it is vital that clinicians be aware of the potential impact of their verbal assessments and nonverbal expressions, such as facial expressions, on the injured person's experience. The tone with which information is communicated is valued tremendously and received intently by the athlete. This exchange will dictate the patient's mood for the rest of the day and will set the tone for the rest of the rehabilitation process. With experience, the clinician will become more apt to communicate honestly while minimizing dramatization, depending on the individual characteristics of the patient.

As the patient progresses through the rehabilitation process, the thought of returning to participation evokes emotions of enthusiasm as well as apprehension and hesitation. The fear of reinjury is not a predominant concern for most people; rather, the injury has become a learning experience and has taught them to be more cautious. They have learned to take care of themselves and not to take anything for granted. It is important for the clinician to realize that the conservative behavior demonstrated upon return to activity is not from fear or lack of motivation.

Assessment of Fear

A plethora of tools and instruments are available to assess psychological well-being and overall health; some are generic, while others are oriented to disease, anatomic region, or a specific dimension of health, such as fear. Depending on treatment setting and patient characteristics, assessment of fear may not be universally appreciated and practiced. Athletic trainers in traditional settings (competitive athletics) generally do not encounter athletes who experience fear. In contrast, clinicians working with adolescent or elderly patients may need to address fear of reinjury or pain from their patients. Nevertheless, the assessment of fear can play an integral part in developing the treatment plan as well as being an effective means of demonstrating treatment outcomes.

The Fear-Avoidance Beliefs Questionnaire (FABQ) and the Tampa Scale for Kinesiophobia (TSK) are dimension-specific instruments that are commonly used to assess patient fear level. Many subsets of these two instruments have been developed, and both are available in many languages, including English, Japanese, German, and Norwegian. These items are usually administered in hard-copy form and take approximately 5 to 10 minutes to complete (depending on the version); Internet and computerized versions have also been developed. As with any form of assessment, clinicians should seek information about an instrument's validity, reliability, and population specificity before using it with patients. These instruments are most commonly used to assess fear level in patients experiencing low back pain, but they have also been used with knee and hip injuries. It is beyond the scope of this text to expound upon the specifics for each of these instruments, but we do encourage all clinicians to investigate applications that fit their setting and consider integrating them into their clinical practice. The importance of clinical outcome measures with rehabilitation is discussed in chapter 3.

MAXIMIZING COMPLIANCE WITH A REHABILITATION PLAN OF CARE

The success of any injury rehabilitation program is not just based on the expertise of the clinicians and their use of evidence-based techniques but also on the patients following the prescribed program. A positive relationship has been established between adherence to rehabilitation and clinical outcome. Adherence refers to the degree to which an injured person complies with instructions. This applies to in-person (in the clinic) treatment sessions as well as to prescribed at-home exercises and regimens.

Clinicians presume that patients will behave rationally to maximize their self-interest, but patients may not be the rational individuals we imagine. Athletes have reported frustration and boredom in response to rehabilitation programs that are not challenging or progressing toward their intended outcome. Adherence rates to sport injury rehabilitation have been found to range from 40% to 91% (Brewer 1999). As the process of tissue healing involves a sequence of physiological responses, it is important for the injured person to adhere to the established rehabilitation schedule.

Medical, psychological, and sociological experts have recommended various models to support and enhance patient adherence to rehabilitation and management of chronic diseases. From these models, three approaches have been adapted specifically to rehabilitation from sport injury: (1) protection motivation theory, (2) personal investment theory, and (3) cognitive appraisal models. Information provided in this chapter is not intended to be an all-inclusive instructional manual for each proposed model. Rather, the aim is to present specific concepts from each that can be applied in the rehabilitation setting.

Protection motivation theory is based on two cognitive processes, threat appraisal and coping appraisal, that determine the patient's adherence to health behaviors. Threat appraisal involves patients' perceptions of vulnerability—how severe the threat to their health is and how susceptible they are to the health threat. Coping appraisal involves their perceptions of how likely the course of action will be to reduce or prevent the threat (response efficacy) and how able they are to perform the prescribed health behaviors. Adherence is highest when patients perceive the health threat as significant, consider the treatment effective, and consider themselves able to carry out the treatment. A patient who has undergone ACL reconstruction should be educated on how dysfunctional gait alterations will occur if range of motion is not properly reestablished, while also being shown how the prescribed exercises will restore motion and how others have achieved successful outcomes with these exercises.

Personal investment theory is based on the injured person's subjective interpretation of the meaning of the rehabilitation process, which influences personal investment and in turn her behavior. Adherence behavior is determined by personal incentives, a sense of self-belief, and perceived options (Maehr and Braskamp 1986). Personal incentives are the individual's subjective goals for being involved with a particular activity; this could include task incentives, ego incentives, social incentives, and extrinsic incentives. Sense of self-belief includes a person's thoughts and feelings about their existence (e.g., perceptions of competence and self-reliance, tendency to behave in accordance with personal goals, sense of relationship with significant others). Perceived options are the perceived alternative behaviors that can determine motivation in specific situations (e.g., belief in the efficacy of treatment, knowledge of treatment, plans for future sport activity). According to this model, individuals who are self-motivated are less likely to be deterred from participating in rehabilitation, and those who receive social support are more likely to adhere to the prescribed program.

Cognitive appraisal models suggest that post-injury behavior is influenced by emotional responses to injury, which result from interactions between personal and situational factors. The athlete's response to injury is influenced by her appraisal of whether the injury is a threat to her well-being (primary appraisal) and if she has the resources to cope with the injury (secondary appraisal). Athletes who make negative appraisals of their injuries will tend to experience emotional disturbances that negatively influence their adherence to rehabilitation programs. As we described in the previous section, cognitive appraisals are influenced by both personal and situational factors. Personal factors include characteristics such as self-motivation and pain tolerance. Situational variables include the person's belief in the efficacy of the treatment, the comfort of the clinical environment, the convenience of activity scheduling, social support, and the practitioner's expectations about patient adherence. The practitioner's expectation about the athlete's recovery is an important factor that influences the athlete's cognitive and emotional responses. Positive behaviors and a supportive environment can encourage the injured person to be less nervous, angry, and unhappy, leading to better adherence to rehabilitation activities. In addition, when patients comply with rehabilitation, practitioners will be more energetic and more helpful, and they will offer more personal attention.

As a result, this cyclical response is posited to have a direct impact on the athlete's appraisals and to lead to successful rehabilitation outcomes.

Perhaps the greatest influence on adherence to rehabilitation and a positive psychological and emotional adaptation after injury is the rapport established with the injured athlete's caregivers. Certified athletic trainers are often in a unique position among health care professionals in that a working relationship with the physically active person is established before an injury occurs. In addition, high school and college athletes are usually familiar with the athletic training room environment, and they have confidence in the ability of the sports medicine staff to provide a high standard of care.

One major difference between working in a high school, college, or professional setting and working in a sports medicine clinic is the nature of the initial encounter with the injured person. Because a preestablished rapport between the injured person and the certified athletic trainer is usually absent in the clinical setting, patients are uncertain and anxious about what they will experience. Many general orthopedic patients enter the sports medicine clinic believing that therapy and rehabilitation are unlikely to relieve their condition or that it will be a painful experience. Thus, the initial encounter is especially important. A caring, empathetic demeanor is essential. The certified athletic trainer must learn about the problem in terms of the injury, impairment, disability, and handicap. The injured person should leave with an understanding of these issues, the program that will be used to address rehabilitation goals, and his or her responsibilities in resolving the problem. Conducting a successful initial evaluation in a sports medicine clinic requires practice, refined attention to verbal and nonverbal communication, and portrayal of oneself as a competent, caring health care provider.

Set Goals

The importance of setting obtainable yet challenging short- and long-term rehabilitation goals has been noted by sport psychologists and sport rehabilitation specialists (Gieck 1990; Locke and Latham 1985; Worrell and Reynolds 1994). Often these goals seem obvious to the certified athletic trainers and physical therapists; however, they are novel to the injured person. Figure 2.3 shows short- and long-term rehabilitation goals for the senior golfer with the sore shoulder described earlier.

Short-term goals

- Pain relief at rest and early motion exercises within 5 days

- Independent in-home exercise program within 5 days

- Pain-free golf swing with short irons and putting within 10 days

Long-term goals

- Pain-free golf swing with woods and long irons and putting within 3 weeks

- Return to golf within 4 weeks

Figure 2.3 Short- and long-term goals for an injured golfer.

The injured person and the clinician must agree on rehabilitation goals. Often clinicians establish treatment goals without listening to what the patient views as important. On the other hand, the clinician cannot base a rehabilitation program on unrealistic goals expressed by the patient. Injured athletes tend to look only at the ultimate goal: return to competition. Often their expected time frame for achieving the ultimate goal is unrealistic, and important steps in a progressive plan of care are ignored. By incorporating athletes' ultimate goals into the plan of care, you can educate them on the need to achieve simpler, short-term goals (e.g., achieve full knee range of motion) as part of the comprehensive plan to achieve the ultimate goal (e.g., return to playing varsity soccer after anterior cruciate ligament [ACL] reconstruction).

The injured person may not value the short-term goal until it is placed in the context of achieving the ultimate goal. Adherence to a plan of care and achievement of short-term goals are improved when the goals and values are addressed as the plan of care is formulated.

Establishing short-term goals that are integral to returning to sport has an additional positive influence, especially when the recovery period is lengthy. The person recovering from a surgery such as ACL reconstruction can become frustrated by the perception that day-to-day progress is too slow. This can be countered by the positive reinforcement provided when short-term goals are achieved. Short-term goals that can be realistically accomplished in 1 to 3 weeks, yet are challenging, seem to work best. The person who is reminded of the short-term goals accomplished can better cope with the frustrations inherent in a long course of rehabilitation.

Share Responsibility

Treatment and rehabilitation are not *done to* the injured person but are *done by* that person. Through active involvement in establishing goals, the patient learns what responsibilities he or she has if rehabilitation is to succeed (figure 2.4). You must remember that the injury is not your problem. Often young clinicians can become overly possessive of the patient and the patient's problem. The duty of all health care professionals is to provide a high standard of care, not to accept all of the responsibility for achieving goals.

Physically active people appreciate supervision by a certified athletic trainer during their rehabilitation (Fisher and Hoisington 1998; Fisher et al. 1993). The presence of a certified athletic trainer or physical therapist during rehabilitation encourages athletes to do what is expected of them. In a busy athletic training clinic, however, daily supervision is not always possible. Furthermore, in the current managed care environment, most people treated in a sports medicine clinic must be

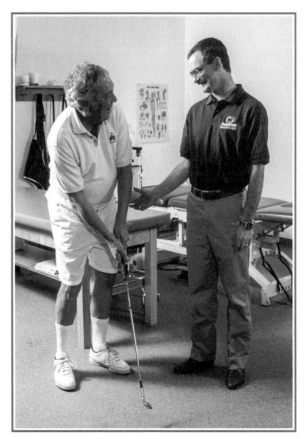

Figure 2.4 The injured person should be actively involved in establishing goals if the rehabilitation plan of care is to succeed.

willing to comply with a program of independent or home-based exercises due to limitations on the number of covered treatment sessions. Thus, you must effectively teach and convey the importance of the exercise program.

To increase adherence to a home exercise program, you can (1) have the person perform each exercise before leaving the sports medicine clinic, (2) provide written instructions as well as illustrations, (3) provide an exercise log to record performance, and (4) have the person demonstrate the exercise program at the beginning of the next treatment session. Proper performance of the exercise program should be positively reinforced. If an injured person cannot complete the exercise program, he or she has not complied with the plan of care. In this situation you must first reconsider the appropriateness of the program. If some exercises increased pain or were beyond the individual's capacity, the exercise program must be modified. However, if the patient has no specific complaints about the exercise program, a nonjudgmental review of the exercise should dominate the treatment session. Failure to have successfully completed the exercise program on the next return visit is strong evidence that the person is unwilling or unable to accept responsibility for getting better. Although such people are frustrating to work with, remember that it is their problem, not yours.

Focus on Today

The more time that is needed to complete a rehabilitation plan, the more imposing the task will appear. Patients can get lost in the big picture of their rehabilitation and lose focus and motivation. Thoughts can become irrational and catastrophic. "I will never be able to play again" is sometimes heard from those who are frustrated by the pace of their recovery and anxious about the future. You can help such patients work through these problems by focusing on what can be accomplished today. Successful rehabilitation requires a lot of small accomplishments, not a miracle cure. Focus the injured person on the short-term goals to be achieved today or this week. Be patient and empathetic. Use thought stopping and positive imagery, as well as examples of successful outcomes, to combat irrational thinking and help the individual during periods of frustration and doubt. For example, after a lateral ankle sprain, a soccer player becomes frustrated by his slow return to full weight bearing. His thought, "I will never be able to play

again," is stopped and replaced with "Rehabilitation takes time; Bobby hurt his knee badly last year but is now playing better than ever." The soccer player is encouraged to stop negative thinking, replace negative thoughts with positive ones, and envision his return to top-level play.

Minimize Suffering

Pain is a universal human experience and a signal that something is wrong. Pain is usually what causes people to seek medical care. Although nearly everyone experiences pain, the psychological and emotional responses are very individual. One of the challenges in health care is understanding each person's response in relation to the severity of the injury or illness.

Pain control is almost always the first goal in a comprehensive rehabilitation plan. Many of the therapeutic modalities discussed in this book have analgesic (pain-relieving) effects. With a professional and empathetic demeanor and effective initial treatment (including pain control), the certified athletic trainer can build a bond of trust with the injured person. If the clinician fails to decrease the person's pain during the first one or two treatments, adherence with the rehabilitation program may decline or the patient may seek care elsewhere.

Physically active people often have a different perspective on pain than nonactive people, which has important implications for the certified athletic trainer. Physically active people view the pain experienced in training and conditioning as a challenge to be overcome. Thus, during rehabilitation, they may have difficulty distinguishing the pain caused by irritation of healing tissues (bad pain) from the pain of strenuous effort (good pain), and they may be too aggressive in rehabilitation. You must help them interpret whether the pain they are experiencing during and after rehabilitation indicates further tissue injury, which will ultimately slow their recovery.

Physically active people are very attuned to their bodies. The self-inflicted pain of conditioning is expected and tolerated. However, the same is not true of the pain associated with medical procedures and rehabilitation. Byerly et al. (1994) reported that the more pain athletes experienced during their rehabilitation, the less they adhered to their plan of care. Athletes, however, reported that pain during therapeutic exercise was less of a deterrent to rehabilitation adherence than athletic trainers perceived it to be (Fisher and Hoisington 1998). Thus, you must monitor the rehabilitation plan closely and make modifications when self-reported pain affects compliance. Athletes and athletic trainers agree that an accurate appraisal of the pain to be experienced is important to adherence with a plan of care. Discuss issues related to pain with your athletes honestly and with empathy. Those who feel they are suffering unnecessarily will not comply with a plan of care and will often seek treatment elsewhere.

Finally, although each person responds differently to pain and injury and these differences should be respected, physically active people are generally more willing to begin and progress through a rehabilitation plan. This is important for the certified athletic trainer who is used to working with highly competitive athletes; he or she may encounter less-active people in a clinical environment. Physically active people like to exercise, want to exercise, and feel comfortable with exercise. There are great differences between physically active and sedentary people. The sedentary person often struggles to learn therapeutic exercises, views exercise as a chore rather than a means of recovery, and stops at the slightest discomfort or exertion. These patients require more instruction and supervision as well as patience on the part of the health care provider. You must be sensitive to the lower tolerance for pain and effort as well as the greater need for positive reinforcement and encouragement in less-active people.

BARRIERS TO SUCCESSFUL REHABILITATION

Injured physically active and relatively nonactive people present for care with personal and psychological issues that can affect their successful completion of rehabilitation. Sometimes you can help physically active people overcome these barriers by building a bond of trust and simply caring and listening. Sometimes you can identify someone who would benefit from psychological or psychiatric care. Unfortunately, there are some barriers to successful rehabilitation that you cannot change. It is important to remember that the patient has the problem and not to become physically and emotionally exhausted trying to change what you cannot. This section identifies some of the barriers to successful rehabilitation that are common to physically active as well as nonactive people.

Secondary Gain

A physically active person whose performance has not lived up to expectations may find solace in the fact that he or she tried to play while hurt but could not. Someone else may avoid the wrath of a boss, or coach, or, in professional sports, the media through a slow recovery. Others may use an injury to gain freedom from a sport in which they no longer wish to participate. In some cases, the individual may perceive that there is more to be gained by not getting better.

Secondary gain relates to tangible and intangible rewards received after injury. The notion of secondary gain is more commonly associated with automobile accident victims with pending civil litigation or injured workers receiving nearly full salary while away from a job they dislike. However, there are many forms of secondary gain. Illness and injury can change how others interact with a person. The injured person may gain additional attention from parents and others; may be relieved of some responsibilities at home, work, or school; or may experience other "positive" responses to injury. In some situations, the rewards of being ill or injured outweigh the rewards of returning to health.

The pursuit of secondary gain may be a poorly disguised conscious effort or a more subtle behavioral pattern. There is no single solution to treating the person who can gain from slow progress or failure. Most work their way through the system. You must not label someone as a malingerer without thoroughly reviewing the case (see chapter 5), yet you must also guard against self-doubt and a sense of failure when those with more to gain by being injured do not respond to appropriate care.

Substance Use and Abuse

Alcohol and drug abuse continue to be significant problems in our society. The media have reported on many athletes who have substance abuse problems. Collegiate athletes also tend to consume more alcohol than the average nonathletic student. Substance abuse decreases adherence to rehabilitation in general and especially affects performance of self-care and home exercise programs. Substance abuse is a sensitive issue, and few certified athletic trainers and physical therapists receive adequate training in the recognition, not to mention treatment, of this problem. It is a problem most certified athletic trainers do not want to confront. Drug and alcohol use increases the risks of, and impairs recovery from, injury. Thus, all members of the health care team should be trained to identify substance abuse, and a plan for physician involvement and appropriate referral for treatment should be implemented to help those with substance abuse problems.

Social and Environmental Barriers

Injuries require adjustments in daily routine. Rehabilitation that occurs in both the athletic training room and the sports medicine clinic uses special equipment and requires a time commitment from the physically active person. Some people will find it difficult to adhere to a rehabilitation plan because of personal commitments, time demands, and lack of access to equipment and facilities. Certified athletic trainers and physical therapists in professional, college, and high school settings may be less affected by these barriers to successful rehabilitation than clinic-based providers, but all patients present with unique circumstances that favor or deter successful rehabilitation.

Patients living in rural areas may have to travel considerable distances for care. Athletes may find that their local schools have very limited training facilities. Because they have to travel long distances to the health care clinic, they may be unable to attend formal therapy sessions as often as they and their physicians would like. Creative home exercise programs must be developed for these people to overcome the lack of equipment, facilities, and hands-on care (figure 2.5).

Similarly, those with family and work responsibilities may be less compliant with rehabilitation because they lack support from others who can assume some of their responsibilities. You must account for these limitations as you develop a plan of care. Sometimes you will have to modify a program to meet the person's needs and accept that the rate of progress may be slower. The injured person must believe that she or he will be able to complete the rehabilitation program. If the plan of care conflicts with the time and energy available, the person probably will not adhere to the rehabilitation plan.

In the traditional setting, injury often also results in separation from a team and the loss of social support. The certified athletic trainer and the injured athlete's coach should explore ways to keep the athlete involved with the team, which will maximize

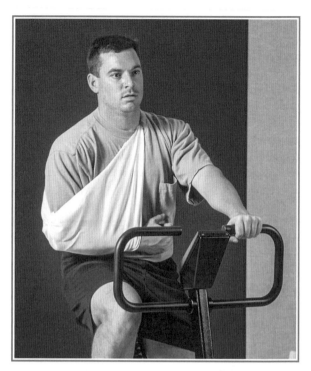

Figure 2.5 Some physically active people find it difficult to adhere to a rehabilitation plan of care. Creative plans must be developed to fit the person's needs, such as prescribing exercises that can be done at home or with limited equipment.

support from peers and minimize disruption of the athlete's daily routine.

Depression, Anxiety, and Sleep Disturbances

People who suffer serious injuries may develop concomitant problems related to depression and anxiety. These problems and persistent pain alter sleep patterns, and this further depletes the athlete's energy and coping resources.

Depression affects many people at some time in their lives. It is estimated that 9.5% of those over 18 years of age will suffer from depression in a given year, with 5% of the general population suffering a major depressive disorder (National Institute of Mental Health 2001). This rate is increased in injured persons and in patients after spinal cord injury, stroke, and heart attack. Depression is not a normal stage in the psychological response to injury, but it can be a significant barrier to successful rehabilitation (Wegener 1998/1999).

Signs and symptoms of depression are discussed in more detail in chapter 5 in relation to persistent pain and somatization. The certified athletic trainer usually interacts with the injured person more than do other members of the sports medicine team and is, therefore, in a position to recognize these signs. Depression is a treatable psychological illness that deserves medical attention. However, there is a stigma in our society regarding psychological conditions. When depression affects a person's rehabilitation efforts, the sports medicine team must strive to provide the psychological care needed. Failure to recognize and treat depression will delay or prevent successful recovery from injury and a return to sport participation.

Anxiety disorders are characterized by excessive worry. The incidence of anxiety disorders is believed to be less than that of depression, and the effect of injury on the incidence of anxiety disorders is unknown. It is normal for an injured person to be anxious about the impact of the injury on her or his ability to participate, advancement on a team, or potential for a scholarship or professional opportunities. However, extreme and unfounded worry can lead to sleep disturbances and can adversely affect rehabilitation adherence. Informal counseling and relaxation techniques can be very effective in controlling anxiety. However, if someone continues to struggle, referral for psychological care is essential.

Depression, anxiety, and pain affect sleep. Anxiety is most often associated with sleep onset problems, pain with midsleep awakening, and depression with early awakening (Wegener 1998/1999). Regardless of the cause, a sleep disturbance affects a person's mood and general vitality.

PSYCHOLOGICAL IMPACT OF PERSISTENT AND CHRONIC PAIN

When musculoskeletal pain persists, the health care team must consider the possibility that the source is not exclusively connective tissue. Psychological disorders can also cause pain that mimics or exacerbates musculoskeletal pain. Depression and somatization can cause persistent pain. Depression is a common health condition. Not all patients who suffer from depression report pain or experience increased sensitivity to painful stimuli, and not all patients who suffer persistent or chronic pain are depressed. However, there is overlap in the chemical imbalances associated with depression and sensitization to painful stimuli. Serotonin and norepinephrine are important modulators of pain signal transmission in

the **dorsal horn**. Depleted pools of central nervous system serotonin and norepinephrine are a component of clinical depression, and medications used to treat depression increase levels of these mediators of neural activity. Effective treatment of depression requires a diagnosis and targeted intervention just as the successful care of an injured knee does.

While clinicians treating patients with musculoskeletal pain may not be trained to treat depression or somatization, recognition and referral for care is within their scope of practice. One in six (16.5%) people in the United States will suffer from a major depressive disorder in their lifetime. The 12-month prevalence is 6.7%; only about half of people with a major depressive disorder receive treatment. Up-to-date statistics are available at the website for the National Institute of Mental Health (www.nimh.nih .gov/health/statistics/index.shtml). It is likely that many patients reporting musculoskeletal pain suffer from a depressive disorder that contributes to their symptoms or is the result of an injury or illness. The close working relationship between athletic trainers and physical therapists and their patients often provides the opportunity to identify pain caused or exacerbated by psychological conditions. However, a brief screening with the following questions was found to be more accurate than physical therapists' impressions for identifying patients with low back pain who suffered from depression:

1. During the past month, have you been bothered by feeling down, depressed, or hopeless?
2. During the past month, have you been bothered by little interest or pleasure in doing things?

Patients answering yes to both questions were more than four times more likely to suffer from depression than those who answered no to these questions (Haggman, Maher, and Refshauge 2004). Clinicians often recognize the signs and symptoms of depression and somatization listed in the sections that follow, but they should not rely only on their impression of the patient to suspect that a psychological disorder might be contributing to persistent pain.

Recognizing a Major Depressive Disorder

A major depressive disorder is diagnosed by the presence of at least five of the symptoms listed

Signs and Symptoms of Major Depressive Disorder

- Depressed mood
- Markedly diminished interest in or pleasure derived from almost all activities
- Significant weight loss or weight gain
- Insomnia or hypersomnia
- Psychomotor agitation or retardation
- Fatigue or loss of energy
- Feelings of worthlessness or guilt
- Impaired concentration and indecisiveness
- Recurrent thoughts of death or suicide

Features most associated with younger individuals include the following:

- Overeating
- Oversleeping
- Mood that responds to events
- Extreme sensitivity to interpersonal rejection
- Complaints of heaviness in the arms and legs

(Depression Guidelines Panel 1993; Peppard and Denegar 1999). One of the first two must be present. The symptoms must be present almost daily, for most of each day, for 2 weeks.

Somatization Disorder

Somatization is the presentation of somatic symptoms by someone with psychiatric illness or psychological distress (Lipowski 1998). A diagnosis of somatization disorder requires a history of many physical complaints including four pain symptoms, two gastrointestinal symptoms, one sexual symptom, and one pseudoneurological symptom that are not explained by medical conditions or intentionally caused. Undifferentiated somatoform disorder (somatization) is defined as one or more physical complaints, without identifiable cause, that last for more than 6 months (American Psychiatric Association 1994). The region and nature of the symptoms often mimic those of musculoskeletal injury. When a rehabilitation plan of care is initiated but the individual fails to improve, and other causes of persistent pain are ruled out, a diagnosis of somatization should be considered.

Persons with somatization disorder can be very demanding and difficult; however, recognition and appropriate care are to everyone's benefit. In treating somatization, the care provider should (1) provide care for a bona fide injury, (2) develop a sound relationship to prevent the person from fleeing and entering a pattern of "doctor shopping" (seeking care from one doctor after another in search of a physical cause of symptoms), and (3) avoid doing harm by dismissing the person as a malingerer or symptom magnifier.

You should not provide psychological counseling unless qualified to do so. However, many physically active individuals have benefited from informal counseling from members of the sports medicine team. The young physically active person often needs to talk to someone who will listen without prejudging. Listening to young athletes and reassuring them that their fears and concerns are common can help them cope with a difficult situation.

The skilled and appropriately trained certified athletic trainer can help athletes to control their stress response through such techniques as biofeedback, muscle relaxation, thought stopping, deep breathing, and imagery (Peppard and Denegar 1994, 1999). Proficiency at these techniques requires formal instruction and practice, and you should not use techniques at which you are not proficient.

Regardless of your attempts to provide excellent care, patients may fail to progress toward recovery as expected. Not all injured people get better. Physical causes of the problem should be sought; however, it is often easier to continue to search for physical causes than confront psychological ones. The search for psychological causes begins with communication. Listening and interpreting nonverbal communication require training, skill, practice, and patience.

Somatic pain of psychological origin is a symptom, a crying out. The sports medicine team is well prepared to treat the pain of physical injury and illness, but detecting emotional pain requires skill as well. Sometimes all that a person needs is a sympathetic ear and reassurance that the stresses he or she is experiencing are normal. Sometimes the skilled clinician can help patients cope with stress and uncertainty. Definitive psychological care, however, is often required. Patients suffering from depression and somatization warrant medical and psychological attention. The sports medicine team must develop the skills to identify these problems and refer patients to appropriate resources.

Indications of Somatization

Indications that somatization may be present include the following (American Psychiatric Association 1994; Lipowski 1998):

- Increased demand on the athletic trainer's time, including lengthy visits, frequent appointments, and multiple telephone calls
- Frequent requests for treatments that require special attention
- Behaviors that demonstrate a need for special attention
- Anger when the athletic trainer indicates that the condition has improved sufficiently to warrant discontinuation of treatment and a return to sport
- A history inconsistent with the physical exam

A WORD ABOUT PLACEBO

The vast majority of people treated for musculoskeletal conditions believe that treatments with therapeutic modalities and other interventions recommended by their care providers will enhance their recovery from injury. This observation can be explained by the natural history of most musculoskeletal injuries and the known benefits of treatment with therapeutic modalities and exercise. There is, however, another influence that the clinician can use to help the injured patient: placebo. The term *placebo*, derived from the Latin "I shall please" (www.oxforddictionaries.com/us/definition/american_english/placebo), refers to a powerful influence on therapeutic interventions that is difficult to measure. Placebo is often thought of as a positive response to an inactive intervention such as providing a sugar pill in lieu of a real medication. However, bona fide interventions have a **placebo effect**. Believing that a medication or treatment will help can benefit the individual.

Placebo is not a treatment effect on gullible or unstable patients. It is a very real, positive mind–body response. The clinician who can alleviate the injured person's anxiety by accurately assessing the nature and severity of an injury and establishing a plan for recovery builds a bond of trust. When the clinician and the patient believe in the chosen treatment course, there is a high probability of success. How much of an individual response is due to treatment and how much to placebo? We do not know and can only say that a placebo effect is surely at work to some degree. Is a placebo effect bad? Absolutely not; the placebo effect helps people feel better and recover. In fact, today's managed care system, with its lack of personal touch and empathy, suffers from the loss of placebo.

Certainly, those who treat musculoskeletal injuries should continue to study the effects of treatments and rehabilitation programs. However, we should also remember the power of placebo and view it as a positive influence on recovery.

SUMMARY

The mind–body relationship is complex and strongly influences response to injury as well as recovery, and a single chapter is not sufficient to cover all related issues. This chapter discussed the psychological and emotional responses to injury. The responses are individual and do not proceed through a series of stages as was once believed. The members of the health care team can facilitate adherence to rehabilitation, and they should try to identify and address barriers to successful rehabilitation. Certainly not all of a person's problems lie within the expertise and scope of practice of each provider. The health care team should be prepared to use teamwork and appropriate referral to provide injured people with the care they need. Finally, the chapter addressed the placebo response, a poorly understood but positive influence on recovery that can be used to the injured person's benefit.

1. *Compare and contrast the contemporary stage model and the biopsychosocial model of psychological response to injury.*

The psychological response to injury has been described as occurring in stages, based on Kübler-Ross' work on death and dying. More recent literature suggests that the psychological response to injury is highly individual. People often do not experience all of the psychological responses described by Kübler-Ross, nor does their response progress in ordered stages.

2. *Discuss the impact that cognitive appraisal can have on the physically active patient's psychological and emotional responses to injury.*

The biopsychosocial model of psychological response to injury holds that a person's understanding of the nature of the injury, its severity, and the prognosis, as well as other factors, alter the psychological response. Thus, cognition, or knowing about and understanding the injury, modifies the psychological response after that injury.

3. *Identify influences on one's ability to cope with a musculoskeletal injury.*

Many factors influence one's ability to cope with a musculoskeletal injury. Some, such as the tendency to worry and overreact, are intrinsic. Others, such as stresses from work, school, family, and athletic responsibilities and support from friends, family, teammates, and caregivers, are extrinsic. The health care team cannot control all of these influences but can help individuals cope more effectively by identifying those who are struggling and the factors contributing to their stress.

4. *Identify factors that improve an athlete's adherence to a rehabilitation plan.*

Adherence to a rehabilitation plan can be enhanced by building rapport with the injured person, setting appropriate short- and long-term goals, establishing the injured person's responsibility to the rehabilitation program, focusing on the task at hand rather than the long haul, and minimizing the person's suffering.

5. *Identify common barriers to successful completion of rehabilitation.*

Multiple factors are barriers to successful rehabilitation. Secondary gain, in terms of money or avoidance of situations or responsibilities, affects the rehabilitation process. Substance abuse, depression, anxiety, and sleep disturbances also impede rehabilitation. Family and work responsibilities and inconvenience of location or timing of appointments deter the progress of many individuals, especially those outside of high school and university settings.

6. *Discuss the assessment of treatment outcomes in the context of natural history, placebo, and "true" treatment effect.*

It is very difficult to determine the true effects of treatments with therapeutic modalities. Most musculoskeletal injuries sustained by physically active people heal with time, allowing return to full athletic participation. In addition, a placebo response is common after treatment by medical and allied medical professionals. Extensive investigation is needed to identify which therapeutic modalities facilitate the achievement of treatment goals and speed the rehabilitation process.

chapter 3

Evidence-Based Application of Therapeutic Modalities

OBJECTIVES

After reading this chapter, you will be able to

1. define the term *evidence-based health care*;
2. discuss the role of outcomes assessment in advancing evidence-based health care;
3. describe how clinical trials are conducted;
4. identify the components of well-designed randomized controlled clinical trials;
5. describe how a systematic review is developed; and
6. identify resources for locating clinical trials of treatments in which therapeutic modalities were used.

An active 25-year-old patient presents with a history of recurrent right ankle injuries. The most recent occurred 2 weeks ago during a basketball game with some friends. Although the patient can walk comfortably and run with only mild discomfort, he is seeking advice on prevention of further injuries, particularly during a hiking vacation planned next month. He also asks about how to best manage his ankle if reinjury should occur.

Examination and evaluation reveal chronic ankle instability secondary to a severe ankle sprain suffered while playing high school basketball. How can this patient's needs best be met? Clinical preparation and experience suggest that a progressive balance training program and the use of an ankle brace, especially while hiking, will reduce the risk of injury. However, how effective will the plan of care be? What is the risk of reinjury while hiking? Some answers exist in the research literature, but the information must be located and appraised. The integration of the available research and your clinical experience with this patient's unique presentation and values (for example, canceling the hiking vacation would be unacceptable) embodies the practice of evidence-based health care. This chapter is devoted to locating and appraising clinical research that guides sound clinical decision making.

The practice of evidence-based health care requires the integration of the best research evidence with the unique presentation of each patient (medical history, history of current condition, signs and symptoms), the clinician's training and expertise, and the patient's preferences and values. In chapters 1 and 2, the sequelae to injury and the challenges of lasting pain are presented. This background is provided so that the therapeutic modalities that are to be discussed can be applied with an understanding of the physiology of injury and repair and an appreciation for the impairments, functional limitations, and disabilities experienced by injured athletes. In later chapters, the physical principles and application techniques of contemporary modalities are presented. Issues of safety and contraindications are highlighted. After the introduction of the modalities, discussion turns to the when and why of modality application. These issues are further summarized in chapter 19, in which principles of clinical decision making are applied.

The answers about the why and when of therapeutic modalities, as well as other medical interventions, have been and often continue to be based on practice traditions and theory. Increasingly, health care providers are being called on to seek out and provide evidence that the interventions they recommend *enhance recovery and improve the outcome of treatment.* This search for evidence may challenge our assumptions, but it allows us to integrate the best available research into our clinical decision-making process.

In chapters 7 through 15, as well as 17 and 18, the issues of **efficacy** and **effectiveness** of therapeutic interventions are addressed. We provide references to clinical trials and make practice recommendations based on our reviews. Reading these sections should not substitute for individual effort. Each clinician is responsible for the decisions he or she makes based on the information available. Reviewing, analyzing, and applying the evidence found in the existing literature have several potential benefits for the patient, clinician, and health care system. First, critical review may lead to the discontinuation of treatments that may do more harm than good and of ineffective treatments that only delay appropriate care. Furthermore, such efforts identify how effective treatments may be rendered in the most cost- and time-efficient manner. This process also helps focus attention on what is really important: Did the patient get better, and if so, was this really the result of the treatment?

NEED FOR EVIDENCE-BASED PRACTICE

Health care is complex, costly, and essential. The cost of health care can be assessed not only in terms of money spent but also in terms of time required of patients and providers. The challenge across health care is to provide the care needed to optimize treatment outcomes in the most efficient manner. The challenges facing the health care system of patients, providers, and payers are no less a concern in athletic training than in other health care disciplines. To meet these challenges, treatment regimens need to be analyzed and compared based on the outcomes and costs of care. Those treatments not demonstrated to improve outcomes should be abandoned from general practice. For example, Deyo et al. (1990a) reported that transcutaneous electrical nerve stimulation (TENS) as a sole intervention is ineffective in the management of chronic low back pain. This does not mean that a particular modality like TENS is of no value. Further study of some treatments may be warranted to identify medical conditions, circumstances, or populations (patients without contraindications treated for pain associated with acute rib fracture) for which the treatments are effective (Oncel et al. 2002). New evidence should be evaluated and, when appropriate, should change how clinicians practice. Moreover, new research and systematic reviews of existing research may also result in new practice recommendations for all clinicians.

Many tools have been developed to assess the outcomes of treatment with medications and surgery as well as modality application and therapeutic exercises. Assessment of treatment outcomes often includes clinician-derived measures such as changes in range of motion and strength. However, information provided by patients about levels of pain, functional limitations, and perceived disability is also vital. Reports of treatment outcomes based on clinician assessments and patient self-assessments are increasingly available to guide the clinician's selection of effective treatments with therapeutic modalities and exercises. Clinicians must be able to identify pertinent literature, assess the validity of the conclusions drawn by investigators, and judge the extent to which the results of **clinical trials** generalize to the people they treat.

At this point you may question why published clinical trials are important to modality use specifically and health care in general. When a patient under your care reports improvement, can you not be certain that your treatment was beneficial? *Unfortunately not!* Many factors can lead to improvements. Often improvement occurs with the passage of time (natural history of the condition). Simple reassurance that a condition is not serious and that recovery is nearly certain, along with other efforts to reassure and empathize, can result in perceived improvement. True placebo and the effects of other interventions such as exercise may also explain the perceived benefits of modality application.

Given that many things may contribute to reports of improvement and demonstrable functional recovery, how do we decide the best course of treatment? Searching the literature for clinical trials on various treatments can yield valuable information, and this process is introduced in the next section. The literature, unfortunately, is lacking in many areas of athletic health care. For example, evidence may exist for the effectiveness of a treatment in managing nonathletic patients but generalization of the research to an athletic patient in your care may not be appropriate. Clearly a great deal of research is needed to better define those treatments that are truly beneficial in the management of specific patients. This is not laboratory research but rather research that must be conducted in the practice setting and must involve the clinicians providing care.

FINDING AND ASSESSING THE EVIDENCE

The widespread practice of evidence-based health care was made possible by advances in information technology. Years ago, the identification and retrieval of research in a library might have taken days; now thanks to the Internet we can conduct searches on a personal computer, tablet, or phone in a matter of minutes. Searching the databases, however, is a skill, and the clinician has many choices in where to search. Following are selected databases that we use to find research and practice guidelines related to the diagnosis and treatment of musculoskeletal conditions and the effectiveness of therapeutic modalities.

- PubMed (aka Medline via PubMed) (www.ncbi.nlm.nih.gov/pubmed) is supported by the U.S. National Library of Medicine and provides links to abstracts and full-text papers in scholarly journals concerning health care and medicine.

- Scopus (www.scopus.com/home.url) is an international database of research from more than 20,000 publications, including research in health care and medicine.

- PEDro: The Physiotherapy Evidence Database (www.pedro.org.au) is produced by the Centre for Evidence-Based Physiotherapy at the George Institute for Global Health; it offers access to systematic reviews, clinical practice guidelines, and original research related to therapeutic interventions.

- CINAHL Plus with Full Text (https://health.ebsco.com/products/cinahl-plus-with-full-text) is a database that provides access to scholarly journal articles in nursing and allied health.

- National Guideline Clearinghouse Comprehensive is a database of full-text evidence-based clinical practice guidelines and related documents.

While some research can be found in multiple databases, you need to search several to develop an exhaustive list of research papers devoted to a clinical question. For routine searches that rapidly yield results we most commonly search PubMed first. Identifying a database is only the start. All searches require that a key word or words be entered into a query. The key words are found in the question being asked; thus the starting point is to explicitly state a clinical question.

For example, a clinician might ask "Is massage effective in reducing low back pain?" The search engines do not care about words such as "Is" or "in." Moreover, words such as "effective" and "reducing" are the outcomes of interest and do not relate to the intervention or the patient problem or population. The "massage" and "low back pain" provide the search terms. The rules for combining terms varies between databases. In PubMed, Boolean maneuvers that include operations based on the words AND, OR, and NOT as well as " " marks and * are used to direct the search. In this case we can develop a

search string of ("massage" AND "low back pain"). The words such as AND are always capitalized. The use of the quotation marks keeps the words in a phrase so that individual words such as *pain* are not included. Including "pain" as a single term would yield all papers related to massage and pain and force the clinician to sort through more titles than is desirable or necessary. If one wanted to exclude a type of low back pain, such as pain related to pregnancy, the addition of "NOT pregnancy" could be included. If *pregnant* appears rather than *pregnancy*, the paper would not be excluded from the search. The judicious use of * allows the search engine to find all derivatives such that pregnan* would not exclude papers with *pregnant* or *pregnancy* in the title or abstracts.

The use of medical subheadings or MeSH terms allows for the capture of papers germane to the question that did not include the specific key words. For example, if you wished to learn about the treatment of poison ivy, you might not consider the term "Toxicodendron," which includes shrubs, trees, and vines that produce allergenic oleoresin, which causes the dermatitis commonly known as poison ivy. Practice is required to make the most out of database searches, but once developed, the skills provide rapid access to the literature that supports the practice of evidence-based health care.

The literature search provides the titles and abstracts of papers containing the key words. Often these can be quickly scanned to find the papers of greatest interest. Now the work of critically appraising the research and making judgments about the applications to one or more patients in your care begins.

ASSESSING

The improvement of an individual patient may or may not be due to the care rendered or be attributable to a particular treatment. The body has an incredible capacity to repair damaged tissues and fend off pathogens (bacteria and viruses). Thus, in many cases improvement in, or resolution of, a condition may be expected over time. In the treatment of musculoskeletal injuries, patients may be exposed to an array of interventions including medications, instructions in rest, therapeutic exercises, and modality applications. Are all aspects of the plan of care necessary or even helpful? Answers about what treatments are effective may lie in the clinical literature. Once a successful search is completed, new questions emerge as each paper is considered.

Initially it is important to consider the subjects of the research and the outcomes measured. One may wish to learn whether a combination of superficial heating and stationary cycling improves mobility in the community for a senior with knee osteoarthritis. A search may include papers on community mobility following total knee arthroplasty or research into changes in quadriceps strength following a 6-week cycling program. Both research projects are related to the primary question but do not directly address the clinical question. A quick scan of titles and abstracts is often needed to find the most relevant research. The more similar the subjects and outcomes measures in a research report are to your situation, the greater the likelihood you will be able to apply the data to clinical decisions.

Research data that can guide clinical decision making can be collected by clinicians or provided by patients. The biopsychosocial model presented in chapter 2 should be considered when appraising clinical research and practice guidelines. Measurements of impairments (other than pain) and some aspects of function can be obtained by clinicians, but these "objective measures" do not correlate well with participation restrictions and quality-of-life perceptions that are important to patients. After knee surgery, for example, the strength of the quadriceps and hamstring muscles is often assessed on an isokinetic dynamometer. While strength recovery is important, just having strength does not mean that an athlete will be able to run, cut, jump, or perform in his or her sport. In general, the clinician will find a mix of outcome measures that include objective measures obtained by clinicians and patient-generated self-reports that are useful in guiding recommendations and planning care. When reviewing a clinical trial, consider whether the measures assessed are really of interest.

Patient Self-Report Instruments

Patient self-report instruments have been developed and validated for several situations. The most basic are visual analog scales of pain perception (e.g., 0 = no pain, 10 = worst possible pain). While valuable, learning the patient's perception of the pain being experienced does not provide a more global assessment of health. More comprehensive instruments provide information related to physical and social functioning and sense of well-being. The SF-36

(www.sf-36.org/tools/SF36.shtml) is a commonly administered patient self-report of general health and function. The eight scales of the instrument provide summary measures of physical and mental health. The United States National Institutes of Health provides several assessment instruments through the PROMIS system (www.nihpromis .org), including some specifically designed for and validated in pediatric and adolescent patients.

The SF-36 and PROMIS instruments provide a global assessment of health but lack information specific to particular conditions or structures. Condition-specific instruments have also been developed to help clinicians better understand the impact of conditions such as low back pain and knee osteoarthritis on patients and learn more about the outcomes of clinical care. The Knee injury and Osteoarthritis Outcome Score (KOOS) (www.koos .nu) is a patient self-report that addresses symptoms, pain, stiffness, function, and quality of life in patients suffering from osteoarthritis or other knee conditions. The Oswestry Low Back Pain Scale (aka Oswestry Low Back Pain Questionnaire) assesses pain and function in patients with low back pain in 10 subsections. The KOOS and Oswestry instruments (figures 3.1 and 3.2) illustrate condition-specific patient self-assessment instruments.

Efforts continue in developing instruments specific to injured athletes such as the Disablement in the Physically Active Scale (Vela and Denegar 2010). Self-report instruments provide the clinician an opportunity to understand the consequences of injury and illness as the patient views them from a biopsychosocial perspective. The information gathered also permits assessment of whether the treatments provided by health care providers really make a difference in the outcome after injury or illness. The development and validation of self-report instruments is time-consuming and costly. However, the data provided are critical to the advancement of evidence-based health care.

Clinical Trials on Effectiveness and Efficacy

After considering the characteristics of patients studied and the data collected in a clinical investigation, you should consider the study's validity and whether the results can be generalized into your practice. Clinical trials can address the efficacy or the effectiveness of health care procedures. Effectiveness is defined as the result of interventions applied

Koos Knee Survey

Today's date: _____ / _____ / _____   Date of birth: _____ / _____ / _____

Name: _____

Instructions: This survey asks for your view about your knee. This information will help us keep track of how your feel about your knee and how well you are able to perform your usual activities.

Answer every question by ticking the appropriate box, only one box for each question. If you are unsure about how to answer a question, please give the best answer you can.

SYMPTOMS

These questions should be answered thinking of your knee symptoms during the **last week**.

S1. Do you have swelling in your knee?

NEVER	RARELY	SOMETIMES	OFTEN	ALWAYS
☐	☐	☐	☐	☐

S2. Do you feel grinding, hear clicking or any other type of noise when your knee moves?

NEVER	RARELY	SOMETIMES	OFTEN	ALWAYS
☐	☐	☐	☐	☐

S3. Does your knee catch or hang up when moving?

NEVER	RARELY	SOMETIMES	OFTEN	ALWAYS
☐	☐	☐	☐	☐

S4. Can you straighten your knee fully?

NEVER	RARELY	SOMETIMES	OFTEN	ALWAYS
☐	☐	☐	☐	☐

S5. Can you bend your knee fully?

NEVER	RARELY	SOMETIMES	OFTEN	ALWAYS
☐	☐	☐	☐	☐

STIFFNESS

The following questions concern the amount of joint stiffness you have experienced during the **last week** In your knee. Stiffness is a sensation of restriction or slowness in the ease with which you move your knee joint.

S6. How severe is your knee joint stiffness after first wakening in the morning.

NONE	MILD	MODERATE	SEVERE	EXTREME
☐	☐	☐	☐	☐

S7. How severe is your knee stiffness after sitting, lying or resting **later in the day?**

NONE	MILD	MODERATE	SEVERE	EXTREME
☐	☐	☐	☐	☐

PAIN

P1. How often do you experience knee pain?

NEVER	MONTHLY	WEEKLY	DAILY	ALWAYS
☐	☐	☐	☐	☐

Figure 3.1 Koos Knee Survey.

Reprinted from Knee injury and Osteoarthritis Outcome Score (KOOS). Available: www.koos.nu/koos-english.pdf

What amount of knee pain have you experienced in the **last week** during the following activities?

P2. Twisting/pivoting on your knee

NONE	MILD	MODERATE	SEVERE	EXTREME
☐	☐	☐	☐	☐

P3. Straightening knee fully

NONE	MILD	MODERATE	SEVERE	EXTREME
☐	☐	☐	☐	☐

P4. Bending knee fully

NONE	MILD	MODERATE	SEVERE	EXTREME
☐	☐	☐	☐	☐

P5. Walking on flat surface

NONE	MILD	MODERATE	SEVERE	EXTREME
☐	☐	☐	☐	☐

P6. Going up or down stairs

NONE	MILD	MODERATE	SEVERE	EXTREME
☐	☐	☐	☐	☐

P7. At night while in bed

NONE	MILD	MODERATE	SEVERE	EXTREME
☐	☐	☐	☐	☐

P8. Sitting or lying

NONE	MILD	MODERATE	SEVERE	EXTREME
☐	☐	☐	☐	☐

P9. Standing upright

NONE	MILD	MODERATE	SEVERE	EXTREME
☐	☐	☐	☐	☐

FUNCTION, DAILY LIVING

The following questions concern your physical function. By this we mean your ability to move around and to look after yourself. For each of the following activities please indicate the degree of difficulty you have experienced in the **last week** due to your knee.

A1. Descending stairs

NONE	MILD	MODERATE	SEVERE	EXTREME
☐	☐	☐	☐	☐

A2. Ascending stairs

NONE	MILD	MODERATE	SEVERE	EXTREME
☐	☐	☐	☐	☐

For each of the following activities please indicate the degree of difficulty you have experienced in the **last week** due to your knee.

A3. Rising from sitting

NONE	MILD	MODERATE	SEVERE	EXTREME
☐	☐	☐	☐	☐

Figure 3.1 *(continued)*

A4. Standing

NONE	MILD	MODERATE	SEVERE	EXTREME
☐	☐	☐	☐	☐

A5. Bending to floor/picking up an object

NONE	MILD	MODERATE	SEVERE	EXTREME
☐	☐	☐	☐	☐

A6. Walking on flat surface

NONE	MILD	MODERATE	SEVERE	EXTREME
☐	☐	☐	☐	☐

A7. Getting in/out of car

NONE	MILD	MODERATE	SEVERE	EXTREME
☐	☐	☐	☐	☐

A8. Going shopping

NONE	MILD	MODERATE	SEVERE	EXTREME
☐	☐	☐	☐	☐

A9. Putting on socks/stockings

NONE	MILD	MODERATE	SEVERE	EXTREME
☐	☐	☐	☐	☐

A10. Rising from bed

NONE	MILD	MODERATE	SEVERE	EXTREME
☐	☐	☐	☐	☐

A11. Taking off socks/stockings

NONE	MILD	MODERATE	SEVERE	EXTREME
☐	☐	☐	☐	☐

A12. Lying in bed (turning over, maintaining knee position)

NONE	MILD	MODERATE	SEVERE	EXTREME
☐	☐	☐	☐	☐

A13. Getting in/out of bath

NONE	MILD	MODERATE	SEVERE	EXTREME
☐	☐	☐	☐	☐

A14. Siting

NONE	MILD	MODERATE	SEVERE	EXTREME
☐	☐	☐	☐	☐

A15. Getting on/off toilet

NONE	MILD	MODERATE	SEVERE	EXTREME
☐	☐	☐	☐	☐

For each of the following activities please indicate the degree of difficulty you have experienced in the **last week** due to your knee.

A16. Heavy domestic (moving heavy boxes, scrubbing floors, etc.)

NONE	MILD	MODERATE	SEVERE	EXTREME
☐	☐	☐	☐	☐

Figure 3.1   *(continued)*

A17. Light domestic (cooking, dusting, etc.)

NONE	MILD	MODERATE	SEVERE	EXTREME
☐	☐	☐	☐	☐

FUNCTION, SPORTS, AND RECREATIONAL ACTIVITIES

The following questions concern your physical function when being active on a higher level. The questions should be answered thinking of what degree of difficulty you have experienced during the **last week** due to your knee.

SP1. Squatting

NONE	MILD	MODERATE	SEVERE	EXTREME
☐	☐	☐	☐	☐

SP2. Running

NONE	MILD	MODERATE	SEVERE	EXTREME
☐	☐	☐	☐	☐

SP3. Jumping

NONE	MILD	MODERATE	SEVERE	EXTREME
☐	☐	☐	☐	☐

SP4. Twisting/pivoting on your injured knee

NONE	MILD	MODERATE	SEVERE	EXTREME
☐	☐	☐	☐	☐

SP5. Kneeling

NONE	MILD	MODERATE	SEVERE	EXTREME
☐	☐	☐	☐	☐

QUALITY OF LIFE

Q1. How often are you aware of your knee problem?

NEVER	MONTHLY	WEEKLY	DAILY	CONSTANTLY
☐	☐	☐	☐	☐

Q2. Have you modified your life style to avoid potentially damaging activities to your knees?

NOT AT ALL	MILDLY	MODERATELY	SEVERELY	TOTALLY
☐	☐	☐	☐	☐

Q3. How much are you troubled with lack of confidence in your knee?

NOT AT ALL	MILDLY	MODERATELY	SEVERELY	EXTREMELY
☐	☐	☐	☐	☐

Q4. In general, how much difficulty do you have with your knee?

NONE	MILD	MODERATE	SEVERE	EXTREME
☐	☐	☐	☐	☐

Thank you very much for completing all the questions in this questionnaire.

Figure 3.1 *(continued)*

Oswestry Low Back Pain Scale

Please rate the severity of your pain by circling a number below:

No pain | 0 | 1 | 2 | 3 | 4 | 5 | 6 | 7 | 8 | 9 | 10 | Unbearable pain

Name _____ Date _____

Instructions: Please circle the ONE NUMBER In each section which most closely describes your problem.

SECTION 1—PAIN INTENSITY

0. The pain comes and goes and is very mild
1. The pain is mild and does not vary much.
2. The pain comes and goes and is very moderate.
3. The pain is moderate and does not vary much.
4. The pain comes and goes and is severe.
5. The pain is severe and does not vary much.

SECTION 2—PERSONAL CARE (WASHING, DRESSING, ETC.)

0. I would not have to change my way of washing or dressing in order to avoid pain.
1. I do not normally change my way of washing or dressing even though it causes some pain.
2. Washing and dressing increase the pain but I manage not to change my way of doing it.
3. Washing and dressing Increase the pain and I find it necessary to change my way of doing it.
4. Because of the pain I am unable to do some washing and dressing without help.
5. Because of the pain I am unable to do any washing and dressing without help.

SECTION 3—LIFTING

0. I can lift heavy weights without extra pain.
1. I can lift heavy weights but it gives extra pain.
2. Pain prevents me from lifting heavy weights off the floor.
3. Pain prevents me from lifting heavy weights off the floor, but I can manage if they are conveniently positioned, e.g., on a table.
4. Pain prevents me from lifting heavy weights but I can manage light to medium weights if they are conveniently positioned.
5. I can only lift very light weights at most.

SECTION 4—WALKING

0. I have no pain when walking.
1. I have some pain on walking but it does not Increase with distance.
2. I cannot walk more than 1 mile without increasing pain.
3. I cannot walk more than 1/2 mile without increasing pain.
4. I cannot walk more than 1/4 mile without increasing pain.
5. I cannot walk at all without increasing pain.

SECTION 5—SITTING

0. I can sit in any chair as long as I like.
1. I can sit only in my favorite chair as long as I like.

Figure 3.2 Oswestry Low Back Pain Scale.

Reprinted from Spine Research Institute of San Diego.

2. Pain prevents me from sitting more than 1 hour.

3. Pain prevents me from sitting more than 1/2 hour.

4. Pain prevents me from sitting more than 10 minutes.

5. I avoid sitting because it increases pain immediately.

SECTION 6—STANDING

0. I can stand as long as I want without pain.

1. I have some pain on standing but it does not increase with time.

2. I cannot stand for longer than 1 hour without increasing pain.

3. I cannot stand for longer than 1/2 hour without increasing pain.

4. I cannot stand longer than 10 minutes without increasing pain.

5. I avoid standing because it increases the pain immediately.

SECTION 7—SLEEPING

0. I get no pain in bed.

1. I get pain in bed but it does not prevent me from sleeping well.

2. Because of my pain my normal nights sleep is reduced by less than one quarter.

3. Because of my pain my normal nights sleep is reduced by less than one half.

4. Because of my pain my normal nights sleep is reduced by less than three quarters.

5. Pain prevents me from sleeping at all.

SECTION 8—SOCIAL LIFE

0. My social life is normal and gives me no pains.

1. My social life is normal but it increases the degree of pain.

2. Pain has no significant effect on my social life apart from limiting my more energetic interests, e.g., dancing.

3. Pain has restricted by social life and I do not go out very often.

4. Pain has restricted by social life to my home.

5. I have hardly any social life because of the pain.

SECTION 9—TRAVELING

0. I get no pain when traveling.

1. I get some pain when traveling but none of my usual forms of travel make it any worse.

2. I get extra pain while traveling but it does not compel me to seek alternate forms of travel.

3. I get extra pain while traveling, which compels me to seek alternative forms of travel.

4. Pain restricts me to short necessary journeys under 1/2 hour.

5. Pain restricts all forms of travel.

SECTION 10—CHANGING DEGREES OF PAIN

0. My pain is rapidly getting better.

1. My pain fluctuates but is definitely getting better.

2. My pain seems to be getting better but improvement is slow.

3. My pain is neither getting better nor worse.

4. My pain is gradually worsening.

5. My pain is rapidly worsening.

Figure 3.2 (continued)

during routine daily practice. Efficacy is best established through randomized controlled clinical trials (RCTs) in which efforts are made to control for all threats to the validity of the data. In simpler terms, RCTs try to link the differences observed within a group or between treatment groups to the manipulation of the treatment variables. For example, if an investigator wished to learn if TENS reduces pain following a rib fracture, patients might be assigned to receive functional TENS or a sham treatment. All care of the patients would be identical in all other aspects. Thus, any differences in pain relief between the groups would only be attributable to the application of TENS.

RCTs are not the only clinical research design. Cohort studies, case control studies, and case series reports are critical to clinical research. Sometimes it is not ethically or practically possible to randomly assign patients to treatment groups. If a condition is uncommon it may not be reasonable to try to assemble a sample large enough to conduct a useful RCT.

Clearly, well-designed RCTs account for the effects of multiple factors, including the passage of time (natural history), placebo, investigator bias, and subject bias that can compromise the validity of data. However, the application of therapeutic modalities rarely occurs as an isolated treatment. Following a rib fracture, patients may need medication for pain relief, and the type and amount of medication consumed will affect our ability to attribute a portion of pain relief to TENS unless all patients receive the same medication regimen. Studies that compare cohorts of patients exposed or unexposed to TENS may be more readily generalized to everyday clinical practice, where multiple treatments (medication, taping, therapeutic modalities, etc.) are often applied. The limitations of cohort designs can best be understood by examining the best approaches to conducting an RCT.

In an RCT, patients or subjects are randomly assigned to treatment groups. All patients within a group receive the same treatment (e.g., TENS), but the treatment will differ between groups (e.g., patients in one group may be treated with a sham or inoperable TENS device). To the greatest possible extent, subjects, clinicians, and evaluators are all kept in the dark about which group receives which treatment. Natural history (improvement over time exhibited by patients receiving a sham or control) and placebo effects (improvement due to belief that a sham treatment is effective) can bias the data; they must be controlled in order to truly

assess the effect of therapeutic modality application on treatment outcomes. High-quality RCTs on the care of active populations have become more numerous and more easily accessed in the past decade.

We can turn to the management of lateral epicondylitis (tennis elbow) for an example of the process. Iontophoresis, discussed in detail in chapter 8, is often administered by certified athletic trainers and physical therapists in the treatment of lateral epicondylitis. Each of the authors of this text has done this procedure. Our collective observation has been that some athletes treated for lateral epicondylitis with iontophoresis get better, suggesting that the treatment is, to some extent, effective.

However, when the hypothesis that iontophoresis with a steroidal medication is effective in the treatment of lateral epicondylitis was tested in a high-quality randomized controlled clinical trial, the result was that the treatment did not improve outcomes (Runeson and Hacker 2002). Such studies provide far stronger evidence of benefit, or the lack thereof, than individual observations. It is quite possible that benefits we have observed in response to iontophoresis were attributable to factors other than that intervention, factors we could not control for at the time of treatment.

Interestingly, some of the third-party health insurance providers we work with, including Medicare, no longer reimburse for iontophoresis treatment because of the lack of evidence of efficacy. Evidence-based medicine is a strategy not only for improving patient outcomes, but also for guiding public health policy. This is a dynamic process. As new RCTs and other studies are published, clinical practice guidelines (discussed later) and health care policies can be revised. Ultimately, the most beneficial treatments will become the standard for care, and ineffective treatment will be abandoned. Studies of the therapeutic modalities discussed in this text are particularly needed.

Table 3.1 presents a hierarchy of study designs in order of control of confounding variables (see MacCauley and Best 2002 and Domholdt 2005 for greater detail). The criteria for grading the methodological quality of clinical trials were developed by the Physiotherapy Evidence Database. While it is mainly used to grade or appraise RCTs, the instrument also gives us insight into the threats to data validity that exist when studies lack random assignment. These guidelines identify those factors that minimize the risk of falsely attributing

Table 3.1   Hierarchy of Study Designs in Order of Control of Confounding Variables

Type of study	Important characteristics
Randomized controlled clinical trial (RCT)	Prospective assignment of subjects/patients to two or more treatment groups
Cohort study (may be prospective or retrospective)	Investigates the outcomes following exposure to an intervention (may be prospective or retrospective)
Case control study	Identifies an outcomes and then seeks to understand the interventions associated with the outcome (retrospective)
Cross-sectional study*	Documents health status at a single point in time seeking to compare groups
Case study, case report, and case series*#	Reports on one or more cases including condition, treatments, and outcomes (retrospective)

*Studies lack prospective random assignment and generally have less control over factors that threaten validity of study results.

#In cases of relatively rare and more chronic conditions, case series reports may be useful in identifying effective treatments, especially when variables of interest are objective and highly reproducible.

favorable treatment outcomes to specific interventions or exposing data to bias.

These issues are of particular interest in assessing the efficacy and effectiveness of therapeutic modalities used to treat musculoskeletal injuries. In the research conducted by Runeson and colleagues noted previously, the investigators were able to blind the patients, the clinicians providing the treatment, and the investigators assessing change as to whether the patient actually received active medication. Exposure to therapeutic modalities such as superficial cold or heat cannot be hidden from either the patient or the provider. Thus, the belief that the treatment is beneficial, rather than the effects of the treatment, may result in perceived improvement. As noted

previously, prospective cohort studies may better address the effectiveness of health care by examining the association between exposure (receiving a treatment) and an outcome of care. When an RCT is not conducted, the validity of data may be threatened by the same issues addressed in the PEDro instrument, and the potential for bias must be considered. The critical appraisal of the research requires more than grading of methodological quality. Clinicians must consider the patient characteristics, the outcomes measured, threats to data validity, and the generalizability of findings to their practice. Issues of how data are analyzed and reported are beyond the scope of this chapter, but they also warrant consideration. Such appraisal requires training in statistics, which

Assessing the Methodological Quality of RCTs

The 11 points identified permit a critical appraisal of the quality of controlled clinical trials. When there is conflicting information about an intervention, higher-quality studies are much more likely to reflect the truth. Readers should be careful, however, not to dismiss a study due to the absence of one or more of the criteria listed. In some cases it is not possible, even under ideal circumstances, to meet all criteria. This guide will help you to sort out those studies most likely to support sound clinical decisions.

1. **Eligibility criteria were specified.** Investigators should include specific information about criteria for entry into and exclusion from a study. This is critical when the certified athletic trainer ponders whether the results of a study can be generalized to an individual case.

2. **Subjects were randomly allocated to groups.** Studies in which subjects are assigned to groups by investigators and studies involving self-selected group membership introduce the potential for bias on the part of the researcher or subject.

(continued)

3. **Allocation was concealed.** Treatment group assignment should not be shared among participants, providers, and evaluators.

4. **The groups were similar at baseline in the most important prognostic indicators.** Investigators should adequately describe the composition for each of the treatment groups. For most characteristics there is a normal distribution across the population, and this distribution is reflected in all treatment groups. Random chance can, however, result in unequal distributions and should be identified and, when possible, controlled for.

5. **There was blinding of all subjects.** When subjects are unaware of whether they received a "real" or placebo treatment, subject bias is eliminated. Blinding subjects to treatment may sound simple and in some cases may be. One could provide real and placebo magnets that look identical. In other cases, however, such as with TENS (discussed in chapters 7 and 8), it may not be possible to adequately blind subjects to the treatment they receive. This issue is discussed in detail by Deyo et al. (1990b).

6. **There was blinding of all clinicians who administered therapy.** When possible, the clinician providing the treatment (e.g., instructing the subject in the application of a flexible magnet) should not be aware of whether the magnet is active or placebo. This process prevents the clinician from introducing bias into the study. As with blinding of subjects, blinding of clinicians is easily accomplished in some studies and impossible in others.

7. **There was blinding of all assessors who measured at least one key outcome.** When assessors—whether they are taking measurements such as range of motion or collecting self-report information—are unaware of the treatment received, the potential of the assessor to bias the results is removed.

8. **Measures of at least one key outcome were obtained from more than 85% of the subjects initially allocated to groups.** Loss of subjects to follow-up or dropout can occur for a number of reasons. When dropout exceeds 15%, however, the validity of the results is threatened. For example, suppose that 100 subjects are randomly assigned to receive ultrasound or sham ultrasound treatments for Achilles **tendinopathy**. The authors indicate that at follow-up, 20 of 24 in the treatment group reported significant improvement while 20 of 40 in the sham group improved. The investigators conclude that the 80% recovery in those treated is significantly better than the 50% in the sham treatment group and that ultrasound enhances recovery in athletes suffering from Achilles tendinopathy. A closer look, however, reveals that 20 of 50 in each of the original treatment groups are improved. Did dropout bias the results?

9. **All subjects for whom measures were available received the treatment or control condition as allocated.** Or, where this was not the case, data for at least one key outcome were analyzed by intention to treat.

10. **The results of between-group statistical comparisons are reported for at least one key outcome.** Statistical analysis controls for random fluctuations in the populations and provides estimates of the extent to which outcomes attributed to treatment effects were due to chance. A low probability that results were chance events strengthens the validity of study conclusions.

11. **The study provides both point measures and measures of variability for at least one key outcome.** Reports of clinical trials should provide information about change over time and estimates of variability in outcome measures and thus responses to treatments.

is essential for clinicians seeking to integrate the best available research into clinical decision making.

SYSTEMATIC REVIEW AND PRACTICE GUIDELINES

The ability to search and critically appraise the research literature is an essential skill for the practicing clinician. Individual clinicians cannot, however, devote the time to collecting and critically reviewing the literature on each diagnostic test performed or each therapeutic intervention rendered. This is reality for all health care professionals.

It is also important to understand that the results obtained from the study of a sample of patients may not reflect the response that would be obtained from the study of the entire population from which the sample was drawn. This is one of the reasons that two clinical trials addressing the same intervention on similar patients may come to different conclusions. In general, results obtained from the study of a large sample are more likely to reflect the truth than those from the study of a smaller sample provided that the methodological quality is similar.

The fact that multiple articles on the same topic offer different conclusions further adds to the challenge of evidence-based clinical practice for the busy clinician. How many articles must be retrieved and appraised to ensure the integration of the best available evidence? Relief to the burdened clinician is sometimes found in the availability of a systematic review or clinical practice guideline.

Systematic reviews are research efforts in which data are acquired from existing literature through a planned and thorough search process. Data acquired through systematic review may undergo statistical analysis through a process called meta-analysis. Because data from multiple studies are combined, one can have greater confidence in the conclusions drawn from the analysis. Remember the benefits of larger samples. Thus, when well-conducted systematic reviews are available, the clinician may find powerful evidence in a single article and be able to avoid a detailed search and careful appraisal of multiple articles. Recall the discussion at the beginning of this chapter about the management of an ankle sprain. There have been several studies on the effects of balance training following ankle sprain. However, a systematic review such as the one by McKeon and Hertel (2008) may provide the evidence you need to help the patient in question. Essentially, the hard

work of appraising individual articles is completed by the authors of such reviews, permitting more time for the integration of the best available research into one's clinical practice.

Systematic reviews are research efforts and, as with RCTs, the methodological quality can affect the conclusions drawn. The research methods of a systematic review are presented in the methods section of the article as is typical of other types of research reports. Appraising the methodological quality of a systematic review is beyond the scope of this chapter, but the PRISMA (**P**referred **R**eporting **I**tems for **S**ystematic Reviews and **M**eta-**A**nalyses) guidelines available at www.prisma-statement.org provide an excellent tutorial. Systematic reviews need careful appraisal, especially since the subjects or patients included may be diverse, and generalization of results needs careful consideration. However, a growing number of high-quality systematic reviews can be applied to everyday clinical practice.

In an effort to apply and disseminate new information, several professional groups have authored evidence-based practice guidelines. Evidence-based practice guidelines are developed by groups of authors with recognized expertise in the professional organization. Like the authors of all systematic reviews, these groups assemble and evaluate the existing literature using preestablished criteria. The Cochrane Collaboration (http://www.thecochrane library.com) is an example of this process. A team of authors reviews available clinical research and develops recommendations for the use or discontinuation of specific interventions and identifies areas where further research is needed. Similar processes are used to develop practice guidelines for many professional groups and organizations.

The number of evidence-based practice guidelines in sports medicine and athletic training has increased, but few if any address the application of therapeutic modalities in the treatment of active and athletic populations. New guidelines are important to the evolution of evidence-based practices. Recalling the framework of evidence-based practice, however, remember that guidelines are not complete truths, recipes, or protocols. A consensus of experts independently reviewing the available literature does offer a strong measure of credibility, but, as noted previously, each patient requires unique and personalized care, and guidelines are dynamic. New research may emerge that will cause clinicians to change how they practice before practice guidelines can be revised. This takes us back to the primary issue addressed in this chapter: Be prepared to integrate, and base your decisions on, the best currently available evidence.

Clinical practice will never be based exclusively on practice guidelines and the critical review of clinical trials. To conclude this chapter, we again return to the definition of evidence-based practice: *The integration of the best research evidence with clinical expertise and patient values.* Each patient and each clinician is unique. Patients vary in terms of health histories, coexisting conditions, and personal preferences. Clinicians vary in experiences and skills. Ultimately each clinician has a responsibility to provide care that best addresses the patient's condition and needs while avoiding treatments that add to the costs but do not improve outcomes. The integration of the best available evidence into daily practice facilitates the achievement of these objectives.

In later chapters we refer to some of the published clinical trials, systematic reviews, and practice guidelines available. It is not possible to complete a thorough analysis of all of the available literature within a single volume. Furthermore, new studies have been published since the revisions to this text.

Most important, you should not rely solely on our interpretations. What is vital is that the student and practicing clinician use the literature, engage in evidence-based health care, and provide the most effective treatments available.

SUMMARY

This chapter introduces key concepts linking evidence-based practice to the application of therapeutic modalities. An overview of evidence-based practice precedes discussion of the role that current evidence should play in recommending the application of a therapeutic modality. Strategies for locating and appraising the methodological quality of clinical research are then presented to provide a foundation for exploration of research related to the modalities and treatments discussed throughout Parts III, IV, V and VI. The sources of data that guide clinical practice include both clinicians and patients. Patient self-reports are discussed to emphasize the outcomes that are most important to patients. The focus then shifts to the types of clinical research available to the clinician and important considerations for a critical appraisal of the research.

1. *Define the term evidence-based health care.*

Evidence-based health care, as defined by Sackett et al. (2000), is the integration of the best research evidence with clinical expertise and patient values.

2. *Discuss the role of outcomes assessment in advancing evidence-based health care.*

Outcomes assessment is necessary for determining whether the treatments rendered to patients result in greater or more rapid recovery or reduce the incidence of reinjury. Some outcomes measures can be obtained by clinicians, but patients' self-reports provide important insights into the effects of the treatments they receive.

3. *Describe how clinical trials are conducted.*

Clinical trials involve the study of patients with specific conditions and their change in health status over time. Randomized controlled clinical trials (RCTs) randomly select patients into one or more treatment groups. One or more groups usually are treated with a placebo or serve as a no-treatment control.

4. *Identify the components of well-designed randomized controlled clinical trials.*

The methods of a randomized controlled clinical trial can introduce bias that may ultimately affect the conclusions of the investigators. Potential bias can be minimized through true random assignment to treatment groups; blinding of subjects, clinicians, and assessors to the treatment delivered; analysis of data as though all subjects completed the study; assessment of differences between groups at the start of the study; provision of valid measures of treatment outcomes; and comparison of the results from the various treatment groups.

5. *Describe how a systematic review is developed.*

Systematic reviews are research efforts in which data are acquired from existing literature through *a planned and thorough search process*. Databases to be searched and search terms are identified prior to beginning the search. Papers included in the review are selected based on established criteria. Data acquired through systematic review may undergo statistical analysis through a process called meta-analysis. The search and analysis processes are described in the methods section of a well-developed systematic review.

6. *Identify resources for locating clinical trials of treatments in which therapeutic modalities were used.*

While there is a need for more high-quality randomized controlled clinical trials in sports medicine, several databases can assist the certified athletic trainer in the practice of evidence-based health care. These include, but are not limited to, CINAHL (nursing and allied health cumulative index), EMBASE (a comprehensive bibliographic database covering the worldwide literature in biomedical and pharmaceutical fields), Physiotherapy Evidence Database (an Australian-based initiative to catalog systematic reviews and clinical trials and grade the methodological quality of clinical trials), Cochrane database (the Cochrane Collaboration is a multicenter international project providing high-quality systematic reviews and analyses of clinical trials across a broad spectrum of medicine), and SPORTDiscus (database of published articles related to sports medicine).

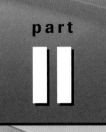

Physiology of Pain and Injury

The body's immediate response to injury and the process of tissue repair are complex. The appropriate management of musculoskeletal injuries requires knowledge of how the physiological events leading to repair and remodeling are regulated. Pain is another complex phenomenon. Pain is associated with tissue damage, but it can persist beyond the initial inflammatory response to injury. Pain can also occur in the absence of tissue injury or inflammation.

Part II of this text provides a strong foundation in inflammation, repair of musculoskeletal tissues, pain perception, and the clinical management of pain. These topics are recurrent themes in subsequent chapters as specific therapeutic modalities and exercise are discussed in the context of alleviating suffering, promoting repair, and restoring the ability of tissues to resist the forces generated through sport and physically demanding work.

Tissue Healing

OBJECTIVES

After reading this chapter, you will be able to

1. describe the role of the inflammatory response in tissue healing;

2. identify key events in the acute inflammatory, repair, and remodeling phases of tissue healing;

3. describe the events and controlling chemical mediators of the acute inflammatory response;

4. discuss the relationship between the signs and symptoms and the physiological events characteristic of an acute inflammatory response;

5. discuss the physiological events responsible for swelling associated with tissue injury, as well as treatment strategies for swelling; and

6. discuss the similarities and differences in repair of muscle, tendon, bone, and ligament.

A soccer player is assisted into the sports medicine clinic. You find that she has a grade II sprain of the tibial collateral ligament. In consultation with a team physician the athlete-patient is informed that she likely will be able to safely return to soccer participation in about 6 weeks. Initially the patient is placed in a knee immobilizer and instructed to partially bear weight using crutches. She is advised to use ice several times each day to control pain. Using pain as a guide, gentle active range of motion (ROM) exercises and quadriceps setting with straight leg raises are initiated. Biofeedback with **electromyography (EMG)** is used to improve neuromuscular control of the quadriceps while the muscle is exercised isometrically. After a few days, joint and soft tissue mobilization assists in regaining ROM and provides mechanical stimulus to the healing tissue. Once active, pain-free range of motion is restored, open- and closed-chain resistance exercises as well as functional exercises are added to the program. After 4 1/2 weeks, the patient has full motion and strength, and stress testing of the injured ligament reveals no pain or laxity. The athlete is cleared to begin an aggressive, sport-specific program of exercises in preparation for return to top competition in a stepwise fashion. What physiological events take place over this time period as the injury is repaired? Can treatment interventions speed tissue healing? When does the tensile strength of the injured ligament return to normal?

As illustrated in the soccer player's case, understanding the physiology of **inflammation** and applying therapeutic modalities accordingly will best meet the needs of physically active people and facilitate their return to activity. Tissue injury triggers an elaborate response by the body to remove injured tissue and repair the damage. Inappropriate treatment can delay or even halt repair. This chapter provides an overview of events from the time of tissue damage until tissue repair and maturation are completed.

An understanding of the healing process is essential for all medical and rehabilitation professionals. Knowledge of the healing process, the relative time frames in which healing events occur, and tissue-specific healing characteristics will help in attaining optimal outcomes. Choosing appropriate interventions based on the status of healing tissue as time passes will help avoid disruption of the healing process and poor outcomes.

There are several prerequisites to developing this skill set. Identification of the injured structures and extent of damage is crucial. To that end, a thorough medical history, a history of the current condition and physical examination, and, when indicated, diagnostic imaging are necessary. In the postoperative case, knowledge of the individual's presurgical status, understanding of the surgical procedure and the tissues involved in repair, and early contraindications to activity help determine an optimal course of rehabilitation. These decisions are based largely upon time frames of tissue-specific healing events.

We must first acknowledge some challenges in understanding the complexity of the healing process. The number of cells, molecules, and simultaneous interactions involved can easily muddy the waters of understanding. Coordinated repair actions involve plasma proteins and **leukocytes** that infiltrate damaged tissues. The quality of repair can be quite variable depending upon the extent of injury, vascular status of tissue, function of resident cells, and the person's overall health. That is to say, not all tissues heal similarly, and different patients' healing capacity depends on many local and systemic factors.

Healing "stages" are often described and typically include the inflammatory, proliferative, and remodeling stage, each with approximate time frames ascribed to them (figure 4.1). The inflammatory phase usually lasts 48 to 72 hours, with the proliferative stage accelerating as inflammation subsides, peaking about one week post-injury. The remodeling stage may last for months and even years.

For optimal healing, all stages of the continuum must occur in a coordinated fashion. During healing, bouts of recurrent inflammation or even an absence of inflammation may be observed, and the process may not be stepwise and orderly. Nonetheless, knowledge of the healing process and relative time frames in which significant events occur is necessary, as is the ability to recognize signs that the healing process has been disrupted. There is great potential for rehabilitation professionals to either disrupt or optimize the healing process, and this has a direct influence on outcomes.

This chapter presents a working description of healing. The primary phases and events of the healing process are described and associated with clinical signs that healing is progressing (or not progressing). This foundation leads into the introduction of strategies to optimize healing for successful restoration of function and safe return to sport and work participation. The chapter concludes by reviewing repair of specific musculoskeletal tissues including muscle, tendon, bone, and ligament.

TISSUE AND INJURY

Often healing is described in three overlapping stages of acute inflammation, proliferation of cells and tissue, and remodeling. A general sequence of events that occur within the stages of healing is shown in figure 4.1.

Forces are imparted on the body from our interaction with the environment, and they impose stress on tissues. Musculoskeletal tissue responds and adapts to stress placed on it. A simplistic definition of injury is excessive stress on a tissue, either in one episode or over time. Because force has both a mass and an acceleration component ($F = MA$), an excessive force delivered at high velocity often results in a traumatic injury and rupture of tissue (macrotrauma). Injury due to the accumulation of stress and resultant microtrauma over time is considered an overuse injury. Overuse of tissue may occur asymptomatically, and it can predispose the athlete to traumatic injury.

Mechanical Basis of Overuse in Viscoelastic Tissues

Viscoelasticity is the mechanical property of tissue that exhibits elasticity, or the ability to elongate and return to normal length in a time-dependent manner. Time dependency refers to the manner in which the duration or rate of exposure to force affects tissue response. Musculoskeletal tissues exhibit viscoelastic characteristics of mechanical creep. When a constant force is applied to a tissue over time, the tissue will continue to elongate, which is called "creep." Likewise if a tissue is held at a constant amount of elongation, over time less force will be required to maintain elongation, which is called force/relaxation (figure 4.2). From a mechanical perspective, overuse injury in viscoelastic tissue is the result of accumulated elongation and decreased resistance to stress that make it more susceptible to injury. Accumulated creep or elongation has been shown to last for more than 7 hours after 60 minutes of low-intensity activity. (Kubo).

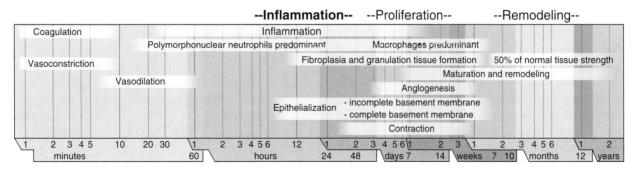

Figure 4.1 The stages and corresponding events of the healing process.

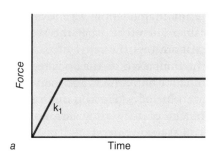

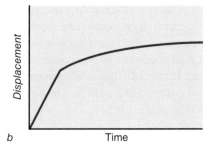

Figure 4.2 Mechanical creep. *(a)* Constant force (rather than constant elongation) is applied. *(b)* Displacement measured under a constant force for a given amount of time.

Often a tissue subjected to chronic stress will fail acutely, requiring the clinician to determine if a traumatic injury is rooted in overstressed, weakened tissue or is simply the result of a sudden and overwhelming force leading to tissue rupture. This phenomenon can be observed when degenerative changes lead to ultimate failure and rupture of a tendon and when overstressed or osteoporotic bone suddenly fractures. This clinical determination is paramount in understanding the distinct healing processes and potential for reinjury in many musculoskeletal conditions.

Tissue Composition

Musculoskeletal tissues are composed of cells (**fibroblasts**, including **osteocytes** in bone, **myocytes** in muscle, **tenocytes** in tendons, and **chondrocytes** in cartilage) and **extracellular matrix** (ECM). Cells maintain the ECM through remodeling and production of new ECM components. The ECM is composed of fibrillar proteins and polysaccharide complexes. ECM integrity directly influences cell function, and the cell-ECM symbiosis results in tissue homeostasis. Structural damage to tissue results in cell death and disruption of the ECM. Damage to the ECM results in inappropriate signaling to surviving cells and to resident cells that

can mature into fibroblasts and repopulate tissue, thereby compounding the effects of injury over time. Damage to tissue provides a potent stimulus to initiate healing through the activation of cells and chemical mediators. Repair processes can be further stimulated by therapeutic exercise and by some therapeutic interventions. The art of caring for musculoskeletal injuries involves the selection, timing, and extent of interventions. Inappropriate care can slow or halt repair as effectively as optimal management will facilitate repair and remodeling of injured tissues.

IMMEDIATE RESPONSE TO INJURY

Immediately following injury, the body mounts an acute response to limit blood loss. When injury occurs, small-diameter vascular structures (capillaries, arterioles, and venules) are damaged. Epinephrine and substances released from platelets, especially thromboxane A2, produce vasoconstriction. Thus, immediately following tissue damage, the body's defense mechanisms are at work to repair damage to blood vessels and prevent further blood loss (figure 4.3).

Larger vascular structures (arteries and veins) may also be injured, which can result in a loss of blood volume. Arrest of hemorrhage is crucial for survival.

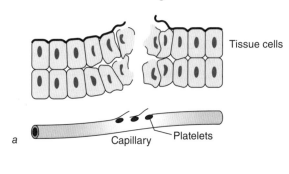

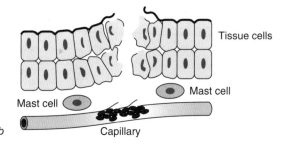

Figure 4.3 Early response to tissue damage. *(a)* Tissue injury and damage to capillaries and tissue cells. *(b)* Platelet and fibrin repair of capillary damage.

If large vessels are damaged, the patient will go into **hypovolemic** shock. The neurovascular status of the injured limb should be assessed after any acute traumatic injury. Fortunately, most musculoskeletal injuries do not damage the large vessels. When large blood vessels are injured and bleeding is present, external compression and elevation can stabilize blood pressure. Hypovolemic shock can also occur without external signs, particularly with visceral injuries. The clinician must recognize the signs of shock regardless of the cause and immediately act to stabilize the patient and activate an emergency response plan.

Signs of Shock

- Rapid, weak pulse
- Low blood pressure
- Rapid, shallow breathing
- Cool, clammy skin
- Lethargy

Previously, clinicians were taught to immediately apply ice to an injury to control bleeding and thus prevent swelling. Although the application of cold has a place in the management of acute musculoskeletal injuries, cold has little effect on blood loss. The body's own mechanisms control blood loss. It is more important to carefully examine the injury than to rapidly apply cold.

Most musculoskeletal injuries sustained by physically active people do not damage large blood vessels. Damage to the small vessels is plugged very rapidly. The events that limit the loss of blood from small vessels begin within seconds and end in minutes. The lining of blood vessels is composed of a monolayer of endothelial cells. Within seconds after injury to soft tissues (ligaments, tendons, muscle) or bone, platelets adhere to the site of damage in the small blood vessels in response to disrupted endothelium and exposure to underlying basement membrane (supporting connective tissue). Platelets activate the coagulation cascade, leading to hemostasis. The initial platelet plug recruits other platelets through the release of substances such as prostaglandin and thromboxane, as well as initiating secondary hemostasis through the activation of the clotting cascade of plasma proteins. This cascade of enzymatic activity results in the production of **fibrin** from circulating plasma fibrinogen, which cements platelets and cellular debris together to form the meshlike network of a clot. Once damage to the blood vessels has been plugged, the rest of the acute inflammatory response can begin.

INFLAMMATION

What do we mean when we say something is inflamed? On the surface the area is red, warm to the touch, swollen, and painful. These are the cardinal signs of inflammation. Within the tissue, substances and cells are chemically attracted to sites of damage to clean and repair. Blood flow increases to the area, and substances similar to bleach and hydrogen peroxide are released by inflammatory cells to clean and remove (debride) damaged tissue. The result is tissue swelling and chemical irritation. Although the cardinal signs emerge and the resulting pain and swelling affect comfort, function, and participation, the inflammatory process is essential to repair. Moreover, even though the signs and symptoms of inflammation resolve, the repair and maturation process continues.

The acute inflammatory response spans the events immediately post-injury through the cleaning and debridement process. The inflammatory response begins within seconds and can persist for several days. The initial activity of the inflammatory reaction is the recruitment of inflammatory cells. This is accomplished through cytokine-mediated chemoattraction and increased vascular permeability, allowing cells and plasma proteins to escape through the capillary walls and migrate toward the wound by the process of **chemotaxis**. Chemotaxis is the process in which cells direct their movement in response to chemicals in their environment. Proinflammatory cytokines, plasma proteins, and damaged tissue are powerful chemoattractants for inflammatory cells.

Cytokines are small signaling proteins produced by cells that have local (autocrine and paracrine) effects. Cytokines may be classified based on their actions; they include **chemotactic** agents (chemokines), mitogens (growth factors), and differentiation factors (morphogens). An individual cytokine may have varying functions depending on the context of its release, and thus it could have more than one classification. As an example, transforming growth factor-β (TGF-β) can act as a morphogen, induce matrix production, and induce inflammation.

Cytokines can also stimulate or repress other cytokines, can be regulated by various binding proteins, and can have different effects based on their interactions with other concurrent molecular activities.

The interleukin family of cytokines consists of 11 proteins that serve multiple roles in immune and inflammatory regulation. IL-1, IL-6, and tumor necrosis factor (TNF) are prominent proinflammatory cytokines present during the early inflammatory process. TNF mediates many of the cellular interactions that occur early in the healing process. In general, proinflammatory cytokines have redundant functions geared toward increasing vascular permeability, attracting cells from circulation to the site of injury, and promoting cellular activity.

Increased vascular permeability is accomplished by a loosening of the connection between vascular endothelial cells. The inside lining of blood vessels is composed of a single layer of endothelial cells that connect in tight junctions of intercellular adhesion molecules. Proinflammatory substances derived from plasma, endothelial cells, and platelets within the vascular compartment, as well as from inflammatory cells and cytokines outside of the vascular compartment, contribute to increasing vascular permeability. It is important to appreciate that the actions caused by various mediators occur simultaneously. An increase in vascular permeability is necessary to allow leukocytes (especially neutrophils), discussed in the next section, to enter into the area of tissue damage. The increase in permeability, however, also allows more plasma proteins to escape from the circulation. Proteins exert an osmotic pressure (attract water). Thus, the increased volume of free proteins in the damaged area attracts water, which is clinically observed as swelling (figure 4.4). The proteins are eventually absorbed by the lymphatic system, and swelling resolves. Compression, elevation, and muscle contractions can encourage drainage from the lymph system and reduce swelling after a musculoskeletal injury.

Three plasma protein cascades are associated with the acute inflammatory response (see table 4.1). The clotting cascade results in a fibrous framework for tissue repair (figure 4.5). The kinin cascade results

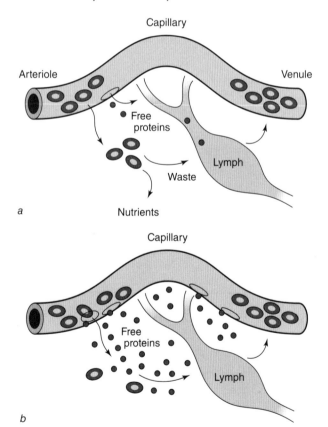

Figure 4.4 (a) Normal capillary filtration pressure balance (b) and an increase of free proteins, which disrupts normal capillary filtration pressure balance.

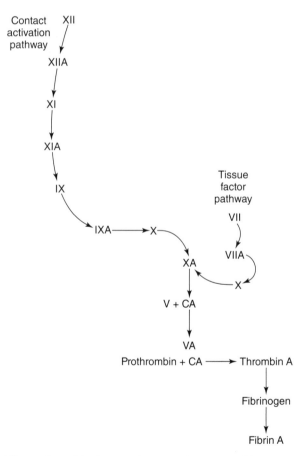

Figure 4.5 Clotting regulates the formation of fibrin. Two pathways lead to a common sequence of events triggering the formation of thrombin and finally prothrombin. A = active form of plasma proteins.

Table 4.1   Plasma Protein Cascades

Mediator	Purpose	Relation to signs of inflammation
Clotting cascade	Prevent loss of red blood cells	No direct relationship
Kinin cascade	Increase capillary membrane permeability	Pain and swelling
Complement cascade	Facilitate all aspects of acute inflammatory response	Increases all signs of inflammation

in the formation of bradykinin. The complement cascade affects all aspects of the acute inflammatory response. These protein cascades interact and occur simultaneously with other events of the acute inflammatory response.

The clotting cascade converts plasma protein fibrinogen to fibrin. Fibrin forms a meshlike web with platelets to temporarily repair damaged **vascularized** tissues. The first protein in the clotting cascade, factor XII, or the Hageman factor, also activates the kinin cascade (figure 4.6), first converting the plasma protein prekallikrein to kallikrein, which then activates the conversion of kininogen to bradykinin. Bradykinin increases capillary membrane permeability and interacts with prostaglandins to stimulate free nerve endings, causing pain.

The complement cascade is a family of plasma proteins that participate in virtually every aspect of the inflammatory response, including lysis (breakdown) of membranes of dead cells, chemical attraction of leukocytes (chemotaxis),

increased capillary membrane permeability, and the facilitation of phagocytosis via opsonization. An opsonin coats bacteria or damaged tissue to facilitate inflammatory cell binding and ingestion. The complement cascade also stimulates mast cell degranulation.

Mast cells, found in the connective tissues adjacent to vasculature, may also initiate the inflammatory response by the release of several substances (table 4.2). Mast cells are activated to release histamine and serotonin from preformed granules upon direct injury as well as upon exposure to bacteria, plasma proteins, and cytokines. Histamine and

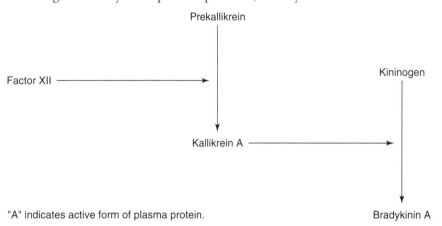

"A" indicates active form of plasma protein.

Figure 4.6   Conversion of kininogen to bradykinin.

Table 4.2   Proinflammatory Substances Secreted by Mast Cells

Mediator	Purpose	Relation to signs of inflammation
Histamine	Vasodilation	Heat and redness
Neutrophil chemotactic factor	Attract neutrophils to phagocytize necrotic tissue	Swelling, indirectly, because increased membrane permeability is required for neutrophil emigration
Serotonin	Increase capillary membrane permeability	Swelling
Heparin	Prevent occlusion of capillary blood flow	No direct relationship
Prostaglandin E2	Increase capillary membrane permeability	Pain and swelling
Leukotrienes	Attract neutrophils to phagocytize necrotic tissue	Swelling, indirectly, because increased membrane permeability is required for neutrophil emigration

serotonin cause **vasodilation** and increase capillary membrane permeability, respectively.

It should be apparent that these cascades interact. An injury or illness activates one or more cascades. If mast cell degranulation occurs first, it will trigger the plasma protein cascades. If the plasma protein system is activated first, other plasma protein systems will be activated and will stimulate mast cell degranulation. Thus, the inflammatory response is said to be nonspecific. The same events occur regardless of the precipitating stimulus.

Prostaglandins, leukotrienes, and lipoxins are metabolic products of arachidonic acid (AA), which is derived from the cell membrane of most cells, and they act as potent regulators of inflammation via multiple mechanisms (figure 4.7). Upon direct injury or exposure to proinflammatory cytokines, AA is liberated from the cell membrane via the enzyme phospholipase A2 (PLA2). Arachidonic acid is then transformed into prostaglandins via the cyclooxygenase enzyme and leukotrienes via the arachidonate 5 lipoxygenase (5-LOX) enzyme. These substances regulate a variety of physiologic functions and are targets for anti-inflammatory and pain-relieving drugs.

The actions of cyclooxygenase on arachidonic acid are not limited to prostaglandin synthesis. During the transformation from AA to stable prostaglandins, **free radicals** are released (Kerr, Bender, and Monti 1996; Ward, Till, and Johnson 1990). These free radicals activate proteases such as collagenase, which break down adjacent cell membranes, liberating additional AA metabolic products (Kerr, Bender, and Monti 1996; Ward, Till, and Johnson 1990). Lipoxins are derived from AA by the 15-Lox enzyme and have important anti-inflammatory functions.

Leukocyte Infiltration

White blood cells (leukocytes) originate from stem cells in bone marrow. Stem cells proliferate and differentiate into granulocytes (neutrophils, eosinophils, basophils), monocytes, and lymphocytes (T and B cells). These cells comprise the total white blood cell count. Nearly 2 billion granulocytes are produced each day, the majority of which are neutrophils (Abramson and Melton 2000). The majority of leukocytes (90%) reside in the bone marrow, where they mature and are released upon stimulation by various cytokines. A small percentage (about 3%) of leukocytes are in circulation and 7 to 8% are dispersed throughout tissues. Once a leukocyte is released from the marrow, it has a short lifespan (1 day–2 weeks), and therefore storage in bone marrow allows for a ready supply of viable cells upon stimulation from injury, inflammation, or infection. Infiltration of leukocytes occurs in an orderly fashion and relates to specific cellular functions (figure 4.8).

The first infiltrating cells on the scene of injury are neutrophils, with concentrations peaking 24 hours post-injury. Neutrophils get their name from their large, multilobed nucleus. The size of the nucleus is related to the ability to rapidly produce and release quantities of caustic substances that degrade bacteria and tissue. Neutrophils, like mast cells, are granulocytes, and they have preformed substances ready for immediate release. Within the neutrophil armamentarium are bacteriocidal oxygen and nitrogen radicals, antimicrobial and proteinase enzymes, and chemotactic agents. Neutrophils not only have potent cleaning capabilities, but they also release chemokines that powerfully attract monocytes, which mature into macrophages to sustain the inflammatory response.

Oxidative Killing

The term *oxidative stress* refers to the overproduction of **reactive oxygen species** (ROS). ROS are a by-product of oxygen metabolism and serve many homeostatic functions. ROS produced in abundance result in damage to cells, including the genetic apparatus, and can induce apoptosis (cell death). Upon activation (interaction with bacteria or damaged tissue) the neutrophil engulfs

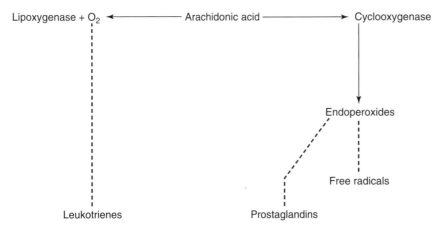

Figure 4.7   Synthesis of leukotrienes and prostaglandins from arachidonic acid.

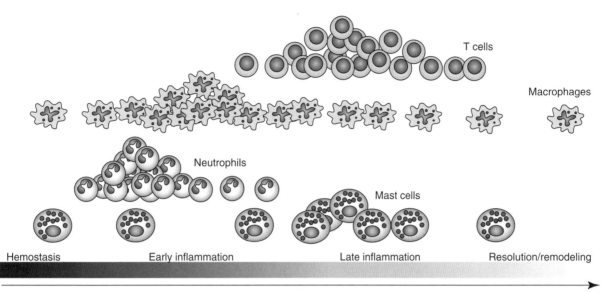

Figure 4.8 Order of infiltrating leukocytes.

T.J. Koh and L.A. DiPietro, 2011, "Inflammation and wound healing: The role of the macrophage," *Expert Reviews in Molecular Medicine* 13: e23, reproduced with permission.

the offending agent or tissue and destroys it. The primary phagocytic enzymatic cascade responsible for the generation of ROS used for cleaning is the NADPH oxidase system (NOX enzymes) or "oxidative burst oxidase." This reaction is characterized by the consumption of oxygen and the production of superoxide and other ROS (Zhang and Mosser 2008). The NADPH enzyme is present in neutrophils, eosinophils, and mononuclear **phagocytes** (macrophages). The enzyme is dormant in circulating neutrophils and is activated upon exposure to microbes, inflammatory mediators, and damaged tissue.

Phagocytic cell membrane receptors for bacteria and damaged tissue include the formyl peptide receptors (FPRs). These receptors bind debris, or opsonins bound to debris, and trigger **phagocytosis** through downstream cell signaling and cytoskeletal rearrangement. Upon phagocytosis, engulfed debris is enveloped in a phagosome. NOX enzymes embedded in membranes of secretory granules are activated and fuse with the phagosome. Activation of the NOX enzymes results in the production of large quantities of ROS, the free radicals (superoxide, hydrogen peroxide, and the hydroxyl radical), and hypochlorous acid (which is a bleach), resulting in the destruction of the offending agent. ROS activate proteases as well, breaking down collagen and other ECM constituents. Due to the large quantities of ROS produced, healthy tissue in the surrounding area may also be damaged.

Neutrophils are also capable of nonoxidative killing through the release of lysosomal enzymes (lysozyme and collagenase), which degrade cell membranes and tissue as well as release phospholipase A2 for the production of AA metabolites (prostaglandins and leukotrienes). These chemical mediators stimulate the complement cascade and the kinin systems. Through the actions of lysosomal enzymes and prostaglandins, the inflammatory response is perpetuated until the damaged tissues are removed. The neutrophil also releases potent chemotactic factors that recruit macrophages (Novak and Koh 2013).

MACROPHAGE FUNCTION

Circulating monocytes are extruded from leaky endothelium, attracted to injured tissue via chemotaxis, and activated by the inflammatory environment to mature into macrophages. These circulating monocytes provide the main source of macrophages after injury, but resident tissue macrophages are quite active as well, and they provide some of the initial signals to trigger the inflammatory process. Macrophage infiltration peaks 3 to 7 days postinjury.

Macrophage activity persists throughout the stages of healing, contributing to removal of damaged tissue, cell recruitment and proliferation, and promotion of angiogenesis, matrix production, and remodeling. Such a diversity of cellular capabilities is remarkable and is made possible by the multiple phenotypes (physiological properties) these cells can assume. Early on (0–4 days), the proinflammatory macrophage (M1) is active. As time passes and inflammation subsides, the M2 or anti-inflammatory macrophage is active. There are several intermediate phenotypes that help direct the abatement of inflammation and promotion of cell and tissue proliferation (Lech and Anders 2013).

Early in the healing process the primary role of the macrophage is to promote inflammatory activity and help remove damaged tissue. In the early inflammatory environment (0–2 days) prominent cytokines present include TNF, interferon gamma, IL-1, and IL-6. These cytokines are produced from a variety of cells, including activated macrophages. These cytokines have prolific proinflammatory actions, including recruitment and activation of the proinflammatory M1 macrophage to the site of injury. TNF promotes several important inflammatory functions in a variety of cells. TNF induces proinflammatory cytokine production, orchestrates chemotaxis, and is responsible for fever via hypothalamic stimulation. Activated M1 macrophages promote the inflammatory process and remove pathogens and damaged tissue.

When musculoskeletal tissue is damaged, prominent components of the ECM are cleaved and bind to macrophages via damage-associated molecular pattern (DAMP) receptors and **integrin proteins** on the macrophage cell membrane. (Note: Integrin proteins are central to the effects of mechanical signals on cell function and are discussed in detail in chapter 16.) Damaged tissue and dead cells are engulfed and destroyed by enzymes and ROS during phagocytosis. Exposure of macrophages to inflammatory stimuli induce the expression of ECM-degrading enzymes that are secreted to further degrade damaged tissue. Among these enzymes are the matrix metalloproteases (MMPs), which cleave molecular bonds of damaged matrix contents, leading to further degradation, as well as stimulate additional macrophage activity. Thus the macrophage perpetuates the cleaning process until the stimuli resulting from injury abate.

Prominent examples of damaged and degraded ECM components recognized by DAMP receptors are fragments of collagen, biglycan, hyaluronan, fibrinogen, and fibronectin. Fibronectin is attached to debris and acts as an opsonin, enhancing binding to macrophages and facilitating phagocytosis. Binding with fibronectin also induces the production of MMPs, leading to further degradation of damaged matrix.

Termination of Inflammation and Early Repair

As debris removal nears completion and the inflammatory environment subsides, macrophages assume an anti-inflammatory role and coordinate the activity of wound repair. The M2 macrophage exerts many anti-inflammatory effects. Through macrophage production of anti-inflammatory cytokines such as IL-10 and TGF-β, proinflammatory cytokine production is inhibited. The source of M1 and M2 macrophages is the subject of debate. It was once hypothesized that M1 macrophages were derived from infiltrating monocytes, whereas M2 macrophages were derived from monocytes in the affected tissues. There is now evidence that cells derived from "infiltrating" monocytes in the tissues switch their phenotype from M1 to M2.

Environmental factors such as cytokine exposure and mechanical forces imparted on a cell help regulate the phenotypic shift to anti-inflammatory cell functions. It is therefore easy to see how inappropriate force on injured tissue early on can directly influence healing through the function of the macrophage. Early application of appropriate force directly influences macrophage activity and thus pro- and anti-inflammatory activity. The rehabilitation professional modulates force on the injured tissue by choosing interventions and activities.

Once the hostile inflammatory environment abates, cell and tissue proliferation begins. The termination of acute inflammation is a complex process involving the activity of over 80 genes. Due to the short lifespan of the neutrophils (a few hours to a day) and the extremely short half-life of most inflammatory cytokines (seconds to minutes), eradication of the offending stimulus should result in the termination of inflammation and the avoidance of "overcleaning" that can damage healthy tissue.

The resolution of inflammation results from the depletion of proinflammatory mediators and removal of dead neutrophils and their secreted products by macrophages. The process of phagocytosis itself helps to regulate inflammation. During phagocytosis, the cell concurrently produces TGF-β and IL-10. TGF-β production by the macrophage stimulates new tissue production and thus wound healing, and IL-10 inhibits proinflammatory cytokine production.

There is also built-in anti-inflammatory regulation within arachidonic acid metabolism through the simultaneous production of lipoxins. These autocrine and paracrine signaling molecules help resolve inflammation through a variety of anti-inflammatory actions. Lipoxins can bind to FPR receptors on leukocytes and inhibit granule release, the production of proinflammatory cytokines, and chemotactic ability.

The lifespan of the inflammatory process depends in part on the extent of damage, but it typically resolves within 1 to 5 days. Activities that excessively stress the injured area during this time will result in further damage and the propagation of the inflammatory process. Inflammation may also recur later in the healing process if excessive stress damages the fragile remodeling tissue.

When the immune system is properly modulated, inflammation resolves, tissue repair occurs, and function returns. An overly robust inflammatory response often results in excess scarring, fibrosis, and diminished ultimate tissue strength. An inadequate inflammatory response results in degenerative, disorganized, and weakened tissue as in the case of tendinopathy. Absence of an inflammatory response, such as in **avascular** tissue like the meniscus or articular cartilage, results in an inability to heal.

Proliferation

M2 macrophage cytokine expression is geared toward activating fibroblasts to produce and remodel ECM, as well as activating **progenitor cells** to replenish the pool of damaged reparative cells. The cell types activated are tissue dependent. We will see, however, that cell type switching in tissue under pathologic conditions readily occurs.

Cellular proliferation peaks around day 6 following tissue injury and persists at low levels for up to 2 weeks. During this time, fibroblasts and other tissue cells are activated, proliferate, and produce ECM. Collagen-producing fibroblast-like cells are the predominant stromal (structural) cell type in musculoskeletal tissue. Fibroblasts are not only present in tissue, they can also derive from circulating monocytes in an immature form termed the fibrocyte (Bianchetti et al. 2012). The fibrocyte is likely an intermediate in the differentiation process between monocytes and mature fibroblasts. Fibrocytes can differentiate into other cells such as myofibroblasts and adipocytes. The overabundance of fibrocytes has been linked to wound fibrosis and suboptimal repair.

Early Repair

Coagulated blood within the tissue from the time of injury forms the beginning scaffold from which the provisional matrix is formed. The provisional matrix is crucial for optimal wound healing because it is a potent chemoattractant and provides attachment sites for cells and growth factors needed for tissue repair. Along with complement, which aids in cleaning and chemotaxis, plasma fibrin and fibronectin are deposited at the site of injury and exist within the coagulated blood in the tissue.

Fibronectin plays a crucial role in wound healing. Fibronectin coats bacteria and damaged tissue, acting as an opsonin. As repair of the injured tissue begins, macrophages and fibroblasts bind fibronectin via **integrins**. There is considerable crosstalk between macrophages and fibroblasts. Like macrophages, fibroblasts have phagocytic capability but are limited to damaged ECM, and they achieve most remodeling through the release of remodeling enzymes such as matrix metalloproteinases (MMPs). Fibroblast and macrophage MMP production is stimulated by macrophage cytokine expression. As phagocytosis commences, macrophages stimulate fibroblasts to make new insoluble fibronectin, which stabilizes the wound.

Concurrent with fibrin and fibronectin removal, the fibroblast produces an abundance of **proteoglycans** and type III **collagen** (2-5 days). The weblike structure of type III collagen serves to stabilize the provisional matrix. Eventually the provisional matrix is removed by a combination of extracellular and intracellular digestion, and the definitive matrix, rich in type I collagen and native tissue, is deposited by fibroblasts and native cells (5 days–weeks). Organization of newly formed matrix is highly dependent upon mechanical force experienced by the tissue during this period. Newly formed tissue tends to align along planes of stress. The clinician directly affects the healing process by choosing the dose of stress newly healing tissue experiences.

Repair

Repair implies the growth of new tissue. Once injury debris is removed and the vascular network to support tissue growth is in place, repair is well under way. The extent of repair possible will depend on the health of the individual, blood supply to the tissue, resident cell type and activity, and degree of injury. Large defects in tissue in which tissue approximation and supporting connective tissue architecture are disrupted usually produce fibrosis. Fibrosis is due to excessive ECM production by fibrocytes and fibroblasts and a concomitant failure of resident cells to synthesize native tissue.

Tissues are classified according to the proportion of cells in mitosis (actively dividing) normally present (Martinez-Hernandez and Amenta 1990). Tissues such as the epidermis contain cells that are continuously being replaced; these are classified as **labile** cells. Bone marrow and the cells lining the respiratory, gastrointestinal, and genitourinary tracts are also labile cells. Tissues made of labile cells have excellent regenerative capacity.

Stable cells have less regenerative capacity. Cells that make up the tissues of the liver, pancreas, and kidneys, as well as fibroblasts, osteocytes, endothelial cells, and chondrocytes, are classified as stable cells. Fibroblasts synthesize collagen and elastin, which are the major components of ligaments and tendons. **Osteoblasts**, which mature into osteocytes, form bone; and **chondroblasts**, which mature into chondrocytes, form cartilage. Thus bone and cartilage can regenerate, but they do so more slowly than tissues made up of labile cells.

Cells that have no regenerative capacity in adults are classified as **permanent** cells. The nerves of the central nervous system, the lenses of the eyes, and cardiac muscle have no regenerative capacity. Advances have been made in understanding why some tissues lose regenerative capacity after birth—work that has special application in the treatment of spinal cord injuries.

Cellular plasticity refers to a cell's ability to alter its behavior or phenotype. Due to the common mesodermal lineage musculoskeletal cells share, inappropriate stress or exposure to inappropriate substances can push a progenitor cell (immature cell) to differentiate away from its native tissue cell type. This has been demonstrated in muscle in response to crush injury and subsequent bone deposition as occurs with myositis ossificans. Tendon fibroblast progenitors can differentiate into chondroblasts, osteoblasts, or adipocytes in response to inappropriate load or exposure to dexamethasone (Zhang, Keenan, and Wang 2013). Further discussion of cellular plasticity is found in the sections on tissue-specific healing.

Because excessive stress on healing tissues disrupts repair and slows recovery, the clinician must understand how damaged tissues are repaired and the time frame over which repair occurs. One difficulty in determining appropriate stress exposure during the healing process is our inability to quantify the stress experienced by tissue during a given activity. Understanding of applied anatomy and biomechanics allows us to infer the progressive loading of a tissue, both in magnitude and volume. In general, immediately after injury during the inflammatory phase, pain will limit activity. Modalities are applied to reduce pain and control swelling. Given the importance of the inflammatory process for adequate healing, efforts toward eliminating inflammation impair healing. After day 3 or 4, as inflammation subsides and injury-specific rehabilitation begins, recurrent bouts of inflammation must be avoided. Signs of recurrent inflammation include reoccurrence of the cardinal signs of inflammation: increasing pain, swelling, redness, and loss of function. Pain at rest and increasing pain during passive ROM activities are also signs of excessive activity during healing. These are very general guidelines, however, and tissue- and injury-specific interventions that do not disrupt healing are needed for optimal outcomes.

Skeletal Muscle Healing

The muscle cell or myofiber contains the contractile elements responsible for force generation. Each myofiber is surrounded by endomysium, a connective tissue envelope composed predominantly of type IV collagen and proteoglycan (see figure 16.7 in chapter 16). Myofibers are bundled together to form fascicles and are surrounded by the perimysium. The entire muscle is encased in epimysium. The connective tissue structure of muscle is responsible for lateral force transmission, with the epimysium running continuously into tendon, which transmits force to bone. Minor activity-related damage to muscle typically involves intracellular protein disruption that is readily repaired; however, more extensive damage involving the connective tissue architecture requires a more involved healing process, and may lead to scarring.

After injury to skeletal muscle, the ensuing healing process resembles the general healing process described previously. Injury results in a hematoma between myofibers, which includes serum fibrin and fibronectin. Proinflammatory cytokines increase permeability and recruit a variety of cells that migrate, proliferate, and attach to the provisional matrix. Macrophages are the predominant inflammatory cell, phagocytosing damaged tissue and activating quiescent progenitor cells residing in the basal lamina (figure 4.9). The inflammatory phase of muscle healing typically lasts about 3 days.

From 3 days to 2 weeks, fibroblasts produce ECM components, growth factors, and remodeling enzymes. Progenitor cells use necrotic basement membrane to correctly orient themselves, ensuring correct myofiber position. With extensive disruption to the connective tissue architecture, disorganized fiber arrangement and poor repair result. As parallel myofibers are repaired, fibroblasts proliferate and migrate, producing ECM for myoblasts to adhere and form myofibers. Macrophages and fibroblasts also produce vascular endothelial growth factor (VEGF) to promote angiogenesis in the new tissue.

Remodeling and Maturation

Remodeling of muscle occurs over months, with the central zone of injury decreasing in size as new tissue is formed. Proper modulation of inflammation is crucial for muscle healing. Interfering with the acute inflammatory response following injury leads to incomplete debridement of damage and often results in fibrosis. In contrast, reducing the chronic inflammatory condition characteristic of dystrophic muscle decreases fibrosis and enhances regeneration (Tidball 2005).

SPECIFIC HEALING OF TENDON TISSUE

Tendon tissue, similar to skeletal muscle, is composed of hierarchical bundles of fibers (figure 4.10). Tendon fibers are composed of type I collagen bundled in endotenon. Endotenon provides attachment sites for tenocytes as well as vasculature and lymphatics. Bundles of fibers are surrounded by epitenon, which forms tendon fascicles. Epitenon is wrapped in paratenon, which is connected to tendon sheath. Not all tendons have a sheath, and the outer layer of paratenon can serve as the tissue that connects to the deep fascia compartment.

Tendon presents several inherent challenges to healing after injury. In tendon, blood supply is derived intrinsically from the bony insertion (osteotendinous junction) and the myotendinous junction. Extrinsic blood supply from existing synovial sheath contributes as well (if present) and supplies superficial portions of the tendon. Injury to these areas significantly affects healing capability. Vascularity in the midportion of tendon is often insufficient.

Upon initial acute injury or laceration, an inflammatory response occurs, resulting in inflammatory cell infiltration from the resulting hematoma as well as from extrinsic sources such as the peritenon and junctional zones (osteotendinous and myotendinous junctions). The inflammatory response of tendon typically persists 3 to 7 days postinjury. The predominant inflammatory cell present

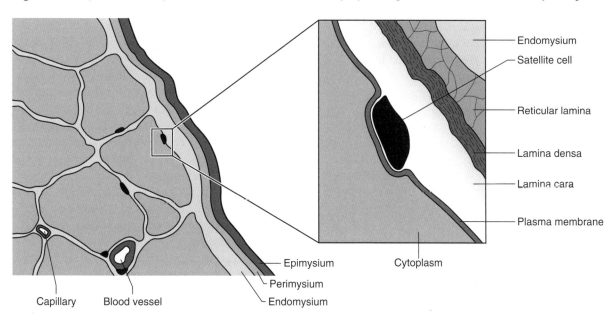

Figure 4.9 Skeletal muscle satellite cell residing in the basal lamina.

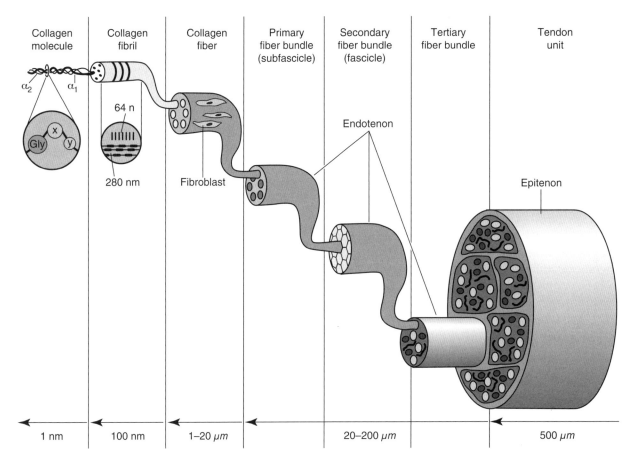

Figure 4.10   The hierarchical structure of tendon from collagen molecules to bundling of fibrils into fascicles.

Reprinted from *Journal of Biomechanics,* Vol 39(9), "Mechanobiology of tendon," J. H-C. Wang, pg. 1563-1582, copyright 2006, with permission from Elsevier.

in tendon is the monocyte-derived macrophage. The proliferative stage of tendon healing lasts for three weeks post-injury and is characterized by the proliferation of ECM-producing fibroblasts. The native tendon fibroblast (tenocyte) initially secretes type III collagen and transitions to type I collagen as the proliferation phase concludes 5 to 8 weeks post-injury. The tenocyte releases VEGF to promote neovascularization to supply repaired tissue. Tendon remodeling persists for up to a year to complete healing. Increased collagen density and fiber organization are achieved through cross-linking of fibrils; however, tendon regeneration never completely occurs and there is always some residual tissue disorganization, hyper- or hypocellularity, and decreased tensile strength. Restriction to the vascular compartment may limit inflammatory cell infiltration. The resident tenocyte is left to maintain the integrity of the tissue. The predominant signaling apparatus of the tenocyte is stimulated through mechanical force transferred through the tendon ECM to the integrin receptor,

resulting in gene transcription, matrix production, and remodeling.

Chronic overuse injury in tendon is often the result of a failed healing response. Overuse injury in tendon (tendinopathy) typically results in degeneration of tendon ECM, variable and dysfunctional cellular activity, and absence of inflammatory cell infiltration. Proinflammatory cytokines are present in the peritendinous tissue, but inflammatory cells do not respond. The result is a painful, or sometimes asymptomatic, tendon that degenerates due to the inadequacy of inflammatory-stimulated remodeling. The histological term for degenerative tendon in the absence of inflammation is **tendinosis**. Tendinopathy is the preferred clinical designation for overuse tendon injury.

The ultrastructural changes of degenerative tendon include collagen disorganization with visible microtearing, decreased density and fiber diameter, and loss of crimp (Järvinen et al. 1997). An increase in collagen type III is prevalent and may represent an attempt at tissue repair. Healthy tendon typically contains little proteoglycan, predominantly the collagen-bound small leucine-rich decorin. In areas of excessive compressive and shear loading, common in areas where tendon wraps around bone, fibrocartilaginous tissue forms and is associated with the large proteoglycan aggrecan. A prolific increase in proteoglycan is often present and may be associated with fibrocartilaginous metaplasia or may be present in streaming bands throughout the tendon midsubstance. Tendon cells surrounding pools of proteoglycan often resemble chondrocytes, which are responsible for the production of large-molecular-weight proteoglycan. It is important to note that the end-stage histological picture of a disease process may not be indicative of the preceding pathologic process. Various pathologic processes may lead to a similar histological picture of tendinopathy.

Ligament Healing

In many extra-articular ligaments, such as the medial collateral ligament (MCL), healing takes place as described, including inflammatory, proliferative, and remodeling phases. Once damaged tissues are removed, neovascularization, resident cell differentiation, and up-regulation of fibroblasts ultimately result in a framework of dense type I collagen and ECM. Collagen will align in response to imposed stresses throughout remodeling, which may continue for more than a year.

Intra-articular ligaments such as the anterior cruciate, however, have a poor healing response. This is largely due to the inability of the disrupted tissue to physically approximate and form a provisional matrix. Without tissue connectivity and provisional matrix formation, the foundation for repair simply does not exist.

Specific Healing of Bone Tissue

Three structural classifications of bones exist: long, cuboidal, and flat (figure 4.11). Generally, flat bones are found surrounding vital structures (such as the skull and ribs), cuboidal bones make up complex joints (like the wrist), and long bones make up the axial skeleton. Bone consists of a hard outer cortex of cortical bone and an inner, more porous medulla containing marrow and trabecular bone. Both cortical and trabecular bone are organized in pillars or osteons. The outer layer of concentric osteons is the lamella.

Bone is composed of type I collagen, hydroxyapatite mineral, and proteoglycan (see figure 16.10 in chapter 16). Bone cells include osteoblasts, osteoclasts, and osteocytes. Osteoblasts synthesize the components of the ECM (collagen and prostaglandin [PG]) and release vesicles of calcium and phosphate to aid in mineralization. Osteoblasts embedded in matrix become osteocytes, which develop a complex intercellular connection network. The osteocyte resides in a cavity or lacuna, and its long cytoplasmic extensions connect with neighboring cells via gap junctions in canals or **canaliculi**.

Fracture healing can be described in three stages as with other tissues: inflammation, repair, and remodeling. During the inflammatory stage, intracellular enzymes from damaged osteocytes trigger the destruction of surrounding ECM, which induces an inflammatory response lasting 2 to 5 days. Bone is a vascular tissue, and therefore hematoma formation and damaged tissues provide a strong chemotactic stimulus for inflammatory cells as well as mesenchymal stem cells (MSCs). Platelets at the site of damage release cytokines, which promote the inflammatory response and attract inflammatory and reparative cells.

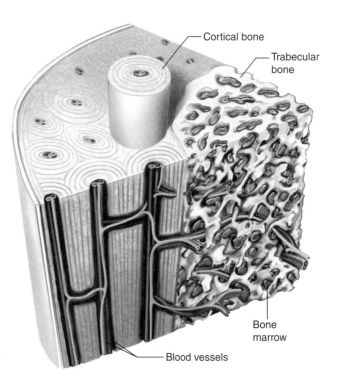

Figure 4.11   The structure of long bones, which are composed of the hard outer cortical and inner spongy trabecular bone. Osteons provide structural integrity due to the interposed lamellar structure.

The provisional matrix in bone healing is called a callus. The bony callus is predominantly type III collagen and PG. Infiltrating stromal cells proliferate and differentiate into bone-forming cells. Angiogenic stimuli result from the release of VEGF from peripheral and infiltrating bone cells. Within days of fracture, MSCs differentiate into cartilage cells (chondroblasts) and produce ECM that is similar to that found in cartilage. A combination of abundant proteoglycan and collagen types II and III are randomly organized and are called woven bone. Woven bone is eventually replaced. Type I collagen and mineralization occur around collagen fibers, adding rigidity to the remodeling tissue. The mineralized callus then undergoes the process of remodeling to form lamellar bone. Lamellar bone obtains strength through an organized yet variable alignment of collagen in successive layers. The repair phase can take 2 to 12 months.

Bone Remodeling

Bone remodels through the coordinated function of osteoblasts, osteoclasts, and osteocytes. Osteocytes embedded in the canalicular network secrete sclerostin, which inhibits the activation of surface stromal cells. When damage occurs, osteocytes at the site of injury apoptose. Osteocytes proximate to the injury secrete nitric oxide (NO), prostaglandin (PG), and other growth factors. Surface lining preosteoblasts pull away and merge with the circulation as they are positioned adjacent to blood vessels. Decreased sclerostin production from embedded osteocytes along with exposure to proinflammatory cytokines induce stromal cell differentiation in preosteoblasts. Preosteoblasts secrete receptor activator of nuclear factor kappa-B ligand (RANKL), which interacts with RANK receptors on preosteoclasts. Interaction of preosteoblasts and osteoclasts results in fusion and enlargement of preosteoclasts into mature osteoclasts. Osteoclasts bind bone via integrin receptors and secrete bone-resorbing acids over a period of 2 weeks and then apoptose. Once damaged bone is removed, mature osteoblasts discontinue secretion of RANKL and secrete osteoprotegrin (OPG). OPG binds to RANKL and inhibits osteoclast formation and activation. Osteoblasts then align along the resorbed bone and secrete new bone ECM. As bone is formed, osteoblasts are surrounded by ECM and become osteocytes. Osteocytes reform the lacuna canalicular connectivity network through which mechanical signal is transduced. Remodeling of the damaged area can last for up to 3 years and is largely dependent upon mechanical signal.

Cartilage Healing

Articular cartilage is avascular, aneural, and alymphatic and thus has very limited repair potential. Optimal conditions for cartilage healing include a source of cellular repopulation, formation of provisional matrix (although the absence of blood severely hinders this), an intact subchondral bone plate for nutrient transmission, and appropriate mechanical stress. Typically, the repair of articular cartilage is accomplished through the deposition of fibrous scar, and damage typically leads to osteoarthritis.

SUMMARY

Chapter 4 is devoted to understanding tissue injury and repair. Tissue damage triggers a cascade of events that result in inflammation. Although inflammation causes pain and swelling, the process is essential for repair. Clinicians caring for patients suffering from musculoskeletal injury must understand the fundamental role of inflammation in recovery, must be able to identify where each patient is in the repair process, and must treat appropriately. The key mediators and the links between early events involved in phagocytosis, cell differentiation, up-regulation of fibroblasts, and ultimate remodeling of tissues to withstand the forces of physical activity are presented to build the foundation for evidence-based clinical decision making, including the judicious application of therapeutic modalities and progression of exercise.

1. *Describe the role of the inflammatory response in tissue healing.*

Inflammation is the process by which the body removes damaged tissues and establishes a blood supply and repairs tissue damage. Once damaged tissues have been removed by the phagocytic cells, surviving cells and newly matured cells produce the proteins and other components of the extracellular matrix. The repair process continues as weaker repair tissues are replaced by stronger, more resilient tissue. Over time, tissue responds to the stresses imposed by activity and remodels. Through remodeling, tissue develops greater tensile strength and resistance to force.

2. *Identify key events in the acute inflammatory, repair, and remodeling phases of tissue healing.*

The acute inflammatory response begins with vasoconstriction and clotting. Vasoconstriction results from the actions of epinephrine and thromboxane. The clotting cascade is activated to minimize hemorrhage. This is a rapid and relatively short process. Once further blood loss is prevented, vasodilation and increased capillary membrane permeability allow for the invasion of neutrophils and later macrophages. The cells attack bacteria and phagocytize damaged tissue. As phagocytosis occurs, a new network of capillaries is formed to support the repair phase. M2 macrophages stimulate new tissue formation by fibroblasts, osteoblasts, or chondroblasts. Progenitor cells differentiate to form new tissue-building cells. Over time, stress to new tissues results in the production of new tissues. The capacity of the tissue to resist force increases as remodeling progresses.

3. *Describe the events and controlling chemical mediators of the acute inflammatory response.*

The acute inflammatory response can be divided into cell-mediated, plasma protein–mediated, and leukocyte-mediated events as well as events mediated by the products of phospholipid breakdown. Cytokines released from the mast cells, including histamine, serotonin, and neutrophil chemotactic factor, collectively promote vasodilation and capillary endothelial permeability and cause pain. Plasma proteins from the clotting, kinin, and complement cascades participate in all aspects of the inflammatory response. Neutrophils regulate inflammation and attract macrophages to the area and perpetuate the inflammatory response. Prostaglandins and leukotrienes formed from phospholipids cause pain in many cells, influence capillary membrane permeability, and attract leukocytes. Ultimately, M2 macrophages and other factors exert an anti-inflammatory action, and repair begins.

4. *Discuss the relationship between the signs and symptoms and the physiological events characteristic of the acute inflammatory response.*

The signs and symptoms of acute inflammation include heat, redness, pain, loss of function, and swelling. Heat and redness occur with vasodilation, which is caused by histamine and complement cascade proteins. Pain is caused by irritation of free nerve endings by prostaglandin E2, bradykinin, and pressure created by swelling. Loss of function stems from pain. Swelling results from the attraction of water to free proteins accumulating in the *interstitium*. Normally, very few plasma proteins pass through the capillary membrane. However, several chemical mediators of inflammation increase the permeability of the capillary membrane, allowing plasma proteins to escape. In addition, the breakdown of the cell membranes of damaged tissue contributes to the pool of free proteins in the interstitium.

In short, injury and acute inflammation disrupt normal capillary filtration pressure balance. Interstitial fluid will accumulate until a new pressure balance is reached. Swelling will resolve when free proteins are removed from the interstitium by lymphatic drainage.

5. *Discuss the physiological events responsible for swelling associated with tissue injury, as well as treatment strategies for swelling.*

   Swelling results from increased permeability of the capillary membrane. Proteins leaking into the tissue attract water (exert an osmotic pressure). The accumulation of proteins and water is observed as swelling. Swelling can be minimized through elevation, which decreases capillary hydrostatic pressure, and external compression, which introduces a counterforce to increased interstitial osmotic pressure. Muscle contractions promote the movement of lymph and resolution of swelling.

6. *Discuss the similarities and differences in repair of muscle, tendon, bone, and ligament.*

   Damage to these tissues results in the initiation of an inflammatory response, but several factors affect how repair and remodeling proceed. Tissues with more blood supply have greater access to neutrophils needed to begin clearing out dead cells and disrupted extracellular matrix. Well-vascularized tissue, such as muscle, is also under greater influence from the endocrine system. Poorly vascularized tissue such as tendon may not repair due to a blunted inflammatory response and a failure to phagocytize damaged tissue and up-regulate tissue repair pathways. Intracapsular ligaments, such as the anterior and posterior cruciate of the knee, will not heal due to their inability to bridge the gap between tissue ends with a provisional matrix. When phagocytosis does occur, repair will proceed under the influence of the endocrine system and cytokines released locally. Ultimately there is enough cell activity to restore the extracellular matrix. Remodeling of repaired tissues occurs in response to forces imposed on the tissues.

Pain and Pain Relief

OBJECTIVES

After reading this chapter, you will be able to

1 describe the multidimensional nature of pain;

2 explain the role of pain in preserving health and well-being;

3 discuss how the pain response can assist in evaluating an injured athlete;

4 describe how pain is sensed and how the pain message is transmitted to the central nervous system;

5 describe the differences between acute and lasting pain;

6 identify common causes for persistent pain in active people, including diagnostic errors and somatic dysfunction, faulty plans of rehabilitation, rest–reinjury cycle, complex regional pain syndrome, myofascial pain, and depression and somatization;

7 discuss the meaning and implications of neuroplasticity on pain and pain modulation;

8 describe alterations in the nociceptive system that may increase pain perception; and

9 discuss the differences between chronic and persistent pain.

A soccer player presents to the athletic training clinic complaining of severe, well-localized back pain. What questions should you ask to determine the nature of the injury? After obtaining a complete medical history and a history of the current condition and completing a physical examination, you conclude that the pain and muscle spasm are resulting from **hypomobility** at one or more lumbar spine facets. In a subsequent evaluation, a team physician agrees with this assessment. How does the dysfunction at the facet result in pain? The perception of pain is a complex neurophysiological phenomenon and will be a focus of this chapter. The soccer player is upset because the physician tells her that her back will take a few days to respond to treatment and she will be unlikely to play in a match this weekend. Is there an emotional response to injury, pain, and dysfunction?

You treat this patient with transcutaneous electrical nerve stimulation (TENS) and superficial heat before performing muscle energy techniques to restore joint mobility, and you instruct her to perform therapeutic exercise. The patient reports much less pain after treatment. What mechanisms would explain such a response? Understanding pain and ways to manage pain is important when you are using modalities.

Pain is critical to human survival. Pain causes the injured person to seek medical attention. However, pain is misery, and it limits function. Clinicians who care for the musculoskeletal system must thoroughly understand pain and the psychological responses to pain and loss of function. In the case study at the beginning of this chapter, the patient's pain brings attention to a joint dysfunction that limits function and her ability to participate in sport. Clinical experience and findings of the physical examination guide the clinician's prognosis about return to competition. Your knowledge of injury, pain, and associated muscle spasm allows for appropriate treatments to minimize suffering and, in this case, speed return to sport. Pain is also used as a guide for therapeutic exercise. If an overzealous patient pushes him- or herself too hard during rehabilitation and exercises to the point of pain, progress is slowed. On the other hand, fear of pain and reinjury can cause the patient to avoid activity, which can also slow recovery and in some cases preclude a return to work or sports.

The application of modalities can modulate pain during the rehabilitation process by allowing controlled exercise that achieves pain resolution while restoring function and promoting a return to participation. Pain relief is often a focus of therapeutic modalities and is the main reason most people seek medical attention. Pain during rest or beyond what is necessary to protect the athlete should be treated with medication, modalities, and activity modification. The goal is to reduce pain so that therapeutic exercise can be performed and function can be restored. Heat, ice, ultrasound, electrical stimulation, and mechanical therapies can all reduce pain.

In chapter 4, pain was identified as one of the cardinal signs of inflammation. However, pain is far more than a symptom caused by the chemical stimulation of free nerve endings. As suggested in the case study at the opening of this chapter, pain is a warning sign that limits function and affects a person psychologically and emotionally. Pain is also a common aspect of athletic performance. The mantra "no pain, no gain" is testimony to the hard work and suffering required to excel. The clinician and athlete must distinguish the normal pain of training and competition from that which indicates a condition requiring medical attention. Pain that is associated with impaired motion and aberrant movement patterns requires evaluation by a health care professional.

This chapter addresses the questions that arise from the case study and provides an in-depth review of the anatomy and physiology of pain and the body's pain-relieving mechanisms. The chapter defines pain; addresses the function, multidimensionality, and physiology of pain; and identifies nervous system structures that carry and receive sensory input. The clinical evaluation and interpretation of pain are reviewed, as are factors that affect persistent or chronic pain. Finally, contemporary theories of pain control are described.

WHAT IS PAIN?

Pain is defined by the International Association for the Study of Pain (IASP) as "an unpleasant physical and emotional experience which signifies tissue damage or the potential for such damage" (IASP 1979, p. 249). This definition points to the complexities of the pain experience, yet it is not comprehensive. Importantly, the definition highlights the fact that pain is not simply a physical experience. Pain affects the entire organism, altering physical and psychological processes. Despite its age, the definition remains standard. The clinician must appreciate the impact of the injury on the athlete and treat from a holistic perspective. Failure to understand the emotional component of pain can affect the relationship between the health care provider and the injured person and can slow recovery.

Pain, however, is not always associated with actual or potential tissue damage. Pain can linger well beyond tissue repair or emerge in the absence of injury. Such pain may result from structural changes in the nervous system that affect how the body modulates pain signals. Pain may also emerge from, rather than simply cause, changes in our psychological state. The root causes of psychogenic pain are complex and well beyond the scope of this text, but they are linked to neurochemical imbalance. The pain felt by patients is real despite the absence of structural injury.

Much of the pain experienced by athletes and other physically active people is related to structural injury. The clinician's goal is to identify that source of pain. Pain changes how we move and makes us miserable. Therefore, early intervention after injury must address the relief of pain. However, despite the unpleasantness associated with pain, it is essential for human survival. Pain protects the body by warning of impending injury, and it is an important guide in the progression of a plan of care. We must also remember that pain signifies that something is wrong. Inflammation, pain, and loss of function are interrelated. Using therapeutic modalities to decrease pain allows the injured person to perform therapeutic exercise that will then facilitate the return of normal movement and function. However, if pain persists, it is essential to reevaluate the patient. It may be that something else is wrong or that the patient is not ready to progress to new challenges in rehabilitation. Pain does not linger without reason.

The skillful clinician incorporates questions about pain into the interview or history portion of the physical exam. Pain also should be quantified so that it will become apparent whether pain is increasing or decreasing over time or after a therapeutic intervention. The answers provided by the patient narrow the diagnostic possibilities and focus the remainder of the physical exam. Thus, although pain relief is usually the first priority of treatment, the pain experience motivates the injured athlete to seek care and helps the sports medicine team make an assessment. Clinical methods of resolving pain are addressed in chapter 6.

TRANSMISSION OF THE PAIN SENSATION

The most common use of therapeutic modalities in the treatment of musculoskeletal injuries is to relieve pain. As clinicians, we need to understand the science behind the pain pathways to develop the best way to interrupt that signal to relieve pain. Any therapeutic intervention has the capacity to alter pain transmission, but the focus of modalities is to use heat, cold, light, sound, or electricity to reduce the transmission or perception of pain so that rehabilitative exercise may be done. The transmission of pain can be affected peripherally where the nociceptors are found, at the spinal cord level and within the brain. Therapeutic modalities such as cold application affect the transmission of signals from the periphery, while TENS affects signal transmission from peripheral nerves to nerves within the spinal cord. TENS may also affect pain transmission by altering the effects of higher brain centers on synaptic transmission in the spinal cord. To understand how modalities can change a pain experience, you must understand the pathways for transmission of painful **(noxious)** and nonnoxious sensory information (touch, temperature, vibration, and proprioception).

Peripheral Sensory Receptors

All information about our environment and the relationship of our bodies to the environment is transmitted to higher brain centers from peripheral sensory receptors. Sensory receptors can be classified as special, visceral, superficial, or deep. Special receptors provide the senses of sight, taste, smell, and hearing and contribute significantly to balance. Visceral receptors perceive hunger, nausea, distension, and visceral pain. These two groups of sensory receptors have little impact on the perception of, and response to, the pain of musculoskeletal injury. The peripheral sensory receptors, however, provide the central nervous system with information about pain, touch, vibration, temperature, and proprioception. These receptors are very important in transmitting information about the status of the musculoskeletal and integumentary systems.

The superficial receptors transmit sensations such as warmth, cold, touch, pressure, vibration, tickle, itch, and pain from the skin (Berne, Koeppen, and Stanton 2010). The deep receptors transmit information about position, kinesthesia, deep pressure, and pain from the muscles, tendons, fascia, joint capsules, and ligaments (Berne, Koeppen, and Stanton 2010). The superficial and deep peripheral receptors transmit the impulses that result in the perception of pain after injury. Table 5.1 identifies the categories and functions of peripheral sensory receptors.

Superficial Receptors

The superficial receptors, also called cutaneous receptors, can be subdivided into three categories based on the types of stimuli to which they respond: **mechanoreceptors**, **thermoreceptors**, and **nociceptors**. Mechanoreceptors respond to stroking, touch, and pressure. Some of these receptors adapt rapidly and perceive changes in stimulation. The hair follicle receptors, Meissner's corpuscles, and Pacinian corpuscles respond to changes in pressure and touch. In contrast, Merkel cell endings and Ruffini endings, which respond to pressure and skin stretch, are more slowly adapting (Berne, Koeppen, and Stanton 2010). These receptors respond to sustained stimuli.

Thermoreceptors respond to temperature and temperature change. Cold and warm receptors are slowly adapting but discharge in phasic bursts when the temperature changes rapidly. These receptors

Table 5.1   Peripheral Sensory Receptors

Receptor	Classification	Function
SUPERFICIAL		
Mechanoreceptors	Meissner's corpuscles Pacinian corpuscles Merkel cells Ruffini endings	Pressure and touch Skin stretch and pressure
Thermoreceptors	Cold receptors Hot receptors	Temperature and temperature change
Nociceptors	Free nerve endings	Pain
DEEP		
Proprioceptors	Golgi tendon organs Pacinian corpuscles Ruffini endings	Changes in muscle length and muscle spindle tension Change in joint position Vibration Joint end range, possible heat
Nociceptors	Free nerve endings	Pain

respond over a large temperature range. However, warm receptors stop discharging at temperatures that damage the skin. The pain of thermal burn results from the stimulation of free nerve endings and **nociceptive** afferent pathways. Cold receptors continue to discharge when tissue cooling is perceived as painful. However, cooling slows the conduction velocity of the nerves between the sensory receptor and the spinal cord (Knight 1995). Thus, tissue injury due to cold (frostbite) is not particularly painful. However, when the frostbitten tissue thaws, there is considerable inflammation and pain.

Nociceptors form the third category of superficial receptor. Nociceptors, also labeled free nerve endings, are stimulated by potentially damaging mechanical, chemical, and thermal stress. It is now recognized that not all nociceptors respond identically. These receptors can be categorized as being mechanical sensitive, chemical sensitive, heat/cold sensitive, or sensitive to a broader range of stimuli (polymodal). There are more polymodal receptors than any other type. The second most common nociceptor is classified as inactive or silent. These nerve endings become active in response to painful events and may explain some of the changes in pain sensitivity throughout life.

Following acute injury, chemical-sensitive nociceptors are stimulated by prostaglandins, bradykinin, **substance P**, serotonin, and other chemical mediators of inflammation. Mechanical-sensitive nociceptors respond to pressure and distension, including that which results from swelling. Polymodal nociceptors conduct painful stimuli that result from mechanical and chemical stimulation as well as extremes of heat or cold, while some nociceptors only respond to extremes in temperature. The body is well equipped to respond to damaging or potentially damaging temperatures, mechanical forces, and changes in the chemical environment. The specialization in the nociceptive system also allows distinctions to be made between pain caused by temperature extremes, pressure, and damaged tissue.

Deep Tissue Receptors

There are receptors in the joints as well as in the ligaments, tendons, and musculature. They are equally complex and provide further sensory information to the central nervous system about pressure (stress and strain), tension, and pain. Ligaments and other deep tissues are supplied by mechanoreceptors (figure 5.1) and nociceptors. The joint receptors include Ruffini endings, which are low threshold, slow adapting and respond to stress; Pacinian corpuscles that are low threshold, rapidly adapting and respond to velocity of movement; Golgi-like receptors that respond to compressive force; and free nerve endings that respond to pain. Nociceptors or free nerve endings signify that motion has exceeded normal limits and that stabilizing structures are at risk of failing or that injury has already occurred. The body's connective tissue or fascial network is also supplied with sensory receptors. Fascia, the "glue" that holds the body together, surrounds the muscles and organs and literally connects the body from head to toe. The innervation of fascia has not

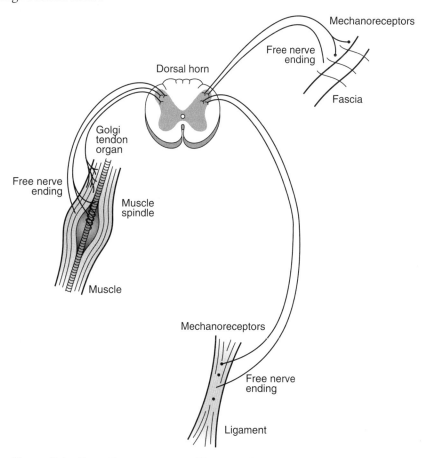

Figure 5.1 Deep tissue receptors. The central nervous system receives information from mechanoreceptors and nociceptors of muscle, ligament, and fascia.

been fully explored. However, input from mechanoreceptors and nociceptors affects the resting length and tension of muscle and is likely the underlying cause of complex pain patterns labeled myofascial pain syndrome, discussed more extensively in chapters 6 and 17. Muscle receptors include the muscle spindles, which respond to changes in the length of the muscle and are responsible for muscle tone, and Golgi tendon organs, which respond to muscle force. It has been proposed that these receptors are reflexively linked to the skin as well as to the surrounding musculature.

Pathways for Transmission of Acute Pain

Acute pain travels along the neocortical tract, which is a fast, three-neuron pathway from the periphery to the cortex. The paleocortical tract is slower and more complex; the pain stimuli travel to the cortex in a manner that can explain the complex emotional components of pain.

Neocortical Tract Pain

Pain is transmitted from the injured area to the brain in a systematic fashion. Acute pain is a rapid, three-neuron sequence that provides accurate information about the location of injury. The nociceptor is the sensory organ in the tissues that is sensitized to the painful stimulation. The information travels to the spinal cord via the sensory nerve, also referred to as a first-order neuron. All sensory nerve fibers have their cell bodies in the dorsal root ganglia and synapse in the spinal cord in the dorsal horn. The second-order pain nerve fiber crosses to the opposite side of the spinal cord (decussates) and transmits the information up to the thalamus. Various sensory inputs (touch, deep pressure, vibration, temperature, proprioception, and pain) travel in organized columns of second-order nerves from the spinal level to the brain. Many second-order afferent nerves carry information about multiple sensations, and they are termed wide-dynamic-range second-order afferent nerves. Some second-order afferent nerves, however, are specific to the transmission of pain. At the thalamus, there is a synapse onto the third-order neuron that carries information to the sensory cortex of the brain where the pain is acknowledged. This three-neuron pathway is called the neocortical system (figure 5.2). It detects the "first pain" (Bolay and Moskowitz 2002), which is well localized, discriminative, and lasts as long as the acutely painful stimulus is applied.

The following neurological components are important in the acute pain pathway:

- Nociceptor (in the skin, soft tissue, and periosteum).

- Sensory nerve (cell body is in the dorsal root ganglion and synapses in the dorsal horn of the spinal cord). This is the first-order neuron. Typically, this is an A-delta fiber.
- Second-order afferent neuron (T cell) "transmits" a signal to the thalamus. The name *T cell* is given to this neuron since pain, temperature, light touch, vibration, and deep touch are carried on different tracts. Therefore T cell is a generic name for the second-order neuron.
- Thalamus: Cell bodies of the third-order neuron are clustered in nuclei organized according to the stimulus and its origin.
- Sensory cortex: Area of the brain that identifies the location of pain.

Paleocortical Tract Pain

"Second pain" is associated with the affective-motivational aspects of the pain experience and is organically connected to various supraspinal areas in the brain. This pain network provides the basis for integrating sensory input with emotional centers of the nervous system and is linked to Melzack's neuromatrix theory of pain (Melzack 2001). The neuromatrix theory describes the brain as the central command center where multiple inputs from memory, various brain centers (nuclei), and interneurons affect the magnitude and overall effect of the pain experience.

As with the neocortical pathway, the initial transmission begins with the receptor. Typically, intense stimuli activate polymodal nociceptors and promote a diffuse, unpleasant, and persistent burning sensation that lasts beyond the acutely painful stimulus. An example of this pain would be the burning sensation of an application of capsaicin, which is the noxious component of hot peppers applied to the skin. The transmission to the spinal cord is similar to that in the neocortical signal, but this pain is carried on C fibers, which are smaller in diameter and have a slower transmission rate because they have less myelin. It is theorized that since the signal is slower, there is more time for a vast, diffuse network of interneurons to be activated in the central nervous system. Wide dynamic range neurons responding to both somatic and visceral stimulation are activated. These signals infiltrate many neurological centers as the input ascends to the supraspinal areas in the brain. The limbic system that is responsible for emotional responses is affected, as are the pituitary gland and hypothalamus, which control vegetative and endocrine functions. Centers for attentiveness, well-being, sleep, and motor activity such as the periaqueductal gray area, the reticular formation, and the raphe nucleus are also activated. These brain centers also have a role in descending pain modulation (see Descending Pathways) when targeted specifically. The second neurological pathway for pain is termed the paleocortical system (figure 5.3).

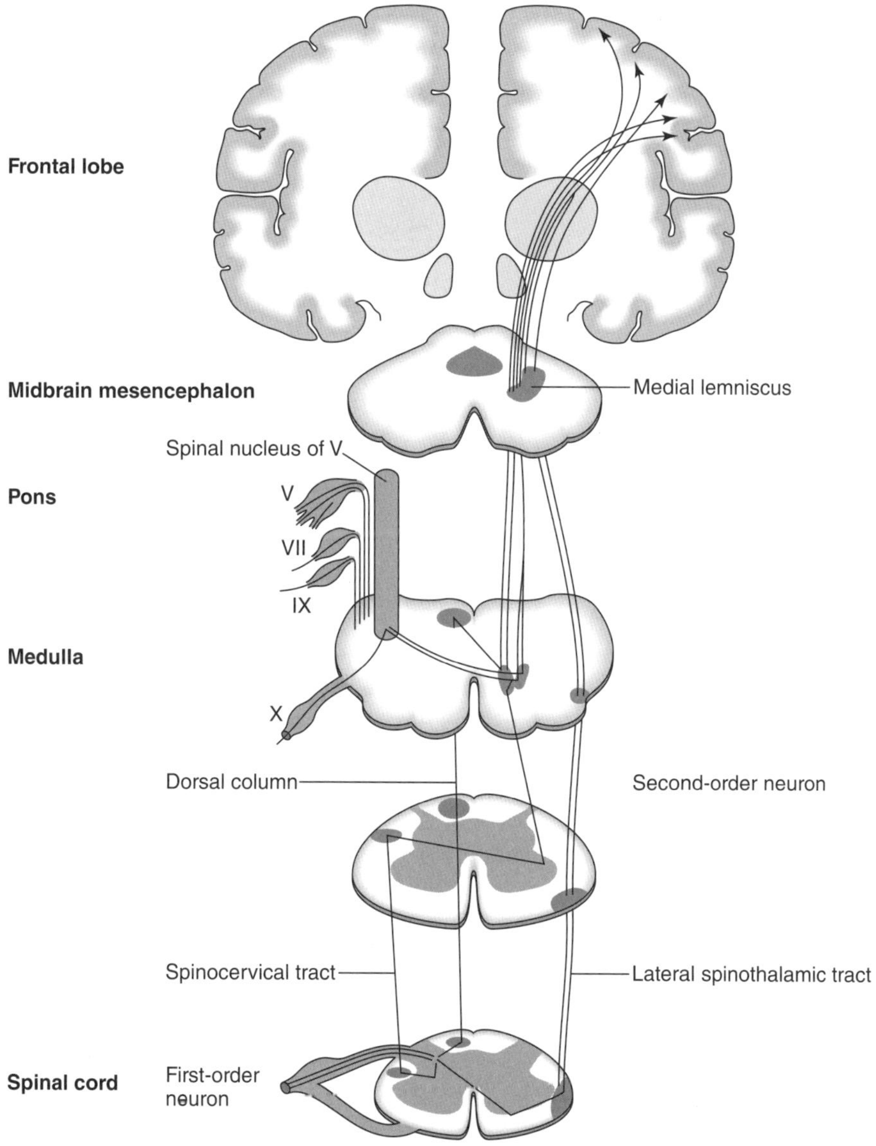

Neurological structures associated with second pain include the following:

• Nociceptors activated (chemical, mechanical, and polymodal).

• Sensory nerve (typically C fiber) or first-order neuron that synapses in the dorsal horn of the spinal cord and activates nociception-specific neurons in lamina I and II.

• The second-order neurons are also transmitted via the T cell but synapse onto multiple centers, including the reticular formation, periaqueductal gray, thalamus, hypothalamus, and pituitary gland.

• Reticular formation: Diffuse network of neurons that mediate motor, autonomic, and sensory functions.

• Periaqueductal gray (PAG): Directs descending inhibition.

• Hypothalamus: Regulates vegetative and endocrine functions throughout the body.

Figure 5.2 Acute pain pathway, the three-neuron pathway that represents "first pain" or the neocortical tract. The painful stimulation travels to the spinal cord from the peripheral sensory organ via the dorsal root ganglion. There is a synapse in the dorsal horn of the spinal cord, and the second-order neuron ascends to the supraspinal levels via the lateral spinothalamic tract after crossing (decussating) to the opposite side. There is another synapse in the thalamus and termination at the sensory cortex.

(continued)

Pathways for Transmission of Acute Pain *(continued)*

- Pituitary: Controlled by hormonal or neuronal signals from the hypothalamus. The pituitary is the master gland of the endocrine system.

- Thalamus: Final gateway/relay center for all afferent input (except olfactory). Specific nuclei direct the function of the thalamus.

- Limbic system: Role in motivational, emotional, and affective behavior. Has input from the thalamus, hypothalamus, and cortex.

- Sensory cortex: Area of the brain that identifies the location of pain. Receives input from all sensory and associated cortical areas and projects to the reticular formation and limbic system. Central processing center.

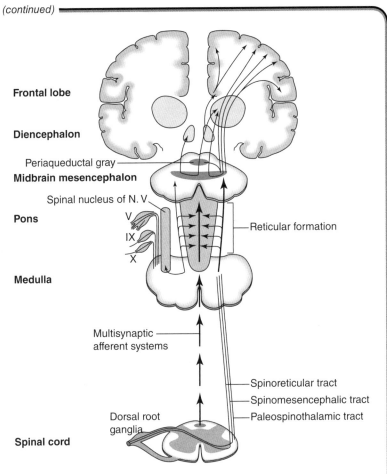

Figure 5.3 The second pain neurological pathway; the paleocortical system.

Afferent Pathways

Impulses generated at the sensory receptors are transmitted to higher centers by **afferent**, or sensory nerves (figure 5.4). A first-order afferent is a nerve fiber in the periphery (outside the central nervous system); it has its cell body in the dorsal root ganglia and synapses in the spinal cord. The afferent nerves are classified according to structural and functional characteristics. Specifically, categories of sensory nerve fibers are grouped by the diameter of the nerve, which reflects the degree of myelination, the conduction velocity, and the nerve's function. The function of nerve fibers determines the type of sensory information carried by that nerve: light touch, pressure, pain, or temperature. Faster conduction velocity occurs in nerves with more myelination. Thus, larger-diameter nerve fibers are more heavily myelinated and are faster-conducting than smaller-diameter, thinly or nonmyelinated nerves. For the

purposes of understanding pain and pain modulation theories, differences in the nerve fibers must be understood. The first-order neurons involved with pain signal transmission or modulation are classified in table 5.2. There are other types of first-order neurons, but these do not have a function in pain and pain modulation, so they are not included.

The **A-beta fibers** originate from hair follicles, Meissner's corpuscles, Pacinian corpuscles, Merkel cell endings, and Ruffini endings. These fibers transmit sensory information regarding touch, vibration, and hair deflection. They are large-diameter, myelinated nerves. These characteristics make the A-beta fiber a fast-conducting nerve fiber. The A-beta fiber has a relatively low threshold, making it easily stimulated. These fibers also accommodate to stimuli quickly. For example, you feel your shirt when you put it on, but it is unlikely that you receive constant sensation about your shirt unless the stimulation changes.

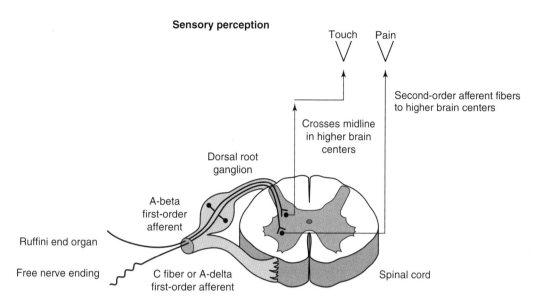

Sensory perception

Touch   Pain

Second-order afferent fibers
to higher brain centers

Crosses midline
in higher brain
centers

Dorsal root
ganglion

A-beta
first-order
afferent

Ruffini end organ

Free nerve ending

C fiber or A-delta
first-order afferent

Spinal cord

Figure 5.4 Primary afferents synapse with second-order afferent fibers in the dorsal horn of the spinal cord. Sensory information is perceived in the opposite sensory cortex; the pain fibers cross at the level of synapsing, but touch and vibration cross in the higher brain centers.

Table 5.2 First-Order Afferents

Type and group	Diameter (μm)	Conduction velocity (μs)	Location	Information transmitted
MYELINATED				
A-beta	6–12	36–72	Skin	Touch, vibration
A-delta	1–6	6–36	Skin	Touch, pressure, temperature, pain
UNMYELINATED				
C	<1	0.5–2	Muscle Skin	Pain Touch, pressure, temperature, pain

Reprinted from *Athletic Training Sport Health Care Perspective*, vol. 2(2), C.R. Denegar and E.F.H. Bowman, "Electrotherapy in the treatment of athletic injuries," pgs. 108-115, Copyright © 1996, with permission from Elsevier.

The **A-delta fibers** transmit information from warm and cold receptors, a few hair receptors, and chemical, mechanical, heat- and cold-sensitive free nerve endings, thus transmitting pain. The free nerve endings supplied by A-delta fibers primarily respond to noxious mechanical stimulation such as pinching, pricking, and crushing. The A-delta fibers are myelinated, but they are smaller than A-beta fibers and thus have a slower conduction velocity. It generally takes more sensory information to send a signal as pain rather than touch. For example, a light or even deep pressure is transmit-

ted as touch, but firm, high pressure is transmitted as pain.

The **C fibers** are the smallest afferent peripheral nerves that are associated with pain. They are unmyelinated and also include the **efferent** postganglionic fibers of the sympathetic nervous system. Those fibers that originate at deep receptors are primarily mechanoreceptors and nociceptors. A few peripheral type C afferents are thermoreceptors, but most are mechanosensitive or polymodal. The C fibers are the slowest of the sensory nerve fibers in conduction and require a greater stimulation than the others to elicit a response.

Supraspinal Centers

The primary target for the second-order neuron in both pleasant and noxious sensory input is the thalamus, just above the brainstem in the diencephalon. The cell bodies of the third-order neurons are located in clusters, or nuclei, of the thalamus. Here the sensory information is organized, and the thalamus becomes a relay center with facilitatory and inhibitory circuits. Figure 5.5 represents the organization of the thalamus. The ventral posterior lateral (VPL) and ventral posterior medial (VPM) nuclei are identified as the most significant for pain transmission and pain modulation (Berne, Koeppen, and Stanton 2010). The fibers ascending from the body synapse in the VPL, whereas the fibers from the head and face synapse in the VPM. The thalamus modulates input from the ascending nerves before transmitting it to the somatosensory cortex. Ultimately, the localization and discrimination of pain occur in the postcentral gyrus of the cortex of the brain. The thalamus also relays input to the limbic system, which regulates the emotional, autonomic, and endocrine response to pain. Thus, the thalamus relays sensory input that provides for the sensory-discriminatory and affective-motivational aspects of pain.

Descending Pathways

Pain transmission is afferent, meaning that it travels in an ascending fashion to the sensory cortex, where the signal is processed. However, because of the paleocortical tract and the influence of interneurons, various pathways that can interrupt the pain signal have been identified. Any activity that occurs after the cortex has received the input is described as occurring along the descending pathways. The descending tracts ultimately have an excitatory or inhibitory action on new impulses that are being transmitted in the spinal cord.

The paleocortical tract describes the diffuse ascending pathways of noxious stimulation. Some of the second-order neuron afferents terminate directly in the periaqueductal gray (PAG) formation in the midbrain. The noxious stimulation causes specific neurotransmitters to activate other brain centers such as the reticular formation and the raphe nucleus. The reticular formation is in the brainstem and helps to control autonomic functions, has some motor function, and helps to provide collateral sensory signals to higher brain centers. The raphe nucleus is an area that controls the level of arousal and affects the individual's perception of well-being. These brain areas—the PAG, the reticular formation, and the raphe nucleus—all have the potential to affect the perception of pain through a descending mechanism. For example, in a painful situation, continual impulses are sent from the receptor to the spinal cord and then to the cortex, where the pain is acknowledged consciously. Inflammation and its chemical mediators sensitize receptors, increasing the pain impulse. When the PAG is activated, a network is initiated that can calm the person and help to filter out some of the pain signals by exciting the reticular formation and the raphe nucleus. The pituitary gland also produces hormones and neuropeptides that help regulate the signals at the spinal cord level. These brain centers ideally lessen the impulses to the cortex. Evoking these descending modulation areas is the goal of pain management, through either medication, modalities, or stress relief. The neuroanatomic representation of these important relay centers is depicted in figure 5.6.

The diffuse network of messages and the activation of brain centers during a painful event may exacerbate the situation. The hypothalamus, pituitary, reticular formation, and raphe nucleus control subconscious, vegetative functions such as respiration, heart rate, attention, sleep, and general feelings of impending doom. When these areas are not inhibited, the affective-emotional response to pain is similar to shock. Painful stimulation continues to flow to the cognitive areas, and the perception of pain increases. It becomes more difficult to concentrate on other activities, and the patient's functional capacity is limited. These areas of the brain respond neurochemically and are strongly affected by medications. They are

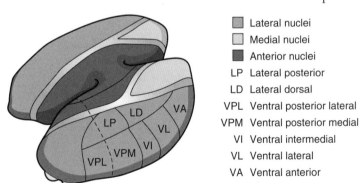

Lateral nuclei
Medial nuclei
Anterior nuclei
LP   Lateral posterior
LD   Lateral dorsal
VPL Ventral posterior lateral
VPM Ventral posterior medial
VI   Ventral intermedial
VL   Ventral lateral
VA   Ventral anterior

Figure 5.5   The organization of the thalamus.

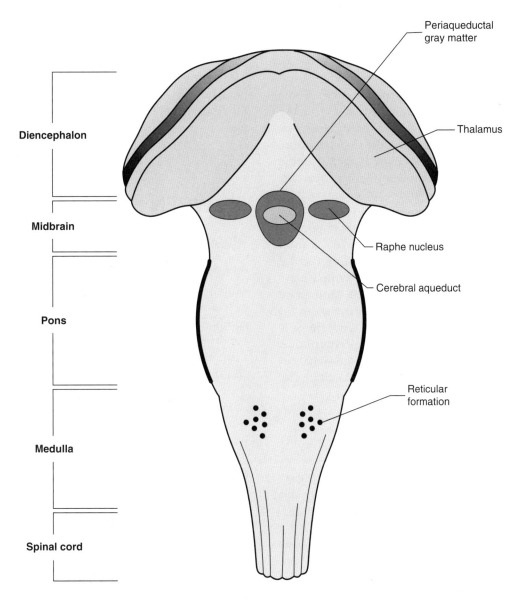

Figure 5.6 Brainstem structures involved in pain perception and modulation.

not controlled by consciousness, although calming, reassuring techniques are often helpful. A phenomenon known as "windup" describes how noxious stimulation can spiral out of control, resulting in a pain syndrome that exceeds its benefit of alerting the injured person to potential harm. The presence of peptide neurotransmitters such as substance P, combined with the release of the excitatory amino acid glutamate in central nociceptive nerve terminals, results in temporal summation. This alters the response characteristics of the second-order cells in the spinal dorsal horn, resulting in a sustained C fiber input. The sensitization of the postsynaptic nerves to such sustained input results in a state of hyperstimulation.

Efforts should be made to control pain with activity modification (rest, splinting), pharmacological agents if needed, stress reduction to prevent neurogenic shock, and therapeutic modalities. Proper treatment usually prevents the hyperstimulated state in an acute injury. However, windup may occur insidiously with persistent pain syndromes that are discussed later in this chapter.

Synaptic Transmission and Transmitter Substances

Communication from one nerve fiber to the next takes place at the **synapse** between the two nerves. Impulses from a presynaptic nerve may stimulate depolarization of the postsynaptic nerve by releasing a **transmitter substance**. When this occurs, the transmitter substance is facilitatory. However, not all substances released from presynaptic nerves stimulate depolarization from postsynaptic nerves. Some transmitter substances are inhibitory and block the depolarization of the postsynaptic nerve. Neuroscience has significantly advanced the understanding of transmitter substances. Many biogenic amine transmitters, amino acid transmitters, and neuroactive peptides have been found to influence synaptic transmission at various locations in the nervous system. Acetylcholine and glutamate are important facilitatory transmitters. Acetylcholine is involved with the transmission of signals at neuromuscular junctions and the functions of the sympathetic and parasympathetic nervous systems. Glutamate plays a role in most excitatory activity in the central nervous system. However, glutamate is not the only transmitter of pain signals. Substance P contributes substantially to the transmission of pain signals in the dorsal horn, which may be further facilitated by nitrous oxide.

Glycine and GABA are inhibitory neurotransmitters. Glycine is predominant in the spinal cord while GABA is found both in the spinal cord and in the brain. Understanding the role of these chemicals helps us determine the best method for applying physical agents or pharmaceutical agents for pain modulation.

Beta endorphin, dynorphin, methionine enkephalin, and leucine enkephalin are classified as opioid peptides because they bind to the same sites as the **opiate** drugs. Because these neurochemicals are produced by the body, they are considered *endogenous* opioids, and they inhibit the transmission of pain impulses. Beta endorphin is a large peptide chain found in distinct locations within the central nervous system (Jessell and Kelly 1991). Beta endorphin has a half-life of about 4 hours, so it can produce long-lasting pain modulation. Dynorphin and the enkephalins are smaller amino acid chains and are more widespread. They have a much shorter half-life, ranging between 45 seconds and 20 minutes. **Enkephalins** play an important role in counteracting the effects of substance P in the dorsal horn. Substance P promotes the propagation of pain signals to second-order afferent nerves, while the release of enkephalins blocks or modulates signal transmission.

In the central nervous system, endogenous opioids occupy the same receptor sites as narcotic medications. Endogenous opioids are important to maintaining homoeostasis and managing the painful stimuli experienced in daily life. Narcotic medications are very effective at controlling severe pain, but when a patient is prescribed narcotic pain medication, pain modulation through endogenous mechanisms is often inhibited. Thus, when a patient is taking narcotic pain medicine, it increases the difficulty of reducing pain with therapeutic agents.

WHEN PAIN PERSISTS

Fortunately, most people who suffer musculoskeletal injuries recover and resume pain-free activity. However, not all musculoskeletal conditions are acutely painful, and some patients fail to respond to treatment. Moreover, some patients present with complaints of pain without an identifiable pathology. These situations challenge the clinician to find the sources of the persistent or chronic pain and challenge the patient to understand and cope with the condition.

Persisting pain is a complex subject and requires some operating definitions. In this book "persistent pain" and "chronic pain" define different problems. Chronic pain has been defined based on a duration of pain such as 3 or 6 months, or the effects of lasting pain on ability to participate and quality of life (ICSI 2009). Chronic pain can also be linked to chronic health conditions such as arthritis, nerve injury, and cancer. Chronic pain has also been defined in the context of response to treatment. An International Society for the Study of Pain (IASP) task force defined chronic pain as "persistent pain that is not amenable, as a rule, to treatments based upon specific remedies, or to the routine methods of pain control such as non-narcotic analgesics" (Merskey and Bogduk 1994, p. 209). The etiology of chronic pain is discussed in the last section of this chapter, but from this definition we learn that the treatments and exercise programs discussed in this book do not provide meaningful relief for those who suffer true chronic pain.

Persistent pain, by contrast, lasts beyond what is expected when tissue is injured and an acute inflammation ensues but is amenable to treatment with therapeutic modalities, including exercise and medication. A patient may present with persisting pain (e.g., "my shoulder has been bothering me for more than a month. I thought it would get better, but now I can't even sleep through the night") or with an apparent acute injury only to have symptoms persist.

From these definitions it should be clear that the distinctions between persistent and chronic pain are not absolute. Duration of symptoms, limitations in function, participation restrictions, and diminished quality of life due to pain do not preclude meaningful improvement through effective care. Similarly, a structural lesion such as an arthritic knee does not equate with prolonged, unremitting pain. Prolonged pain can truly be labeled chronic only when relief requires narcotic medications. The first step in treating patients with persistent pain is identifying the source or sources of their symptoms. The failure to respond to a plan of care that may include nonnarcotic medications, the application of therapeutic modalities, exercise, and the use of assistive devices and orthoses strongly suggests that the pain being reported is intractable and chronic. Without seeking relief through these treatments, however, one cannot be certain of the possibilities.

Finally, the association of persistent pain and psychological factors must be considered. Pain will often affect patients' health-related quality of life, thus affecting their social life and overall feeling of worth. Factors that relate therapeutic modalities, assessment, treatment, and referral are addressed in chapter 2.

SOURCES OF PAIN

The causes of persistent pain span a spectrum from physical or structural to principally psychological. First, and *very importantly*, recognize that symptoms consistent with injury to connective tissue may not emanate from the musculoskeletal system. Cancer is of particular concern. Cancer affecting the vital organs (liver, pancreas) as well as the prostate, as examples, can cause persistent low back pain, sometimes before other signs and symptoms emerge. Cancers affecting bone may mimic the symptoms of stress injuries. All clinicians should consider nonmusculoskeletal sources of persisting musculoskeletal pain and be familiar with the signs and symptoms of cancer.

Once serious medical conditions are ruled out, the next steps are to systematically consider the source or sources of persistent pain. While there is no single approach to evaluating these complex cases, we propose that clinicians first try to identify or rule out structural and biomechanical sources of persistent pain (figure 5.7). Much can be learned from the history of the presenting condition and physical examination. Patients who report immediate pain resulting from trauma need to be evaluated for sprains, strains, and fractures. Those who cannot identify a distinct incident are more likely to suffer from tendinopathy, stress fracture, pain radiating along a compressed nerve, or "syndrome" such as patellofemoral pain or glenohumeral impingement. The pain associated with syndromes and stress fractures likely results from repeated loading and stimulation of sensitized mechanical and polymodal free nerve endings. Pain resulting from pressure on nerves (radicular) often has a sharp, burning quality and may manifest quite distal to the site of compression. For example, pressure on the sixth spinal nerve caused by a cervical disc herniation may cause thumb and forearm pain but not neck pain. Tendinopathy is an enigma. It is not clear why some people with tendon degeneration suffer pain while others do not or whether all tendon-related pain has the same cause. The good news is that with appropriate medical care involving the judicious use of medication and therapeutic modalities combined with exercise, these conditions can be effectively treated. Unfortunately, some patients present having failed to respond to previous treatment efforts.

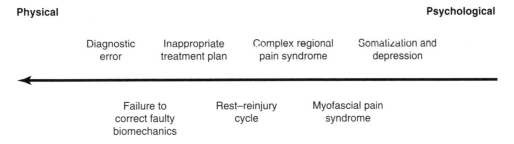

Figure 5.7   Persistent pain spans a spectrum from physical to principally psychological.

Reprinted, by permission, from C.R. Denegar and A. Peppard, 1997, "Evaluation and treatment of persistent pain and myofascial pain syndrome," *Athletic Therapy Today* September 2(4): 40.

Reevaluation

When recovery is not progressing as anticipated or a new patient presents reporting that previous plans of care failed to resolve symptoms, a detailed reevaluation is needed. Important elements of the patient's medical history and a history of the current condition should be confirmed and new questions asked when more information is needed. A complete physical re-examination is also warranted. The presentation of patients changes over time, and the clinician is seeking to learn why symptoms are persisting. Once the examination is complete the data are evaluated against several possibilities. First, the failure to improve may involve a diagnostic error or a treatment plan than is inappropriate for the condition. Persisting symptoms may result from faulty biomechanics. In some athletes and workers the resolution of pain is interpreted as full recovery resulting in a cycle of rest and reinjury.

Diagnosis

Accurate diagnoses are essential for effective intervention; you can't treat what isn't identified. Patients with persisting pain may seek care after a period of time, thinking or hoping their symptoms will resolve. In most cases these patients cannot identify a single precipitating event. While such a history usually rules out traumatic injury to bone, muscle, ligament, and tendon, the clinician must sort out the array of potential causative and contributing factors. Plans of treatment may involve activity modifications, specific therapeutic exercises, taping or bracing, the application of therapeutic modalities, and medication. Plans of care must be individualized to address the unique presentation and needs of the patient.

The failure to respond to a plan of care adds another dimension to the challenge of persisting pain. When appropriate improvement does not occur, or when a patient seeks another opinion, the health care team must reevaluate the injury and the complaint as though it were a new problem. Sometimes persistent pain stems from a problem that was not recognized on initial examination. It is important to remember that the source of pain may not be musculoskeletal structures. Thus, the first step in reevaluation is to reconsider the original diagnosis through a comprehensive review of systems. The process of examination and evaluation continues in order to establish a new diagnosis or confirm one made previously. If the diagnosis is confirmed, then detailed evaluation is needed to identify how the plan of care must change to promote the resolution of symptoms and return to work and sports. Reevaluation may reveal the need to address movement mechanics more comprehensively. Persisting symptoms may be related to dysfunction along the kinetic chain that is remote from the site of pain. For example, lateral knee pain related to iliotibial band syndrome is often attributable to hip and sacroiliac mechanics. When these issues are identified in reevaluation, the plan of care must be changed to resolve the patient's complaints.

It is also essential to recognize that pain may emanate from changes in how pain is transmitted and pain signals modulated. Complex regional pain syndrome (CRPS), myofascial pain, and true chronic pain represent different diagnoses related to unrelenting pain or pain associated with non-noxious stimuli. These neurogenic sources of pain must be considered in the evaluation of patients presenting with persisting pain. CRPS and chronic pain warrant particular consideration when the severity of reported pain exceeds what one would expect if symptoms were solely related to musculoskeletal tissue injury.

Rest–Reinjury Cycle

Athletic excellence requires participants to put forth maximum effort and push through pain in their training. When injured, physically active people will generally accept a period of rest until the pain subsides. The absence of pain, however, is often interpreted as a sign that the tissue is healed and that the athlete can return to unrestricted practice and competition. If the tissue is not ready, reinjury occurs, and the **rest–reinjury cycle** begins (Peppard and Denegar 1994). Rehabilitation extends beyond specific treatments and therapeutic exercises and must include a gradual return to functional exercises.

When clinicians find that persistent pain is due to a rest–reinjury cycle, they can educate patients about the differences between conditioning and reconditioning after injury. Reconditioning requires careful control of exercise intensity, frequency, and duration. The exercise program must allow the person to stay within the exercise tolerance window. Exercise that results in pain severe enough to alter movement patterns must be avoided, and intensity and duration must be limited to avoid postexercise pain.

Exercise associated with conditioning and training for sport after injury begins during the remodeling phase of recovery. If someone is too sore to repeat yesterday's therapeutic and functional exercises, the exercise tolerance limit was exceeded and the rehabilitation process slowed. As a well-structured rehabilitation program progresses, the exercise tolerance window widens, and the athlete becomes more tolerant of exercise-induced pain. Training should be specific, structured, and, when possible, supervised. Coaches and strength and conditioning specialists can help the injured athlete progress in gradually more demanding sport-specific exercises and general reconditioning. The clinician should carefully evaluate the use of therapeutic modalities in all cases of persistent pain. This is especially important when a rest–reinjury cycle is involved.

Physically active persons often respond well to modality application for pain control, but they may continue to seek the treatments that allowed them to return to practice and competition after the initial injury. A rest–reinjury cycle may be perpetrated by continuing **palliative care** without educating the injured person and his or her coaches about the problem and restricting the athlete's exercise program.

Plan of Care

A rehabilitation plan of care is developed based on the diagnosis, medical history, history of the current condition, and comprehensive physical examination. Even in the presence of a specific diagnosis (e.g., postoperative care for an anterior cruciate ligament tear), an examination may reveal somatic dysfunction and patterns of movement that may slow recovery, pose a risk of injury to other structures, or increase the risk of reinjury upon return to sport and work. Often we cannot recognize all of the contributors to persistent pain after evaluating the patient's information and examination findings. When pain persists or new problems emerge, such as patella tendinopathy after patellar bone-tendon-bone anterior cruciate ligament reconstruction, the plan of care must change. Rehabilitation following musculoskeletal injuries requires more than a plan to resolve symptoms and impairments and regain function. The physical demands of sport and many occupations require return to a high level of fitness. The demands of the task dictate the training goals. A football lineman will focus on power, while a marathon runner must build endurance. Plans of care must be individualized and the patient fully prepared to resume participation to minimize the risk of reinjury.

Complex Regional Pain Syndrome

Complex regional pain syndrome (CRPS), formerly labeled reflex sympathetic dystrophy (RSD), is a symptom complex characterized by pain that is markedly disproportional to the injury. CRPS can result from injury to nerve (type II CRPS) but is more commonly caused by a musculoskeletal or soft-tissue injury that does not involve nerve tissue (type I CRPS). In many respects CRPS does not fit into a discussion of persisting and chronic pain. CRPS develops rapidly, with significant changes occurring across a few hours to a couple of days. However, clinicians must recognize CRPS as a serious complication of musculoskeletal injury or orthopaedic surgery with the potential to result in severe, permanent pain.

Severe pain is the hallmark of CRPS, but patients commonly experience hypersensitivity to touch and movement, joint stiffness, muscle guarding, edema, erythema, hyperhidrosis, and ultimately tissue **atrophy** and osteopenia. The etiology of this condition is not fully understood, making treatment a challenge. CRPS may occur after even minor injury and may emerge several days after an injury or surgery. Ladd et al. (1989) introduced the term *reflex sympathetic imbalance (RSI)*, which highlighted the importance of attending to pain that is out of proportion to the injury. Patients suffering from CRPS are not magnifying their symptoms, but rather are suffering from a condition in which the pain-modulating systems of the body are overwhelmed. Disproportional pain is the hallmark symptom of CRPS, and other signs and symptoms may not be present at first. Ladd et al. emphasized that RSI (and now CRPS) can be diagnosed based only on the presence of disproportional pain, thus expediting recognition and treatment. Early recognition increases the likelihood of successful treatment. If disproportional pain exists, clinicians must not wait until other symptoms appear before considering a diagnosis of CRPS and initiating appropriate treatments.

Myofascial Pain

As previously noted, when pain persists beyond the time frame for tissue repair, clinicians must review the situation systematically and thoroughly, looking for diagnostic and treatment errors. If this review does not identify the cause of persistent pain, **myofascial pain syndrome (MFPS)** or somatization must be considered. Myofascial pain syndrome is characterized by pain emanating from the muscles and connective soft tissues. It is commonly associated with the cervical and lumbar spine; however, persistent joint pain can result in myofascial pain patterns in the extremities as well.

There is no single cause of MFPS, making the condition difficult to diagnose and treat. Several factors can contribute to its development, including posture, stress, fatigue, and trauma or repetitive microtrauma with recurrent painful episodes. In sport, repetitive microtrauma can trigger MFPS. For example, physically active people with long histories of knee and shin pain, such as medial tibial stress syndrome or patellofemoral pain, can develop secondary, or type II, MFPS (Denegar and Peppard 1997). In these cases patients will continue to report

pain in the affected region despite appropriate treatment for the primary injury. MFPS is characterized by soft tissue tightness and a pattern of local areas of tenderness called **trigger points**. While trigger points are highly sensitive to palpation and pressure, patients typically describe a diffuse, aching pain. Trigger points manifest bilaterally, and those on the contralateral side may be more sensitive than those on the injured side. Figures 5.8 and 5.9 depict common trigger points associated with knee, hip, elbow, back, shoulder, foot and ankle, and forearm and upper extremity pain.

MFPS can result from traumatic injuries and accidents. Patients injured in motor vehicle accidents may develop shoulder pain and headaches several months after the accident. Often the only injury sustained was a "minor" whiplash or low back strain. Acute pain that resolved within 3 weeks and a lingering, aching pain that worsens with fatigue are common findings. Pain while using a keyboard, driving, or performing other activities that place the

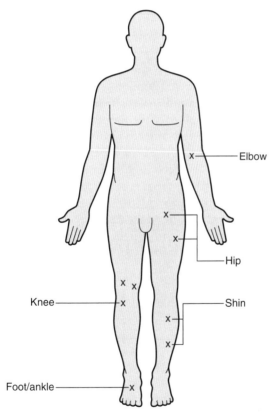

Figure 5.8   Common trigger points associated with knee, hip, elbow, shin, and foot and ankle pain.

Reprinted, by permission, from C.R. Denegar and A. Peppard, 1997, "Evaluation and treatment of persistent pain and myofascial pain syndrome," *Athletic Therapy Today* 2(4): 42.

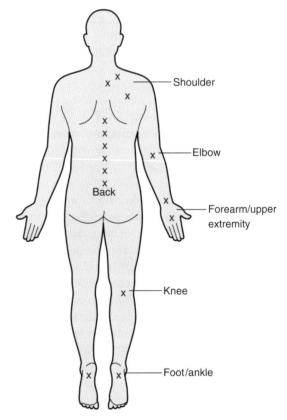

Figure 5.9   Common trigger points associated with shoulder, elbow, back, knee, foot and ankle, and forearm and upper extremity pain.

Reprinted, by permission, from C.R. Denegar and A. Peppard, 1997, "Evaluation and treatment of persistent pain and myofascial pain syndrome," *Athletic Therapy Today* 2(4): 42.

person in a forward-head position and stress the paraspinal musculature is a common complaint. Neck and shoulder pain are often accompanied by headaches. The pain often affects the person's ability to participate in sport or work activities. In these cases, MFPS is the primary problem.

Poor posture, faulty movement mechanics, and stress play a role in the development of MFPS. A general lack of fitness and occupations that lead to postural deficits are associated with type I MFPS affecting the trunk and neck (Denegar and Peppard 1997). Some sports such as cycling and swimming can also lead to muscle imbalances and poor posture. Often people alter movement patterns in an attempt to avoid pain, and these natural adaptations stress tissues that are not well conditioned, exacerbating the pain. Conversely, faulty movement mechanics can cause repetitive microtrauma injuries that lead to type II MFPS. If excessive pronation is the cause of medial tibial stress syndrome or patellofemoral pain, neither the primary problem nor type II MFPS will resolve until running mechanics are addressed, unless, of course, the person quits running. Thus, clinicians must assess posture and movement mechanics and incorporate therapeutic exercises in all cases of MFPS.

Stress is common in our lives, and it is intensified by the demands of sport and work and the pressure to succeed. Student-athletes strive to balance schoolwork, social life, family commitments, and the demands of sports. Other athletic people squeeze training and competition in between job and family commitments. Everyone responds to the stresses of daily life differently. However, many people treated for MFPS in the back, neck, and shoulders "hold" their stress in the affected area. Many do not appreciate how much tension resides in these areas until it is relieved through treatment. Some learn to manage pain when they appreciate how their responses to life events affect them. Some clinicians are very effective at helping patients understand their responses to stress and helping with stress management. Everyone on the health care medicine team must be able to recognize when physical responses to stress contribute to persistent pain, and they must be able to help patients to manage stress.

Chronic Pain

Although chronic pain has been defined as pain that lasts beyond the normal time frame for healing or beyond a specific length of time (e.g., 6 months), the differences between persistent and chronic pain are defined by time. The distinctions lie in pathoetiology and response to treatments. Chronic pain results from changes in the structure and function of components of the nervous system. The nociceptive system is plastic, meaning that it is changeable. In the case of true chronic pain, increased sensitivity to mechanical and thermal stimulation is perceived as noxious because the systems that modulate pain signals fail or descending pathways that increase pain sensitivity are activated. If these changes are permanent, the patient may be categorized as suffering from true chronic pain, and the condition will not improve through the administration of therapeutic modalities.

No change in the pain modulation system is permanent. Fatigue, stress, illness, and other factors may elevate sensitivity to pain. Understanding what pain is signaling (cognitive appraisal), attention to other activity, rest, and effective coping with stress can decrease pain sensitivity. An athlete may not notice an injury suffered during a contest but might feel pain if the same injury were sustained during a walk in the neighborhood. Aching in the shoulder or back may resolve as an upper respiratory infection resolves. A patient who is anxious that the pain in her knee signals a torn ligament, and potential lost income, may experience relief if she learns that her injury is not serious. Patients with chronic pain may experience fluctuation in the pain they perceive, but pain is always present. Interventions that trigger pain-modulating mechanisms are no longer effective.

WHERE AND HOW PAIN SENSITIVITY INCREASES

Individuals with chronic pain report pain that is unresponsive to medication and the interventions provided by athletic trainers and physical therapists.

In the models presented in this chapter, three potential sources of change in the nociceptive and pain-modulating system can be identified (Asmundson and Wright 2004) that help explain why chronic pain may occur. The first involves increased pain signaling to the dorsal horn from the periphery. Increased pain signaling might result from up-regulation of silent nociceptors. It has been estimated that up to one-third of free nerve endings fall into this category. These nociceptors become sensitized to noxious stimulation through mechanisms that have yet to be fully explained. One cause of up-regulation may be previous pain experiences. The up-regulation of silent nociceptors is likely normal, but with more information to modulate there is an increase in pain signaling to higher brain centers.

A second proposed source of increased noxious input into the dorsal horn is a change in the chemical environment around the free nerve endings. This changed environment has been labeled *inflammatory soup*. Inflammatory soup describes an environment where the persistent presence of chemical mediators associated with inflammation (discussed in chapter 4), along with a lowered pH, sensitize free nerve endings. The sensitized free nerve ending thus has a lower threshold to depolarization and will respond to stimuli previously not perceived as noxious.

Phenotype changes in the primary afferent nerves have been reported. Phenotype changes occur when myelinated fibers assume neurochemical properties associated with unmyelinated fibers. In other words, A-beta afferents transmit nociception. The changes in the periphery essentially sensitize the region, allowing normally non-pain-provoking events to be perceived as painful.

Changes in the dorsal horn may also alter signal processing in one of two manners. First, there may be an increase in sensitivity of the second-order afferent nerves, which would ultimately diminish signal modulation, or second, the actual signal pathway could be altered. Altering the pathway can stimulate an adaptation where the A-beta nerves may branch out to terminate in lamina II of the dorsal horn. Thus not only are more primary afferent nerves nociceptive, but also the signal is delivered directly to the portion of the dorsal horn where synaptic transmission toward the brain occurs. Increased sensitivity has also been attributed to increased glutamate receptor activation and NMDA (N-methyl-D aspartate) receptor activation. Recall that glutamate (along with substance P, neurokinin A, and other substances) is associated with noxious transmission. Increased sensitivity of the second-order afferent nerves to glutamate increases the transmission of the pain message to higher centers. Increased sensitivity to NMDA results from the release of nitrous oxide (NO) due to disruption of calcium channels caused by NMDA receptor activation. NO can cause primary afferent depolarization, causing the release of substance P and inflammatory cytokines in the periphery and creating a vicious cycle within the dorsal horn. The increase in the volume of nociceptive input likely overwhelms modulating systems and elevates pain perception.

There is also a fuller appreciation of the role of descending neural pathways in dorsal horn signal modulation. Projections from the raphe nucleus and pons onto the dorsal horn are serotonin- and norepinephrine-mediated pathways that are believed to play an important role in blocking the transmission of pain messages to higher centers. These pathways, however, are only two of many descending influences on dorsal horn activity. Millan (2002) provides a detailed description of pathways descending on the dorsal horn that inhibit and facilitate the transmission of pain messages. The balance in the activity of these pathways likely explains, at least in part, situational changes in pain sensitivity. Most of us would probably agree that moods can affect pain sensitivity. It is likely that some alterations in the activity in descending pathways can be long term if not permanent and can contribute to persistent and chronic pain states.

Finally, interplay between the autonomic and somatosensory systems may lead to increased pain perception. Our understanding of this can be linked to efforts to find the causes of CRPS. CRPS, once known as reflex sympathetic dystrophy, is not solely the result of sympathetic nervous system activity (Bruehl 2010). However, in patients not diagnosed as suffering from CRPS, sympathetic efferent fibers may sprout to free nerve endings that express adrenergic receptors. In this way, sympathetic efferent nerves can stimulate the free nerve endings, setting the stage for increased pain signaling to the dorsal horn. High levels of stress can activate the hypothalamic-pituitary-adrenal axis, which in turn perpetuates sympathetic nervous system activity, creating a cycle of arousal and pain.

In summarizing peripheral sensitization, Asmundson and Wright (2004) noted, "It is apparent that the sensitization process is fairly complex and that different forms of sensitization may develop depending on the nature of the injury or disease." In some cases the complaint of pain may be most attributable to changes in nervous system function. Clearly, mechanisms of truly chronic pain are not fully understood, and a more detailed presentation is beyond the scope of this text. It is important, however, to appreciate that new developments are likely to produce more effective treatment for more sufferers of chronic pain. The clinician must also recognize that some people's hypersensitivity to normally non-pain-provoking stimuli is the result of complex changes in the function of the nervous system.

SUMMARY

Chapter 5 is devoted to understanding pain from multiple perspectives. Pain signals the need for care. Information the clinician learns about the pain experience is often the most valuable aspect of the patient interview. Although pain as a symptom is generally recognized, the mechanisms by which pain is transmitted and perceived require foundational information in neuroanatomy and physiology. Neural pathways and mediators of synaptic transmission are presented in some detail in preparation for a discussion of the body's pain-modulating systems. The role of modulation of pain signals at the dorsal horn through ascending and descending neural pathways is presented with reference to the role of contemporary therapeutic modalities.

1. *Describe the multidimensional nature of pain.*

   Pain can be conceptualized as having two dimensions: intensity and affective-motivational. The intensity component is pain sensation. Where does it hurt and how badly? The affective-motivational component relates to how a person responds to pain. For example, is the person angry or withdrawn? Providing care involves more than asking about the intensity of the pain. The athletic trainer must respect each person's response to pain.

2. *Explain the role of pain in preserving health and well-being.*

   Pain signals that something is wrong with the body and is usually the motivation to seek medical care. Without pain, diseases and injuries (could) go undetected and therefore untreated.

3. *Discuss how the pain response can assist in evaluating an injured athlete.*

   Understanding the pain response after injury can help you make an accurate diagnosis. The causes, timing, locations, and severity of pain often narrow the possibilities and allow the sports medicine team to focus on special tests and examination procedures that lead to a rapid and accurate diagnosis.

4. *Describe how pain is sensed and how the "pain message" is transmitted to the central nervous system.*

   Free nerve endings are the body's pain receptors or nociceptors. When free nerve endings are stimulated, impulses are transmitted to the brain by specific nerves and neural pathways. Impulses are transmitted from the free nerve endings to the spinal cord by A-delta and C fiber primary or first-order afferent nerves. A-delta fibers more rapidly conduct pain, but C fibers cause a diffuse, noxious ache. The pain message is carried from the primary afferents up the spinal cord by second-order afferent nerves. The pain message can be carried on wide dynamic range, second-order nerves or on nociceptive-specific nerves. The nociceptive-specific nerves carry only pain information, whereas the wide dynamic range fibers carry all types of neural input. The second-order afferent fibers terminate at multiple brain centers. The thalamus, PAG region, and reticular formation all play important roles in accurate assessment of the pain message and in mediating the individual's response to pain.

5. *Describe the differences between acute and lasting pain.*

   Acute pain, a warning that something is wrong and requires medical attention, is associated with musculoskeletal injury. Pain that persists beyond the normal time required for tissue repair is less well understood. Often, when an individual's pain lasts for weeks or months, it is labeled chronic pain. Because the term *chronic* implies a sense of hopelessness, the term *persistent pain* was introduced to identify situations in which lasting pain is a signal that something is wrong and will respond to appropriate treatment. Chronic pain is complex and very poorly understood; however, the causes of the persistent pain can often be identified and effectively treated.

6. *Identify common causes for persistent pain in active people, including diagnostic errors and somatic dysfunction, faulty plans of rehabilitation, rest–reinjury cycle, complex regional pain syndrome, myofascial pain, and depression and somatization.*

Persistent pain can result from a number of causes. This chapter begins with physical causes and progresses to psychological causes of persistent pain. Physical causes include diagnostic errors and faulty plans of care. Failure to identify the problem or to effectively address identified problems can lead to persistent symptoms. Physically active people often associate the absence of pain with complete recovery, which can lead them to overstress healing tissues and experience reinjury. This phenomenon can repeat, setting up a rest–reinjury cycle. Complex regional pain syndrome, also labeled reflex sympathetic dystrophy, is characterized by pain out of proportion to the extent of an injury as well as hypersensitivity to touch and movement, joint stiffness and muscle guarding, edema, erythema, hyperhidrosis, and osteopenia. Complex regional pain syndrome is progressive, and the prognosis for complete recovery worsens if diagnosis and treatment are delayed. Myofascial pain, which may result from many causes, is a diagnosis of exclusion characterized by tender trigger points, increased tension in muscles, and often a pattern of referred pain. Physical symptoms can result from psychological dysfunction. The somatic pain experienced by those suffering from depression and somatization is a signal that care is needed. Unfortunately, somatic symptoms stemming from psychological dysfunction are more difficult to interpret. If other sources of persistent pain are ruled out, the sports medicine team should consider psychological causes before making the diagnosis of chronic pain.

7. *Discuss the meaning and implications of neuroplasticity on pain and pain modulation.*
    Plasticity implies a system that is changeable. The ability of the body to modulate and dampen neural impulses signaling pain can change, sometimes permanently. Thus, patients may be more sensitive to stimuli because pain signals are not being modulated in the dorsal horn and thus reach higher brain centers, including the sensory cortex. True chronic pain is associated with more permanent changes that inhibit signal modulation and facilitate pain signaling to higher centers.

8. *Describe alterations in the nociceptive system that may increase pain perception.*
    The nociceptive system may undergo changes at the periphery, at the dorsal horn, or in the influence of descending impulses on dorsal horn activity. The major changes in the periphery include an up-regulation of silent nociceptors, change in the phenotype of the neurons (e.g., A-beta nerves take on nociceptive properties and function like A-delta neurons) and an alteration of the local chemical environment described as inflammatory soup. Dorsal horn changes include sprouting of A-beta afferent nerves into areas of the dorsal horn generally reserved for pain perception, an alteration in receptor sensitivity (e.g., NMDA and glutamate), and an increase in nitrous oxide activity. Changes in the activity along descending pathways affecting the dorsal horn may decrease pain modulation or facilitate pain signaling. While these interactions are complex, they probably explain why some conditions (e.g., depression) are associated with an increase in pain sensitivity.

9. *Define the differences between chronic and persistent pain.*
    The principal difference between chronic and persistent pain is that chronic pain will not respond to conventional treatments such as modality application, and at present it can be reduced only with narcotic medications. Chronic pain is the result of changes within the nervous system in the periphery, spinal cord, higher brain centers, or more than one of these. The changes have only recently been identified and have not been fully understood. Hopefully, research will lead to a better understanding and treatment of chronic pain.

chapter 6

Clinical Management of Pain

OBJECTIVES

After reading this chapter, you will be able to

1. identify sources of persistent pain through a medical history and physical examination;

2. develop appropriate rehabilitation plans of care or referral to appropriate health care professionals for individuals with persistent pain due to diagnostic errors, faulty plans of rehabilitation, faulty biomechanics, rest–reinjury cycle, complex regional pain syndrome, myofascial pain, and depression and somatization; and

3. understand contemporary pain modulation theories from a neurophysiological perspective.

The clinician must be prepared to evaluate a broad spectrum of concerns from physically active people. Often a patient presents with a history of long-standing or persistent pain with no single identifiable cause. Consider the following cases and related questions.

A recreationally active financial advisor presents to a sports medicine clinic with a history of many months of intermittent neck and shoulder pain with frequent headaches. She states that driving and working at her desk often trigger her symptoms. She further states that she developed pain after hiking with a backpack for 3 days about 6 months before her appointment. She denies a history of trauma, and a medical evaluation had revealed no structural problems. She states that a course of anti-inflammatory medication did not alleviate her symptoms. What other questions should be included in the medical history? What factors are contributing to the problem? What would you expect to find on physical examination? What are the short- and long-term treatment goals? Will the use of therapeutic modalities help her achieve treatment goals?

A freshman college track athlete with a history of shin splints throughout high school is evaluated in the athletic training clinic. She has very tight fascia in her legs and multiple tender trigger points. She states that recent X-rays and a bone scan revealed normal results. Why has her problem persisted for so long? Is there an underlying cause? How should this athlete be treated?

A freshman high school baseball pitcher presents to a sports medicine clinic complaining of 4 months of shoulder pain that has limited his ability to pitch. He states that he took 3 weeks off from pitching but the shoulder did not heal. He was concerned that he had a torn rotator cuff despite assurances to the contrary by an orthopedic surgeon. Why does this athlete's shoulder pain persist?

The complaints of these physically active people are not uncommon. The questions raised in each case must be answered to develop an effective rehabilitation plan. In some cases therapeutic modalities may help resolve the problem, but in other cases they may be of little benefit. As stated in chapter 1, the application of a therapeutic modality does not constitute a treatment but is part of a comprehensive plan of care. Developing a plan of care requires that you identify the underlying causes of symptoms. This chapter will help you to evaluate and treat physically active people who have persistent pain and identify situations in which therapeutic modalities may help achieve treatment goals.

As discussed in chapter 5, pain is a complex phenomenon that affects each person differently. There are cultural and societal influences on pain, as well as myths about how pain can be managed. Clinicians must understand that it is often pain that drives patients to seek treatment, and the resolution of pain should be a goal for each patient. We must always include a pain assessment in the musculoskeletal evaluation and determine whether the pain is changing over time. The fundamental premise of evidence-based practice is that objective measures and outcomes are obtained to determine and guide the treatment program.

This chapter presents an overview of pain assessment and discusses current mechanisms of pain control from a neurophysiological perspective. Although pain management is complex, the clinician should understand how pain is mediated through physical agents. Many treatments can influence these mechanisms of pain control and thus prepare the patient to perform therapeutic exercise. The exercise is likely to address the root of the impairment, and rehabilitation occurs. Mechanisms to address persistent pain are also discussed in this chapter.

PAIN AND THE PHYSICAL EXAM

Although the physical examination process is discussed in great detail in *Examination of Musculoskeletal Injuries, Third Edition* (Shultz, Houglum, and Perrin 2010), the interpretation of pain warrants review in this chapter. When evaluating an injured person, you should ask many questions to narrow the diagnostic possibilities, since different structures can elicit a range of sensory experiences. The interview should result in a working diagnosis that is then confirmed or refuted by the physical exam and any subsequent medical imaging or laboratory testing.

Questions about when and how the injury occurred are obvious. However, you may need to ask follow-up questions to fully interpret the answers and develop a clinical diagnosis.

Certainly an acute injury with a well-described mechanism of injury will point to a working diagnosis. Trauma leads to fractures, strains, and sprains. The injured physically active person can often describe the instant and the mechanism of these injuries. When the patient cannot identify the moment of injury or a specific mechanism, the clinician needs to use deductive reasoning and to be more discerning of the **etiological factors** leading to the pain.

For example, a distance runner complained of pain at the Achilles tendon but was unable to identify a specific injury or onset of pain. Further questioning revealed that this athlete's pain had started after running on hills for several days while on vacation. Injuries with an insidious onset and a poorly defined mechanism broaden the diagnostic possibilities and should not be ignored. This runner likely developed Achilles tendinopathy as the result of new loading of this tissue due to a sudden transition from running on flat terrain to running on hills. Repetitive microtrauma can injure tendons, cause stress fractures, and lead to conditions such as plantar fasciosis, medial tibial stress syndrome, patellofemoral pain, and, as in this case, Achilles tendinopathy . Thus, when you understand the

P-Q-R-S-T

One approach for asking questions about pain follows a **P-Q-R-S-T** format. This is easy to remember because **P, Q, R, S,** and **T** are the waves of an electrocardiogram.

P is for provocation. Ask how the injury occurred and what activities increase or decrease the pain.

Q is for quality, or characteristics of pain. For example, does the person experience aching shoulder pain, suggesting impingement syndrome; burning pain, suggesting nerve irritation; or sharp pains, suggesting acute injury?

R is for referral or radiation. Referred pain occurs at a site that is distant from damaged tissue and does not follow the course of a peripheral nerve. Pain in the jaw and left shoulder is a common referral pattern during a heart attack. Radiating or radicular pain follows the course of a peripheral nerve. Pressure on a nerve due to a herniated intervertebral disc will result in radiating pain.

S is for severity. Judging the severity of pain is subjective, but sometimes one knows that the problem is serious just from the severity of pain.

T is for timing. When does pain occur? Night pain may indicate cancer or another nonmusculoskeletal problem since provocative activity is minimized during rest. Pain in the sole of the foot with the first steps in the morning is consistent with plantar fasciitis.

onset of symptoms, you can improve the focus of your injury evaluation and physical exam and make better-informed recommendations for a return to sport.

Other aspects of the pain experience also will help in establishing the diagnosis. The quality of pain can be difficult to assess, but with experience you will appreciate the difference between the sharp, localized pain of a fracture and the diffuse pain associated with myofascial pain syndrome. Pain that radiates within a dermatome indicates pressure on a nerve and is often caused by injury to an intervertebral disc or a vertebral fracture.

Referred pain occurs when there is pain in an area separate from the pathology. Referred pain can be mysterious, but it has predictable patterns. Pain in the left shoulder and jaw during a heart attack and left shoulder pain with a spleen injury are two examples of referred pain. Table 6.1 identifies several medical problems with well-established patterns of referred pain. Unlike the skin and soft tissue, the **viscera** have very few sensory organs. When the sensory information synapses at the spinal cord, an activation of interneurons at that level takes place. The interneurons converge on the neurons that localize pain to the dermatome or myotome at the same spinal cord level. The brain interprets the pain as arising from the soft tissues rather than the involved organ. A thorough evaluation of the injury should identify the area of pathology so that the injury, not the pain site, is treated. Referred pain does not change with provocative tests such as resisted movement or a change in position. The

Table 6.1 Common Referred Pain Patterns

Problem	Location of pain
Myocardial infarction	Neck, jaw, and left shoulder
Spleen injury	Left shoulder
Appendicitis	Lower abdomen and right groin
Pancreatic injury or pancreatitis	Left shoulder, low back, and middle left abdomen
Cholecystitis (gallbladder)	Right shoulder and midscapular region
Renal (kidney) disorder	Low back and left shoulder
Stomach and upper small intestine (duodenum) disorder	Left shoulder

severity of pain often indicates the severity of the problem. If you have a close working relationship with athletes, it is easier to interpret their reactions to pain and injury.

Finally, the timing of the pain can yield clues about the problem. The fact that pain occurs with specific movements or at certain times of the day may be significant. For example, a person suffering from iliotibial band syndrome usually complains of pain while climbing stairs or running up and down hills. Plantar fasciosis is almost always very painful upon arising in the morning and with weight bearing on the injured foot. Questioning the individual about these issues usually provides a working diagnosis, which allows you to focus and organize the physical exam rather than randomly conduct a series of tests. Furthermore, finding out what activities cause more pain helps you to determine what activity modifications are needed. If stairs cause pain, then step-ups should not be included in the rehabilitation plan until changes are made in strength, flexibility, and biomechanics. If possible, the patient should avoid provocative activities.

PAIN ASSESSMENT

Pain is difficult to assess because it is a symptom rather than a sign. Quantification of pain is very subjective since it is a sensory phenomenon with an affective-motivational dimension (Melzack and Casey 1968).

Sensory Component of Pain

The sensory component is what the individual feels. To determine whether your treatments are helping the injured athlete, you should try to quantify the pain.

Pain measurement should be reliable and valid. To assess the intensity of pain, you can use a simple pain scale, for instance by asking the person to rate the pain from 0 = *no pain* to 10 = *worst pain ever*. This type of pain assessment, the verbal pain rating, is quick and simple but becomes less effective when the athlete is asked for a score several times throughout the evaluation and treatment. For example, the athlete will remember reporting a 5 before the treatment and will use that figure as a reference for reporting his or her score after the treatment is over.

A visual analog scale (VAS) (figure 6.1) has no demarcations, so the patient cannot use a previous score as a reference point. The VAS uses a 10 cm line with the words "no pain" on one end and "unbear-

No pain   Unbearable pain

Figure 6.1 Visual analog scale.

Based on Denegar and Perrin 1992.

able pain" on the other end. The upper end should imply postsurgical or excruciating pain. The clinician measures in centimeters the horizontal distance from the left to the athlete's mark of the extent of his or her pain to produce a pain score. Some clinicians have used a continuum of descriptors along the visual analog scale to help better describe the degree of pain. These descriptors are "dull ache," "slight pain," "more than slight pain," "painful," and "very painful" (Denegar and Perrin 1992). The VAS is more accurate when pain is assessed multiple times.

More complex assessments involve pain charts (figure 6.2) or a comprehensive questionnaire such as the Pain Disability Index to assess the impact of pain on function (Pollard 1984). An example of the Oswestry Low Back Pain Scale is presented in figure 3.2. These assessments have been validated and can help you categorize how pain is contributing to the athlete's disability. The simpler scales can be used to quickly assess recovery from injury. These patient-reported outcome (PRO) instruments are very important for documenting changes over time and helping quantify pain and functional restrictions. These scales yield valuable insight about persistent and chronic pain and are a key component to evidence-based practice. They are used in studying the effects of therapeutic interventions and in documenting whether the treatment plan is effective. PROs often include a global rating of change where patients are asked to quantify, in a percentage, the change in their function. When a patient uses a percentage of function, it tells the clinician how well that patient is doing based on how the patient feels he or she should be doing. Reporting a function as 65% versus 90% gives the clinician a good idea of how the patient is performing compared to his or her goals.

Sensory and Affective-Motivational Components of Pain

The affective-motivational component of pain relates to the impact of pain on the person. For example, after injury, pain signifies that something is wrong. However, until the person understands the severity of an injury and the impact it will have on her ability to compete, pain may cause considerable anxiety. Persistent pain can lead to withdrawal and depression, responses that compose the affective-motivational aspect of pain.

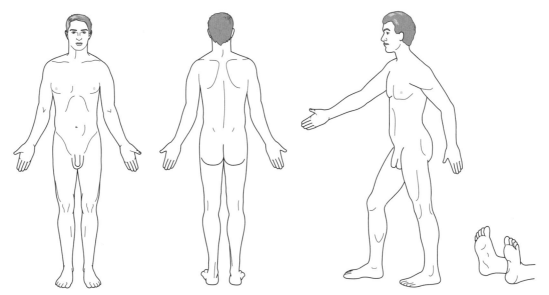

Figure 6.2 Pain chart. The injured person uses the figures to show exactly where the pain is and where it radiates. As precisely and with as much detail as possible, the person uses a blue marker to indicate painful areas, a yellow marker for numbness and tingling, a red marker for burning or hot areas, and a green marker for cramping.

Reprinted, by permission, from S. Shultz, P. Houglum, and D. Perrin, 2010, *Examination of musculoskeletal injuries*, 3rd ed. (Champaign, IL: Human Kinetics), 5.

The response to pain is highly individual and can be influenced by several factors, such as previous pain experiences, family and cultural background, and the specific situation. The clinician must learn to accept individual differences in pain response and help the injured person cope with pain.

When pain persists or becomes chronic, the affective-motivational component of pain becomes even more significant in evaluation and treatment. Lasting pain affects virtually every aspect of day-to-day life, including sleep patterns, the ability to concentrate and study, and social and personal relationships. Persistent pain is discussed in detail at the end of this chapter.

PAIN CONTROL THEORIES

Understanding how pain is perceived is a prerequisite to studying the body's analgesic mechanisms. The pain-relieving effects of touch, acupuncture, and other treatments have been recorded since ancient times. How these treatments alter pain was unknown because of inadequate information about the human nervous system. As recently as the 1960s, pain and pain control theory revolved around the pattern and specificity theories dating to the early 1900s.

The pattern theory denied the existence of pain receptors and suggested that pain occurred when the rate and pattern of sensory input exceeded a threshold. Different sensations were thought to be represented by the pattern of action potentials within the nerve, much like Morse code. The specificity theory suggested that pain was perceived when pain receptors in the periphery were stimulated and that these pain receptors were connected directly to sensory areas in the brain. All sensory input was thought to be directly communicated by a specific receptor to a specific nerve and to a localized area of the brain. Neither theory plausibly explained the pain-relieving effects of treatments long recognized as effective.

In 1965, Melzack and Wall challenged existing theories and proposed a "gate control" theory of pain relief. This theory rationally explained why therapeutic modalities controlled pain, and it led to the development of new treatment approaches, including TENS. Since 1965, more has been learned about the anatomy and physiology of the nervous system than was known before that time, and the theoretical base has expanded. Positron emission tomography (PET scanning) and functional mag-

netic resonance imaging (fMRI) are used to visualize working areas of the brain, and our understanding of neurochemical function is constantly expanding. The theories presented here reflect these advances. However, as our knowledge base continues to grow, the validity of these theories will be challenged, and the scientific basis for clinical application of modalities will continue to evolve.

The scientific basis of clinical practice and the treatment of the musculoskeletal system have advanced considerably in the past few decades; however, they remain incomplete. The rationale behind the use of therapeutic modalities was often based mainly on observations handed down from clinicians to students. With advances in science and clinical research, some of the assumptions about therapeutic modalities have been discovered to be unfounded. The scientific and theoretical basis of clinical care continues to evolve.

One noteworthy step in this evolution is the presentation of the neuromatrix theory of pain, also presented by Dr. Melzack (Melzack, 2001). This theory further explores pain as a multidimensional experience produced by "neurosignature" patterns of nerve impulses that are widely distributed in a diffuse network in the brain. Visual, cognitive, and emotional influences contribute to the neurosignature; thus pain can be generated by sensory input or it can be generated independently by the activity within the brain. The neuromatrix theory emphasizes the brain's control over the cognitive-evaluative, motivational-affective, and sensory-discriminatory systems.

Modulating the Pain Signal

In much the same way pain transmission is organized, pain modulation models reflect the point of intervention. Signals can be slowed or stopped at the periphery, or they can be modulated through activity at the spinal level, at the supraspinal level, and through the pathways that descend from higher centers to the spinal level. Finally, action potential failure is discussed as a mechanism to evoke local and temporary pain management using electrical stimulation.

It is important to understand where pain modulation takes place and how therapeutic modalities and medications act on the transmission of pain. The pain modulation techniques used in therapeutic modalities are named for the type of stimulation used to evoke the **analgesia**. For example, in the gate theory, "sensory" stimulation presynaptically inhibits the pain transmission to the second-order afferent nerves in the lateral spinothalamic tract. In the terminology of contemporary physical medicine, subsensory, sensory, motor, noxious, and action potential failure are mechanisms for modulating pain with electrical stimulation. Pain modulation with electrical stimulation, or electroanalgesia, is discussed in detail in chapters 7 and 8.

Modulation of Peripheral Pain

Pain modulation techniques can target the desensitization of peripheral nociceptors. If the receptor has a higher threshold, or is more difficult to stimulate, then fewer pain impulses are propagated to the spinal cord. The clinician tries to counteract the effects of acute inflammation and mechanical stimuli that sensitize free nerve endings and peripheral nociceptors. Bradykinin, prostaglandin E2, and serotonin in the periphery facilitate nociceptor sensitivity. These chemical mediators are released at the site of inflammation and alter the voltage threshold of ion channels to encourage action potentials (Cesare and McNaughton 1997).

How can peripheral nociceptors be desensitized? We know that cryotherapy, for example, lessens the effects of the chemical mediators and slows the conduction velocity of all sensory input. Applying ice to a painful area eventually leads to superficial anesthesia or numbness, thus minimizing the pain transmission to the spinal level.

Research on the inflammatory process and the peripheral level of pain modulation demonstrates that there is a complex matrix of chemotactic agents, immune cells, and endogenous **opioids** at the receptor sites. In attempts to discover new medications that act at the pain site rather than at the central nervous system, researchers are gathering new information about these mechanisms and the balance of pain and pain control. Although it has been documented that naturally occurring opioids such as beta endorphin modulate pain in the central nervous system, research has shown that intrinsic modulation of nociception can occur at the peripheral terminals of afferent nerves.

One role of the immune system is to interact with peripheral sensory nerve endings to inhibit pain (Stein 1995). Peripheral opioid receptors were identified when exogenously applied opioids were applied to mediate analgesia locally. The analgesic effect was most pronounced during painful inflammatory conditions when the resident immune cells in inflamed peripheral tissue secreted endogenous ligands or opioid peptides (Machelska et al. 1998). When the immune system was suppressed, the peripheral effect of beta endorphin was abolished. Environmental stimuli and endogenous substances, such as corticotropin-releasing hormone and cytokines, can stimulate the release of these opioid peptides. Means of eliciting pain relief with this method are still being explored, but it is also important to recognize that challenges to the immune system can make people more sensitive to pain. Consider the last time you had a cold or influenza. Aching and pain with routine activity are likely due in part to compromised peripheral pain signal modulation.

Subsensory-level electrical stimulation such as with microcurrent application has been proposed to affect pain modulation at the peripheral level. Microcurrent stimulation empirically reduces pain, but the explanation for the pain reduction is perplexing. Microcurrent application has been shown to improve healing in pressure sores (Carley and Wainapel 1985), perhaps due to an increased chemotactic effect of immune cells. This subsensory application of electrical stimulation may also be affecting the peripheral mediators of pain. Likewise, nonthermal ultrasound empirically reduces pain when applied over inflammatory conditions. Laser and other light therapies also have analgesic properties. The energy absorbed in the cells may lessen the sensitivity of the pain receptors. We need further study of the effects of electrical stimulation, nonthermal ultrasound, and laser on peripheral sensitivity and pain perception.

Spinal Level Pain Modulation and the Gate Control Theory

Melzack and Wall proposed the gate control theory in 1965. This point is reiterated because their proposal gave credence to some of the methods used in physical medicine and redirected the research on pain modulation to facilitating the endogenous inhibitory control of pain. According to this theory, a neural mechanism in the dorsal horn of the spinal cord acts as a gate; this gate increases or decreases the flow of nerve impulses from the peripheral fibers to the central nervous system. The extent to which the gate enhances or reduces sensory transmission is determined by the relative activity of the large-diameter (A-beta) and small-diameter (A-delta and C) fibers. When the amount of information passing through the gate exceeds a critical level, it activates the neural areas responsible for pain sensation. Melzack and Wall proposed that the substantia gelatinosa (now referred to as lamina III of the dorsal horn) was responsible for closing the gate. Advances in neuroscience have improved our understanding of the structures and mechanisms involved in modulating the pain signal.

Melzack and Wall's model of presynaptic control has been revised over time. In fact, they published an updated model in which the substantia gelatinosa contains both excitatory and inhibitory cells that project to second-order afferent nerves (aka transmission cells). Melzack and Wall also recognized that not all pain modulation originates from the peripheral and spinal cord levels. They proposed central control mechanisms in the brain that modulate pain, via descending signals to the dorsal horn, and affect the gating mechanism by inhibiting or facilitating the perception of pain. Figure 6.3 depicts the original gate control model. With the identification of endogenous opioids (beta-endorphin, enkephalins, dynorphin), more contemporary models (figure 6.4) have been developed to better define the mechanisms that inhibit the transmission of pain.

In these models the substantia gelatinosa (lamina III) acts as a presynaptic inhibitor. Activity in A-beta afferent nerves stimulates enkephalin interneurons.

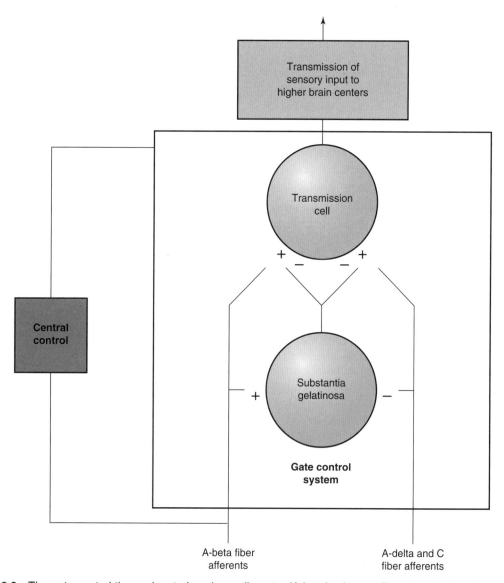

Figure 6.3 The gate control theory. Input along large-diameter (A-beta) primary afferents activates the presynaptic inhibitory influence of substantia gelatinosa on transmission from primary to afferent nerves to a transmission cell (second-order afferent).

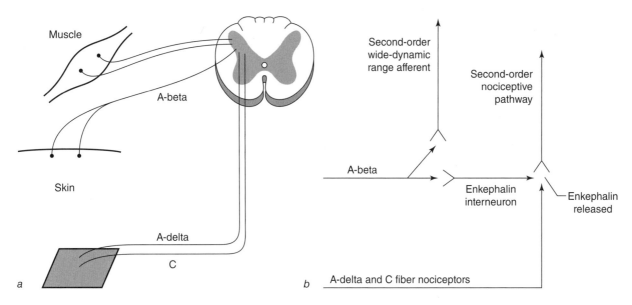

Figure 6.4 *(a)* Ascending influence (level I) model of pain control. *(b)* A-beta afferent nerves synapse with interneurons, which release enkephalins.

The release of enkephalin at the terminus of the interneurons in lamina II blocks transmitter substances intended to depolarize second-order afferent nerves that transmit pain signals to brain centers. The presynaptic influence of enkephalin "closes the gate" and prevents pain signals on the primary afferent nerves from depolarizing the second-order nerve. In other words, the pain signal is stopped, and thus pain is not perceived. As complex as these concepts of neuromodulation are, they are often applied in our daily lives. What is one of the first things you do after you bump your head or get kicked in the shin? You probably rub it, and it feels better. Rubbing your skin activates non-nociceptive touch signals carried into the spinal cord by large nerve fibers (A-beta). The inhibitory interneurons are activated by the A-beta afferent activity, and enkephalin is released, blocking or limiting the transmission of pain signals. These models also explain why "counterstimulation" techniques such as menthol rubs are effective at relieving pain. Electrical stimulators can be applied to activate A-beta afferent nerves. The electrical stimulator (TENS) stimulates the large (A-beta) afferent fibers in a painful region and activates the inhibitory enkephalin interneurons of the dorsal horn and blocks pain transmission. Detailed information on the use of TENS is presented in chapters 8 and 9. Virtually any mechanism that stimulates the large-diameter sensory fibers can trigger the gate mechanism. For example, light touch (massage),

vibration, electrical stimulation, and mild heat are often used in this manner.

Modulation of Supraspinal and Descending Pain

Pain information travels up the spinal cord (ascending) to alert the athlete to a problem and to allow cognitive recognition of the location and nature of the injury. However, pain modulation is complicated and involves both ascending and descending neural components. Anything that occurs above the level of the spinal cord is termed *supraspinal*, and any neurological pathway that travels from the brain to the spinal cord or brainstem is termed *descending*. These pathways do not function sequentially or in isolation.

Noxious Pain Modulation

Pain transmission and modulation occur through a complicated network of interneurons that activates many brain or supraspinal structures. Mechanisms are elicited to help inhibit fear and to contextualize the situation to permit function. These mechanisms strike an intricate balance between alerting the person to a problem and calming the person so that attention can be directed to solving the problem. As discussed previously, the descending mechanisms of pain modulation cause inhibitory signals to decrease the continued propagation of the pain message back at the spinal cord level. Descending pain modulation uses feedback loops that involve several different nuclei in the brainstem reticular formation; specifically, the periaqueductal gray (PAG) and the raphe nucleus are important in controlling pain.

The PAG contains enkephalin-rich neurons that excite the raphe nucleus, which in turn projects down to the spinal cord to block pain transmission by dorsal horn cells. The descending modulation can be either direct, using an enkephalin interneuron, or by presynaptic inhibition. Presynaptic inhibition is caused by neurotransmitter release that blocks postsynaptic terminals. Direct stimulation of the PAG during brain surgery has a remarkable effect on pain control.

A second descending system of serotonin-containing neurons exists. The cell bodies of these neurons are located in the raphe nucleus of the medulla and, as with the noradrenaline-containing neurons, the axons synapse on cells in lamina II and III of the dorsal horn. Stimulation of the raphe nucleus produces a powerful analgesia, and it is thought that the serotonin released by this stimulation activates inhibitory interneurons and thus blocks pain transmission. Serotonin neurons appear to inhibit somatosensory transmission and may have a function in the initiation of sleep. A complicating factor is that serotonin receptors are found in many places in the dorsal horn, including on primary afferents from C fibers. Serotonin may inhibit pain presynaptically by blocking the C fiber terminals for substance P and glutamate. Projections believed to mediate pain signals through the release of norepinephrine in the dorsal horn further contribute to the influence of suprasinal structures and neural networks.

The hypothalamus and pituitary gland are stimulated by pain impulses. These centers base their function on a biofeedback loop to determine the need for neurochemical or neuroendocrine intervention. The pituitary can release precursors to powerful analgesic and anti-inflammatory agents. It is now recognized that not all supraspinal activity suppresses pain transmission and perception. Some circuits facilitate pain signal transmission (Millan 2002), which helps explain why levels of attention, arousal, fatigue, and other factors affect the perception of and response to pain.

The descending pain modulation mechanisms are evoked by pharmacological agents and by various forms of stimulation. Patients with complex pain problems may be prescribed antidepressive agents that affect the serotonin uptake in the central nervous system. Understanding the relationship between serotonin and the descending pathways is important because patients may be confused by information they may read on the Internet about their medications. An informed clinician can explain why the drug was prescribed and how it can help. Helping the patient to understand this is part of a neurocognitive approach to treatment in which explaining the interactions can further elicit the positive effects of descending control.

As far as stimulation techniques are concerned, any treatment that can elicit the activity of C fiber pain can be used. For example, myofascial techniques, some manual therapies, ice, and electrical currents can stimulate these descending mechanisms. This type of pain modulation is termed diffuse noxious inhibitory control (DNIC), and it requires pain fibers to be stimulated to elicit pain relief. The following sections describe the schematic representation of the pain modulation theories, while chapter 8 describes the specific parameters necessary to elicit these responses.

It has been shown that electrical stimulation of the PAG matter of the rat brain and human brain results in profound analgesia (figure 6.5). The raphe nucleus, which is located in the pons and rostral medulla, receives projections from the PAG. A high density of projections from the raphe nucleus to the substantia gelatinosa has been observed. These projections descend through the dorsolateral funiculus of the spinal cord. The analgesia evoked by the stimulation of PAG is dependent on this raphe-spinal pathway.

The raphe nucleus tends to preferentially inhibit A-delta (over A-beta) fibers and contains serotonin-carrying neurons. Serotonergic neurons are heavily concentrated in lamina I of the dorsal horn of the spinal cord and are presumed to have a direct monosynaptic inhibitory effect on the second-order neuron, also known as the T cell.

A second system that originates in the pons also produces dorsal horn inhibition and analgesia. The descending inhibitory system may terminate directly on second-order neurons (T cells) or indirectly by means of an enkephalinergic interneuron.

This conceptual model is "turned on" by elicitation of pain (C fibers) in the affected region. The clinician can use certain types of electrical stimulation to excite C fibers, but a long phase duration is required (see chapter 8 for more information on electrical stimulation). Cryotherapy can also cause

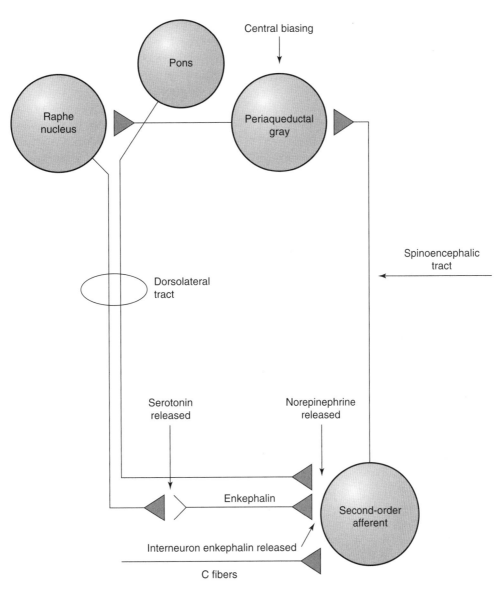

Figure 6.5 Noxious pain control is elicited by very painful stimulation of C fibers, usually using electrical stimulation. This causes an increase in the activity of the PAG and raphe nucleus, producing inhibitory action on the transmission of pain at the spinal level. This type of pain modulation has been examined since the 1970s, when a researcher noted that stimulation of the PAG produced analgesia in unanesthetized rats (Mayer and Liebeskind 1974).

C fiber stimulation. When an ice pack is applied, the injured person will experience sensations of cold, burning, aching, and then numbness. The burning and aching sensations are caused by C fibers and may evoke descending pain modulation. This may explain the powerful analgesic property of ice treatment.

Rhythmical Pain Modulation

Rhythmical stimulation of a type that occurs with joint mobilization, acupuncture, and even gum chewing has been found to have powerful analge-

sic properties through descending pathways. This theory of pain modulation posits that a strong, rhythmical stimulation induces the production of endorphins and produces effects similar to the experience of "runner's high," where the cyclical foot-strikes produce the rhythmical pattern. Endorphins are part of a complex neurophysiological system that decreases pain. They are opioids that are naturally produced (endogenous) in various locations in the body, including the central nervous system. The goal of rhythmical pain modulation is to enhance the production of endorphins.

A precursor to endorphins, a large molecular complex known as beta lipotropin, is primarily produced in the anterior pituitary (figure 6.6). The beta lipotropin molecule is broken down to produce beta endorphin and certain types of enkephalins that have strong analgesic qualities. The rhythmical stimulation also causes adrenocorticotropic hormone (ACTH) to be produced in the pituitary gland and affects cortisol production from the adrenal glands, which lie superior to the kidneys. Variations in cortisol production are normal, and subtle changes in ACTH levels are difficult to measure.

The endogenous opioid production is believed to be enhanced by low-frequency, high-intensity stimulation of peripheral nerve fibers. The frequency of stimulation must be in the 2 to 7 cycle per second range at intensities sufficient to evoke muscular contraction. Furthermore, endorphins have also been shown to exert a powerful influence on the raphe nucleus and PAG that activate the descending control system. Therefore, rhythmical pain modulation with A-delta fibers is linked with the noxious pain modulation (descending tract) as well.

Low-frequency stimulation of trigger and acupuncture points is very valuable in the treatment of chronic and acute pain and injury. Increased corticosteroid levels from the enhanced ACTH production provide analgesic effects as well. Enhancement of pituitary production of hormonal and analgesic factors may also account for the high success rate of low-frequency TENS.

Nerve Block Pain Modulation

The final technique that therapeutic modalities use to decrease pain is nerve block pain modulation or creation of an action potential failure. The application of electrical stimulation creates an "all-or-nothing" response in the nervous tissue to which it

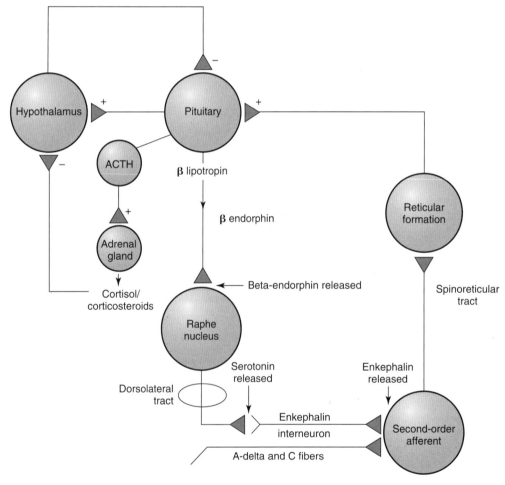

Figure 6.6 Rhythmical pain control. Neuroanatomic structures are stimulated by pulsed motor stimulation to elicit A-delta fiber excitation. Rhythmical pain modulation requires strong but tolerable muscle contractions at 2 to 7 pulses per second and often elicits a motor contraction.

is applied. If the electrical stimulation exceeds the threshold of the resting membrane, if it is applied long enough to overcome the **capacitance** of the tissue, and if it is applied rapidly enough to prevent accommodation to the stimulation, an action potential will occur. This is the **law of Dubois Reymond**, discussed further in chapter 7. Once depolarization occurs, the nerve must "reset" itself with the sodium-potassium pump. This causes a refractory period during which the threshold is increased. If continual impulses are applied to the nerve at a fast pace (over 1,000 pulses per second), the membrane cannot continually fire because of the refractory period. Subsequent stimulation actually hyperpolarizes the membrane further, creating an inhibitory effect. The membrane is unable to keep up, and an action potential failure occurs. This is termed Wedenski's inhibition and is seen with the application of medium-frequency currents such as Russian stimulation or interferential stimulation. The area between the electrodes becomes temporarily anesthetic. This mechanism of pain control may be useful for superficial areas for a brief time period, but the analgesia lasts only as long as the stimulation.

TREATING PERSISTENT PAIN

Pain that lasts beyond its usefulness for identifying the location and protecting the body part is often termed persistent pain. The signs and symptoms associated with injuries, selection of modalities, and decisions about progression of the plan of care were closely linked to the inflammatory response to tissue injury. When symptoms persist, occur in the absence of a history of trauma, or are unrelated to our current understanding of inflammation (e.g., tendinosis), decisions related to modality application must be made on criteria other than the stage of inflammation and tissue repair. Figure 6.7 provides an overview of the diagnostic possibilities and the decisions that the clinician must make in the management of patients presenting with complaints of lasting pain and pain of insidious onset.

Through experience and application of the available research, the clinician's evaluation and treatment of people with persistent pain evolve. In a high school or college athletic training room, most patients treated seek care for acute, sport-related, musculoskeletal injuries. Clinicians caring for those at risk for musculoskeletal injury will certainly be called on to evaluate some athletes with overuse injuries and

persistent symptoms caused by poor mechanics. On occasion, those seeking care will have other causes for their symptoms, and some may be suffering from truly chronic pain. An outpatient sports medicine center is very different. Many patients referred to a sports medicine center for treatment of a musculoskeletal problem, whether they are physically active or not, have experienced pain for weeks, months, and occasionally years. Central sensitization of pain (Latremoliere and Woolf 2009) is a poorly understood phenomenon that explains why some patients continue to experience pain. Often the neurons in the dorsal horn have lower thresholds than neurons in the periphery, making it easier to perceive pain in the areas associated with that spinal level. The pain is real, and a comprehensive approach should be used to address persistent pain.

Preparation to care for patients with persistent pain does not require lots of new skills but rather new applications for existing skills. Patients with persistent pain can make up a large part of the caseload in some outpatient settings. Because persistent and chronic pain can be related to multiple factors, effective management requires a complete health history. During the physical examination the clinician must not forget that the sources of dysfunction may be distant from the area of pain. Decisions about the plan of care—including whether modalities are indicated and which ones—cannot be made without a working hypothesis related to causes, rather than a diagnostic label, for the persistent symptoms.

The rehabilitation plan of care is developed from the medical history and physical examination. Within the plan of care, treatment goals are arranged on a hierarchy from entry into the health care system to full recovery. Therapeutic modalities may facilitate the achievement of one or more treatment goals in the plan of care.

These statements are true whether you are treating an acute injury or persistent pain; however, in the case of persistent pain the medical history and physical examination are more detailed, and the data gathered are analyzed more extensively. All of this information is then combined to develop a progressive plan of care. Unfortunately, when these steps are not fully completed, multiple modalities are often administered in the hope that "something works." On rare occasions the problem resolves despite the lack of a sound plan of care; usually, however, such treatment fails.

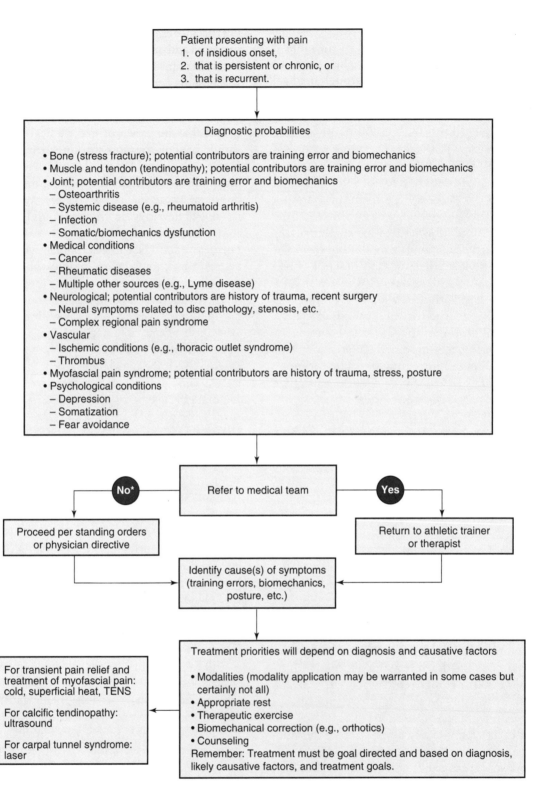

Figure 6.7 Evaluating patients with nonacute pain and selecting those appropriate for treatment with a therapeutic modality.

Medical History

Perhaps the single biggest problem in the clinical management of persistent pain is the failure to obtain, evaluate, and act upon a thorough medical history. Taking a medical history, which is reviewed thoroughly in *Examination of Musculoskeletal Injuries, Third Edition* (Shultz, Houglum, and Perrin 2010), appears to be simple. However, a great deal of practice and attention to detail are needed to maximize the information gleaned from a medical history taken from patients with persistent pain. In college and high school environments, certified athletic trainers know the athletes from day-to-day contact and gain important information from the preparticipation examination. Furthermore, most of the athletes seeking treatment are suffering from acute musculoskeletal injuries, for which the time and often the mechanism of injury are easily identified. Individuals with persistent pain may report an insidious onset of symptoms without an identifiable cause.

Contrast, for example, the medical histories required from two individuals. One is a 17-year-old basketball player for a team you have covered all season who sprained her ankle when she stepped on another player's foot during a practice that you attended. The other is a 38-year-old tennis player, computer programmer, and mother of two small children who has a 6-month history of right shoulder and neck pain of insidious onset. In the first case you know the athlete, her recent injury history, and the nature of her off-court activities, and you probably have established a rapport with her. In the second case you are establishing a plan of care for a person you have never met who may be entering a new health care environment. During the 15 minutes or so allotted for the initial examination, you must collect a lot of information. You need to know when and how the problem started, what seems to make it better and worse, and the impact of work and child care on her symptoms. You must learn what other medical evaluation has been made and what treatment has been administered (and if it helped). While the symptoms are likely of musculoskeletal origin, consideration must also be given to the presence of serious medical conditions and the need for appropriate referral. You must learn about the tennis player's general health and medical history. You must also learn what her goals are in terms of outcome priorities. In short, you need to quickly establish communication with this person so that you can obtain all of the information you need. Furthermore, you must respond to the patient's concerns and questions. As this example illustrates, obtaining a medical history from someone with persistent pain, compared to an athlete you know who has an acute injury, is much more involved, but far more critical to developing an effective plan of care.

At the completion of the medical history, you should have one or more working diagnoses. Developing a working diagnosis requires you to analyze information provided during the history as the interview proceeds. Thus, you must organize the interview, develop the questions, and analyze the responses while listening carefully to what is being said. Completing a thorough, informative medical history requires good clinical skills and lots of practice. A sample format for evaluating musculoskeletal injuries is included here (figure 6.8). Individual items may not be appropriate for all cases (e.g., documentation of gait after a shoulder injury).

Physical Examination

The physical examination should yield information that confirms or refutes the working diagnoses established from the medical history. Conducting a physical exam without a working diagnosis is a time-consuming and usually fruitless endeavor.

The structure of the physical examination will vary based on the medical history and plausible diagnoses. Observation, range of motion assessment, strength assessment, and neurovascular assessment are fairly universal components. However, the order in which tests are performed and the specific tests conducted will differ depending on the nature of the problem. In a well-conducted physical examination you will complete necessary testing in an organized manner while avoiding the tendency to "test for everything" and unnecessarily increase suffering.

Some clinicians complete a physical examination in a cookbook fashion. Rather than focusing on confirming or refuting the preliminary diagnosis, they collect a quantity of data. Unfortunately, the data are not very useful because they were not collected in the context of testing the working diagnosis.

A second common flaw in a physical examination for persistent pain is the failure to examine joint, nerve, vascular, and muscle function throughout the painful region. The screening exams described in *Examination of Musculoskeletal Injuries, Third Edition* (Shultz, Houglum, and Perrin 2010), often yield key findings that confirm the cause and therefore

Evaluation Document

Name: _____   Age/date of birth: _____

Sport/position: _____   Date: _____

Physician ID or medical record #: _____

Diagnosis: _____

Diagnostic tests/medications/surgical procedure: _____

_____

Pertinent medical history: _____

_____

SUBJECTIVE REPORT

Ask about onset, recent improvement, or worsening of symptoms; patterns of symptoms; rating of pain and dysfunction; description of pain; report of radicular or distant pain sites; and previous experience with treatments for musculoskeletal injuries (what seemed to work or not work).

OBJECTIVE FINDINGS

Observation: General appearance; obvious guarding of movement or alteration from normal movement pattern (e.g., limping); presence of swelling; discoloration; and appearance of incisions, wounds, and scars.

Range of motion: Active and passive range of motion.

Circulation, motor function, and sensory function in affected limb or area.

Strength: Results of manual muscle and instrumented resistance tests.

Girth: Swelling at joint or loss of muscle mass.

Gait: Limping, appropriate use of crutches or cane, and evidence of excessive or limited pronation.

Posture: Posture, postural awareness, and postural control.

Results of special tests:

Problem list: Develop a hierarchy of problems that must be overcome to progress the rehabilitation program and return the person to athletics.

Short-term goals and treatment plan: Develop a short list of goals to be achieved in the next few days to 2 weeks and the treatments to be used to achieve these goals.

Long-term goals with criteria for progression.

Figure 6.8 A sample format for evaluating musculoskeletal injuries.

identify the solution to the persistent pain. You must consider and assess for the presence of radicular and referred pain patterns as well as biomechanical causes of persistent pain.

Once you have made a diagnosis and identified the causes of the persistent pain, a plan of treatment can be established. In some cases, therapeutic modalities can be used to achieve goals identified in the plan of care. In other cases, the application of therapeutic modalities may be detrimental because they promote a passive, rather than active, role of the individual in the plan of care.

In chapter 5 the causes of persistent pain were categorized (figure 6.9). The remainder of this chapter reviews treatment strategies, including effective use of therapeutic modalities, in the clinical management of these persistent pain problems.

DIAGNOSIS AND PLAN OF CARE PROBLEMS

When pain persists, the first step in reevaluation is to confirm the medical diagnosis and review the plan of care. A sports medicine team approach to reevaluation is necessary to review the original diagnosis, the response to medications and surgery, and the response to and compliance with the rehabilitation program.

In the context of therapeutic modalities, a failure to improve can provide useful information. Transient (hours or days) relief of pain and swelling after treatment may indicate an underlying structural lesion or a rest–reinjury cycle. For example, persistent knee pain with recurrent swelling may be due to a torn meniscus or a loose body within the joint. Persistent back pain may have many causes, including cancer (see "Case Report and Signs of Cancer"). Thus, the issue of a failure to respond to treatments as expected over a few days or weeks is a serious matter. In these cases, consultation with the patient's physician is warranted so that appropriate care can be rendered.

Interrupting a Rest–Reinjury Cycle

A rest–reinjury cycle develops when damaged tissues undergo excessive stress during the repair and, most commonly, remodeling phases. Some athletes misinterpret the absence of pain as the completion of the healing process. When the level of exercise, work, and athletic activity exceeds the capacity of the remodeling tissue, microtrauma occurs and inflammation and pain result.

A rest–reinjury cycle has some similarities with inappropriate plans of care. For example, consider a middle-aged man seeking treatment after an arthroscopic meniscectomy. He and his surgeon were concerned about a pattern of recurrent pain and swelling in the knee that was always worse after therapeutic exercises. A review of his therapy indicated that he was riding on a stationary bicycle with a very low seat and doing full-range leg extensions with a heavy weight three times per week. The exercise program was aggravating long-standing, mild patellofemoral pain. The treatment consisted of discontinuing the offending activities and starting a simple home exercise program. The pain and swelling were completely resolved at a 2-week follow-up appointment. Problems related to rest–reinjury cycles need to be addressed through a careful review of the individual's activities and education. As with issues related to diagnosis and plans of care, the continued application of the same or different therapeutic modalities is unlikely to facilitate recovery and may delay essential treatments.

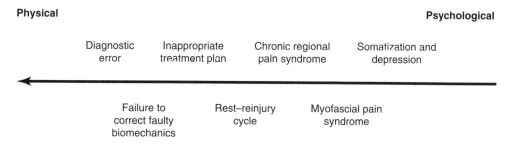

Figure 6.9 Sources of persistent pain.

Reprinted, by permission, from C.R. Denegar and A. Peppard, 1997, "Evaluation and treatment of persistent pain and myofascial pain syndrome," *Athletic Therapy Today* 2(4): 40.

Case Report and Signs of Cancer

An older golfer presented to a sports medicine clinic complaining of back pain. He was treated with transcutaneous electrical nerve stimulation (TENS) and received some short-term relief. His back pain, however, progressively worsened over the next 10 days. The underlying cause of the back pain, identified during this period of treatment, was cancer of the liver. Two lessons were learned: (1) Pain that appears to be orthopedic in nature can be due to organic pathologies, and (2) you must know the signs and symptoms of cancer and explore this possibility in individuals with chronic pain.

Signs and Symptoms of Cancer

You should be aware of signs and symptoms of cancer so you can arrange appropriate medical follow-up. The presence of one or more signs or symptoms associated with cancer does not confirm a diagnosis. The signs and symptoms listed here should not raise alarm but rather should prompt consultation with a physician to identify the cause.

- Persistent, unexplained pain
- Change in bowel or bladder function
- Unusual bleeding or discharge
- A lump or mass in breast or elsewhere
- Obvious changes in a wart or mole or a sore that fails to heal
- Persistent cough or hoarseness
- Night pain or night sweats
- Weight loss
- Difficulty swallowing or loss of appetite
- Jaundice
- Unexplained muscular weakness or loss of coordination
- Fever
- Headaches, memory loss, poor concentration
- Fatigue, increased sleeping
- Onset of seizures

Pain is a warning that the tissues are not ready to withstand the stresses being placed on them. The key to breaking the rest–reinjury cycle is education. The person must accept the responsibility of avoiding activities that reinjure the healing tissues. However, the certified athletic trainer and other members of the sports medicine team need to provide a reasonable rationale for following a plan of care that will safely return physically active individuals to their desired level of performance.

Therapeutic modalities have a limited role in clinical management of a rest–reinjury cycle. Therapeutic modalities can alleviate pain after reinjury, but the pain relief must not be misinterpreted as indicating a full recovery.

Biomechanics

The mechanics of activities are also closely linked to issues of plan of care and rest–reinjury. In this discussion, biomechanics is presented as a subsection to emphasize that improper execution of sport-specific tasks may be the underlying cause of persisting symptoms. Take the case of the freshman baseball pitcher with shoulder pain. A careful history obtained from the baseball pitcher revealed that his pain began shortly after he "learned" to throw a curveball the previous summer. He did not experience pain at rest and was asymptomatic the day he came to the clinic. Physical exam revealed tightness in the posterior rotator cuff, weak scapular stabilizers, and a few mildly tender trigger points. His throwing mechanics, which were evaluated in the parking lot, were poor, especially when he tried to throw a curveball. Fortunately he was to attend a baseball camp at a nearby university in 10 days, and arrangements were made with the coaches to evaluate and correct his mechanical flaws. Two treatments with manual therapy, exercises to condition the scapular stabilizers and rotator cuff, and improved throwing mechanics resolved his shoulder pain. Each component of the plan of care contributed to recovery; however, the correction of the faulty throwing mechanics was essential to the long-term success of treatment. As with other categories of persistent pain, finding the cause sets the stage for successful management.

Evaluation and Treatment of Myofascial Pain Syndrome

The recognition and treatment of myofascial pain syndrome (MFPS) were presented in chapter 5. The concepts from these earlier chapters can now be applied to developing a plan of care for the person with MFPS. Myofascial pain syndrome is complex, and the cause is usually multifactorial. Thus, the first step in developing a plan of care is to complete a thorough medical history and physical examination. Once the diagnosis of MFPS is made and causes are identified, a plan of care can be established (figure 6.10).

Because there is no single cause of MFPS and the condition is not completely understood, there is no single treatment approach. Each injured person is an experiment of one. The plan of treatment must address the primary complaint of pain, provide a progressive plan of therapeutic exercises to improve posture and correct faulty movement mechanics, and help the person recognize when stress and fatigue are contributing to pain. The injured person should become an active member of the sports medicine team as the factors contributing to MFPS are identified and a plan of care evolves.

There are several approaches to pain control in treating MFPS. Myofascial release techniques can be used to alter neural input from painful areas and alleviate fascial restrictions. Conventional modalities including heat, cold, ultrasound, and TENS are effective adjuncts to manual therapies.

Direct stimulation of trigger points often relieves pain. Trigger point massage (acupressure) and TENS over trigger points can result in dramatic, initially transient relief of pain. Deep circular massage of a trigger point can be done with the eraser end of a pencil or an index finger. The massage will elicit a deep burning sensation that is difficult to describe. However, with experience you will be able to help injured persons recognize the difference between pressure and the exquisite sensitivity of trigger points. Generally, trigger points are massaged bilaterally for 30 to 40 s each. The number of trigger points that are sensitive varies depending on the painful region and the individual. However, trigger point stimulation can usually be completed in less than 10 min.

TENS is an alternative to massage and may be somewhat more effective. The stimulus should be intense but tolerable. A low frequency (2 to 4 pulses per second) with a long phase duration (>250 µs) or burst mode should be used. A probe-style electrode (approximately the size of a pencil eraser) such as a Neuroprobe (Accelerated Care Plus, Reno, NV) is ideal. The **intensity** should be adjusted to produce a burning, needling sensation within individual tolerance. Each trigger point is treated for 30 to 40 s. Similarly, the Scenar devices (Grants Pass, OR) deliver a stimulation capable of exciting C fibers.

Pain relief with TENS is usually rapid. Some people experience a dull, numbing sensation after treatment. The initial relief usually lasts for 1 to 2 h, although it can last longer. With subsequent treatments, the duration of relief increases, and complete relief can be obtained in as few as four treatments. In those whose pain continues to return, TENS with conventional parameters may also provide relief. A home TENS unit provides the individual a measure of control over pain.

Myofascial release, conventional heat and cold modalities, and trigger point therapy do not cure

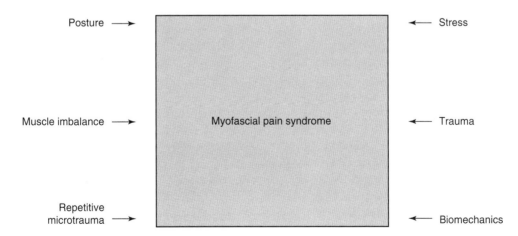

Figure 6.10 Contributors to myofascial pain syndrome.

MFPS. However, these techniques, used individually or in combination, can break the pain cycle. If pain can be controlled, the individual generally will accept therapeutic exercise regimens and will be open to suggestions regarding stress management. Programs of pain-free exercise, improved postural awareness, correction of faulty movement mechanics, and stress management need to be combined with pain control techniques to resolve MFPS.

Although MFPS has multiple causes, there are a few basic components to an effective plan of care. The first is to correct for repetitive physical stresses that aggravate the problem. This may include modifying a workstation, providing an orthotic device, or changing how someone performs a task.

The case studies presented at the opening of this chapter illustrate the challenges of treating MFPS. The initial interview with the financial advisor revealed that she spent much of her workday talking on a telephone while looking up account information on a computer. The risk management office of her employer evaluated her work requirements, provided a headset telephone and a new chair, and rearranged her workstation to decrease the number of repetitive movements during her workday. Without this intervention, her plan of care consisting of pain management, manual therapy, postural retraining, and conditioning of the upper back and paraspinal musculature would not have been effective.

Despite the persistence of the track athlete's shin splints, the ultimate biomechanical cause of her problem had never been identified and addressed. Examination of her foot structure and running gait revealed hyperpronation due to a hypermobile first ray and rearfoot varus. Treatments with cryotherapy and TENS decreased her pain but did not resolve the condition. Orthotic control of hyperpronation, a change in running mechanics introduced by the physical therapist, and a very gradual (5 months) progression to unrestricted training and competition formed the foundation for an effective plan of care. Although carefully controlling her training and doing extensive cross-training were frustrating, she was able to resume her track career, setting a school record in the 100 m hurdles as a freshman.

Each case was resolved primarily because the source of the persistent pain was identi-

fied and addressed. In addition, however, each plan of care contained a program of progressive, pain-free exercise. Therapeutic and conditioning exercises are nearly universal in a plan of care for MFPS. The key to success is pain-free exercise. The neuromuscular adaptations to painful movement were addressed in earlier chapters. To break the cycle of motion, pain, and myofascial adaptation, therapeutic exercises must be pain free; that is, pain must not alter proper movement mechanics, and activities done today can be repeated tomorrow. The role of therapeutic modalities and manual therapies in the management of MFPS is to alleviate pain, desensitize trigger points, and eliminate fascial restrictions; these changes in turn promote pain-free motion.

The benefits of therapeutic modalities and manual therapy in the clinical management of MFPS were demonstrated in the previous case studies. In the case of the financial advisor, moist heat and TENS (figure 6.11) decreased tenderness of the trigger points and decreased muscle guarding. Myofascial release (figure 6.12), includ-

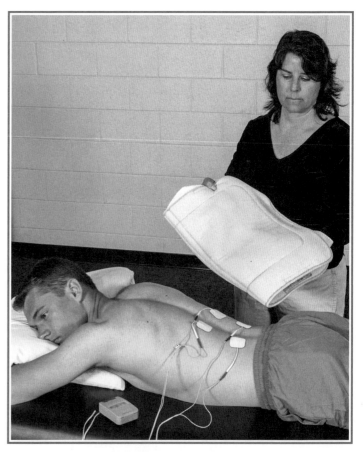

Figure 6.11 Moist heat and transcutaneous electrical nerve stimulation in the treatment of myofascial pain syndrome in the upper trapezius and cervical spine.

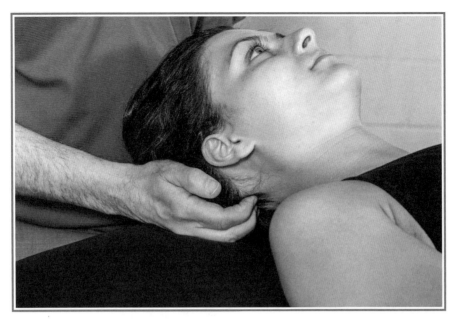

Figure 6.12   Sub-occipital myofascial release technique.

ing suboccipital release and indirect techniques, further decreased the sensitivity and guarding. In theory, the pain–gamma gain cycle has a miscommunication. The relief of pain, fascial restrictions, and muscle guarding fostered compliance with a program of postural exercises. In conjunction with her modified workstation, the plan of care resolved this physically active person's persistent pain within 4 weeks. Although 4 weeks may seem like a long time, the pain pattern had existed for several months and was gradually worsening. The certified athletic trainer and the physically active individual suffering from MFPS must have

patience. Myofascial pain patterns are resolved by breaking the pain–gamma gain cycle, decreasing stresses on affected tissues, building elasticity in tight tissues, and improving endurance and strength in weak muscles. These changes occur over time and require continued compliance with a plan of care after discharge from formal rehabilitation.

Trigger point therapy (figure 6.13) and soft tissue massage broke the pain pattern in the track athlete described earlier. With repeated treatments, the trigger points became less sensitive and her pain decreased. As her pain decreased she was gradually able to tolerate more intense track workouts. Cryotherapy controlled her symptoms when she trained beyond her tolerance. This athlete's coaches supported the efforts of the sports medicine team and were very helpful in developing and monitoring a carefully controlled, progressive reconditioning program. Thus, the routine use of cryotherapy to control postexercise pain was avoided, and the athlete's recovery proceeded at a steady rate with only a few minor setbacks.

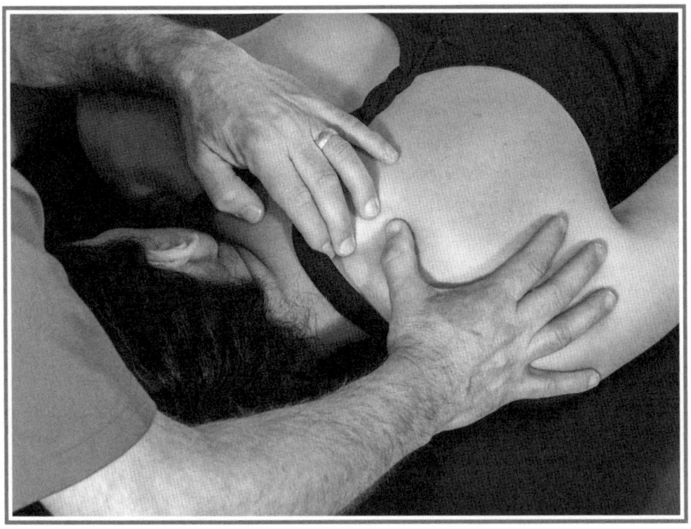

In the case of the freshman baseball pitcher, poor throwing mechanics was the central source of his shoulder pain. Myofascial adaptations, however, were present. He responded well to strain–counterstrain for the posterior rotator cuff and stretching of the external rotators (figure 6.14). He did not experience muscle spasms or pain at rest. In

Figure 6.13   Treatment of trigger point in the upper trapezius.

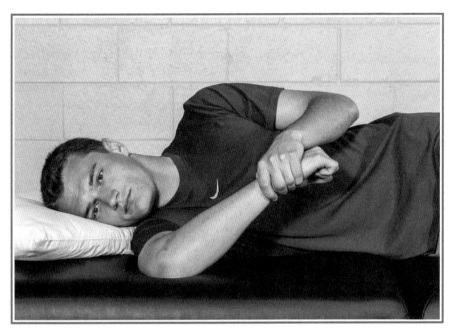

Figure 6.14   Contract–relax stretch of external rotators.

this case, throwing mechanics and posterior shoulder weakness were the primary problems, and treatment goals were established to address these issues. Because other therapeutic modalities would not have helped achieve treatment goals, none were applied. This case reinforces the value of developing manual therapy skills, and it is a reminder that therapeutic modalities should be applied to facilitate specific treatment goals rather than as a habit.

Treating Complex Regional Pain Syndrome

Management of complex regional pain syndrome (CRPS) requires the cooperative efforts of a team of health care professionals. As stated in chapter 5, the most important role of the certified athletic trainer in treating CRPS is recognition. Those with unrecognized CRPS can languish in programs of rehabilitation, delaying comprehensive medical management. Sympathetic blocks and medications are usually needed to prevent the progression of CRPS, alleviate pain, and resolve the condition.

A progressive program of pain-free therapeutic exercise is also needed to allow full recovery from CRPS. Thus, the certified athletic trainer and physical therapist play an important role in treating physically active individuals with CRPS. Therapeutic modalities can exacerbate or alleviate the symptoms of CRPS. In general, modalities that are uncomfortable must be avoided. Cryotherapy should not be used. Sometimes superficial heat or the weight of a hydrocollator pack causes extreme pain; thus, these treatments should be used with caution. TENS, gentle massage techniques, and pulsed ultrasound sometimes can relieve the pain of CRPS. TENS offers the advantage of an adjustable level of sensory stimulus that can be controlled by the individual. Light touch and gentle massage decrease the hypersensitivity of the tissues. In some cases, TENS and massage deliver too much sensory stimulus and increase pain. Pulsed ultrasound offers another alternative; because the cold of the sound head can increase pain, the sound head should be warmed before treatment. Pulsed ultrasound delivers less total energy and is better tolerated than continuous ultrasound. TENS and manual techniques are preferable in treating CRPS; however, no treatment approach has proven universally effective. In treating an individual with CRPS, communicate with that person's physician, be certain that treatments do not exacerbate the condition, and use the resources that afford the greatest relief of pain.

TREATING CHRONIC PAIN

Despite the best diagnostic and treatment efforts, some patients continue to experience pain on a daily basis. As noted in chapter 5, changes in nervous system function may be responsible for pain that is not alleviated by therapies or medications other than narcotics. While there is a definition of chronic pain, medical science is searching for effective treatments. When a patient with true chronic pain is encountered, it is important that the clinician

1. appreciate that chronic pain is the result of altered neural function,
2. appreciate that continued palliative treatment is unlikely to be beneficial, and

3. refer the patient to those best trained in pain management.

Certainly the diagnosis of chronic pain is disheartening; however, the patient must ultimately accept that the lasting pain is due to complex and not fully understood changes in how pain signals are processed and that, at present, no treatment is fully effective. Medicine is devoting greater attention to pain experiences and the challenge of chronic pain, and new, more effective treatments are likely to emerge.

SUMMARY

This chapter addressed the clinical approaches to pain management. A thorough understanding of the neurophysiological mechanisms of pain modulation is needed, as is a systematic method of evaluating pain. Finally, we integrated topics related to the treatment of patients with persistent pain. The medical history and physical examination findings are necessary to identify the sources of both acute and persistent pain and develop an individualized plan of care. The application of therapeutic modalities is not appropriate in all cases, and they should be used to prepare the patient for therapeutic exercise. The implications of modality application for the varying sources of persistent pain were discussed.

There are still gaps in our understanding of the body's pain control systems. Melzack and Wall's notion of a central control of pain continues to intrigue researchers and clinicians. As noted at the beginning of this chapter, there are many influences on the perception of and reaction to noxious stimuli. We all have observed people who can block out pain or alter their pain experience. Relaxation and imagery are but two techniques to facilitate conscious, "central" control of pain.

Placebo responses to treatments are also poorly understood and are discussed in chapter 2. However, a belief that a treatment will relieve suffering may become a self-fulfilling prophecy. The placebo response confounds the investigation of therapeutic modalities used in athletic training and must be addressed by researchers in this area. However, another aspect of the placebo response is often overlooked. Stated simply, a treatment is more likely to be effective if the clinician and patient believe it will be effective. Do not neglect the power of positive thinking in treating an injured athlete, whether you are applying a therapeutic modality or planning a rehabilitation program.

The mechanisms by which we can control our pain through conscious effort and subconscious processes are not fully understood. However, it is clear that the pain control systems described in this chapter are connected to a more complex process of neuromodulation that defines the pain experience.

1. *Identify sources of persistent pain through a medical history and physical examination.*

   Careful questioning of an injured physically active person often reveals the sources of persistent pain and provides direction for the rehabilitation plan. The certified athletic trainer should obtain a history of previous injuries and surgeries as well as information about the onset, location, characteristics, and timing of symptoms. The results of medical testing and responses to medications and other interventions should be reviewed. Thorough questioning may lead to consideration of diagnostic error, treatment error, rest–reinjury cycle, biomechanical flaws, myofascial pain, CRPS, or somatization as the cause of persistent pain.

2. *Develop appropriate rehabilitation plans of care or referral to appropriate health care professionals for individuals suffering persistent pain due to diagnostic errors, faulty plans of rehabilitation, faulty biomechanics, rest–reinjury cycle, complex regional pain syndrome, myofascial pain, and depression and somatization.*

   Diagnostic error must be considered when a physically active person fails to respond to rehabilitation. The sports medicine team must consider the possibility of diagnostic error and should thoroughly reevaluate exam findings and request additional testing as indicated. Faulty plans of care simply require restructuring the athlete's treatment regimen, which may include adding or deleting therapeutic modality application. Rest–reinjury cycles require recognition and education to reverse. The injured physically active person must understand why symptoms are recurring and follow through with a complete plan of care before returning to unrestricted training and competition. Identifying and correcting faulty biomechanics often requires the assistance of experienced coaches and conditioning specialists. Consultation with coaches, as well as the analysis of videotaped performances, may identify and help correct the underlying source of persistent symptoms. Pain out of proportion to that expected after an injury or surgery is usually the first and most telling symptom of CRPS. Swelling, changes in skin color and temperature, and loss of motion also indicate referral to a physician. Early recognition is the key to successful treatment of CRPS. Treating myofascial pain requires identification of contributing factors, desensitization of trigger points, and release of fascial restrictions. Depression and somatization are complex problems, often requiring referral to health care professionals trained to treat psychological and psychiatric dysfunction. The certified athletic trainer should treat existing musculoskeletal dysfunction; however, comprehensive care is beyond the scope of athletic training practice.

3. *Understand contemporary pain modulation theories from a neurophysiological perspective.*

   In 1965, Melzack and Wall published the gate control theory of pain, which proposed that the pain message could be blocked at the spinal cord with appropriate external stimuli. With advances in neuroanatomy and neurophysiology, the basic concept of pain modulation has been refined. Descending modulation of pain is important for pain relief by the application of modalities. The noxious pain modulation model proposes that nerves descending from the raphe nucleus can trigger the release of enkephalin and modulate pain, and that this descending pathway is stimulated by noxious input transmitted in the spinal-encephalic pathway to the PAG. This model offers a plausible explanation for pain relief induced by painful procedures such as acupressure. The motor pain modulation model proposes that pulsed, rhythmic stimulation of small-diameter afferent nerves can trigger the release of beta endorphin by connections between the hypothalamus and the raphe nucleus. Because beta endorphin has a long half-life, this transmitter substance can stimulate the descending pathway for long periods. This model may explain how acupuncture and perhaps superficial heat relieve pain.

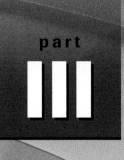
Electrical Modalities and Nerve Stimulation

Electrical currents have been applied in therapy since ancient times. In chapter 7 the physical principles of and physiological responses to electrical currents are presented. Chapter 8 is devoted to integrating knowledge about pain, pain management, and electrical currents. The chapter focuses on the application of transcutaneous electrical nerve stimulation (TENS) to modulate pain via the pathways described in chapter 5. Electrical currents can also be used to stimulate muscle contraction and restore neuromuscular control. Chapter 9 describes the sources of impaired neuromuscular control and the application of neuromuscular electrical stimulation in the management of musculoskeletal injuries. This chapter also introduces electromyographic biofeedback and reviews the applications of biofeedback in facilitating muscle recruitment and relaxing muscle tension. Part III also reviews precautions and contraindications for the application of electrical modalities to assure patient safety.

Principles
of Electrical Modalities

OBJECTIVES

After reading this chapter, you will be able to

1. define *volt, ampere, impedance,* and *resistance;*

2. describe the differences between alternating, direct, and pulsatile currents;

3. define parameters of pulsatile current, including phase duration, amplitude, phase charge, and frequency;

4. describe the capacitance of nerve and muscle tissue and how it affects the strength–duration curve;

5. understand the law of Dubois Reymond with respect to the application of electrical current; and

6. describe the types of electrode configurations used in applying electrical stimulation.

A football player felt a gradual tightening in his low back during a weightlifting session. Although there was no acute injury, the spasms that are developing are limiting motion, and he is unable to continue the workout. He presents to the athletic training clinic with pain at a level of 8/10 and cannot get comfortable. On examination, he has reduced motion in all directions due to pain and has difficulty returning to a standing position after flexion. There is no radicular pain or symptoms, and he has normal strength in the lower extremities (although he remains uncomfortable). You assess palpable spasm in the lumbar paraspinals, but he does not have a stepoff in the lumbar spine.

You want to maximize this patient's pain relief by reducing the spasm. Although you will apply cryotherapy, you feel that the application of electrical stimulation might enhance the relief of his pain and spasm so that you may start a core stabilization program. What type of electrical stimulation should be used, and what do the parameter selections mean? Options available include making decisions about the waveform, amplitude, phase duration, and frequency. This chapter examines these factors by defining the terminology relevant to electrical stimulation and addressing specific parameters used in treatment selection. Further clinical application of electrical stimulation is discussed in chapter 8.

The therapeutic use of electricity dates back to ancient times, when the Greeks used electric eels to treat physical ailments (Kahn 1987). Electrotherapy has continued to evolve and is very commonly applied clinically in many different settings. Electrical stimulation has many uses ranging from pain modulation to assisting muscle contraction. The waveforms and parameters available can be confusing, but it is important to understand how the components of a stimulator affect the tissues. This chapter introduces the principles of electrotherapy and provides a sound foundation for using electrical stimulation in clinical decision making.

BASICS OF ELECTRICITY

Electrical current is the flow of electrons. To have current, there must be (1) a source of electrons, (2) a material that allows passage of electrons or a conductor, and (3) a driving force of electrons (voltage). Current (identified by the symbol I) is measured in *amperes*. One **ampere** (abbreviated A) is equal to the flow of 6.25×10^{18} electrons per second. Amperage is the rate of electron flow past a given point. Because electrons possess a negative charge, a difference in concentrations creates positive and negative polarity. Electrons flow from negative to positive, creating the electrical current.

Electrical *charge* is measured in **coulombs** (C). One coulomb equals 6.25×10^{18} electrons. Thus, 1 A equals the delivery of 1 C of electrical charge per second. Electrical current and electrical charge are both important for an understanding of the principles of electrotherapy. In electrotherapy, the amount of electricity delivered is very small, usually in microamperes (μA or 1/1,000,000 of an ampere) or milliamps (mA or 1/1,000 A).

Voltage (V) is a measure of **electromotive force** and is also referred to as the electrical potential difference. In order for electrons to flow, there must be a difference in the quantity of electrons between two points. The magnitude of the difference between the positive and negative poles is the electromotive force that will drive the current. Think of voltage as a battery. You can hold a battery without delivering a charge because there is potential energy. Once the leads are connected, the power or electrons flow.

Resistance *(R)* is the opposition to the flow of electrons by the material through which the current travels. Resistance is measured in **ohms** (Ω). When the driving force is present (voltage), the amount of resistance determines the amount of current flow (amperage). Thus, current, voltage, and resistance are closely related. An electromotive force of 1 V is required to drive 1 A of current across a resistance of 1 Ω. This relationship, known as Ohm's law, states that current = voltage/resistance, or *I = V/R*. Thus, if resistance increases, a greater voltage is required to drive the same current.

Before voltage can be quantified, **impedance** must be defined. Impedance is often equated with the term *resistance* in that it is the force that resists the flow of electrons. Impedance is the sum of resistance, **inductance**, and capacitance. Resistance is the opposition that a substance offers to the flow of current. Inductance is opposition created by eddy currents that form around materials conducting current. Inductance is of little importance in the discussion of electrotherapy in this chapter, but it is important for understanding how another modality, diathermy (discussed in chapter 12), works. Capacitance is the ability of a material to store an electrical charge. Capacitors are important in the function of many electrical devices. The human body can store electrical charge, and the concept of capacitance will be very important in understanding transcutaneous electrical nerve stimulation (TENS). (You will read about the application of this modality in chapter 8.) Of the three components of impedance, resistance has the greatest influence in the application of electrotherapy.

When a clinician applies electrotherapy, the body becomes part of an electrical circuit as the current travels from one electrode to the other (figure 7.1). The electrical stimulator generates a voltage to overcome the resistance of the wires and tissues, and a current passes through the

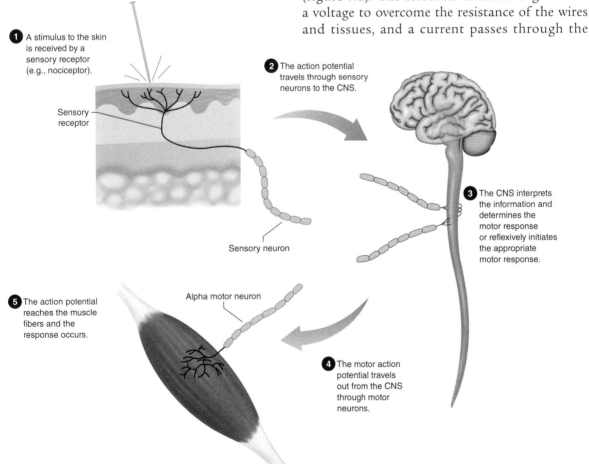

① A stimulus to the skin is received by a sensory receptor (e.g., nociceptor).

Sensory receptor

② The action potential travels through sensory neurons to the CNS.

Sensory neuron

③ The CNS interprets the information and determines the motor response or reflexively initiates the appropriate motor response.

⑤ The action potential reaches the muscle fibers and the response occurs.

Alpha motor neuron

④ The motor action potential travels out from the CNS through motor neurons.

Figure 7.1 Electrical activity in the body is constantly changing depending on the sensory or motor stimulation. When electrical stimulation is added, the signals on the sensory motor system are altered.

Relationship of Current, Resistance, and Voltage

The components of electrical current can be compared to water flowing in a river. The electrons are drops of water (there are *a lot* of water drops in a river, just like electrons in current, and you do not see water drops, just flowing water). The current—the flow of electrons—is like the flow of the river. The voltage is like a dam in the river. The difference in concentration of water between one side and the other creates potential energy. Likewise, as the difference in concentration of electrons increases between two points in a circuit, the voltage becomes higher. Finally, the flow of the river depends on the resistance. If the water is forced through a thin pipe, the pressure is increased, but the total flow of water is lessened. Electrical resistance is affected by the nature of the conductor; it increases with the length of the conductor, the cross-sectional area of the conductor, and the temperature. Resistance is lessened when a short, smooth, and large-diameter pipe is used for water flow.

$$R = \frac{\ell \cdot \rho}{A}$$

where

ℓ is the length (in units of meters),

A is the cross sectional area (in units of m^2); and

ρ is the resistivity (in units of $\Omega \cdot$m) of the material

Ohm's law:

$$R = \frac{V}{I}$$

where

R is the resistance of the object, measured in ohms,

V is the potential difference across the object, measured in volts; and

I is the current through the object, measured in amperes

body along the path of least resistance. Among the various tissues in the body, the skin presents the greatest resistance to current flow. Once the current has penetrated the skin, the electricity has many paths—through the vascular system, through the nerves, and through the adipose, muscle, tendon, and bone tissues. Current travels best through tissues with the least amount of resistance, such as the nerves. When you understand electrical charge, current, voltage, resistance, and capacitance, you can explore the differences between the types of electrical stimulators. Ohm's law states that voltage = current × resistance. As resistance increases, more voltage is required to pass the same current through an electrical circuit. If resistance is held constant, a greater voltage will result in greater current.

TYPES OF ELECTRICAL CURRENT

To understand the different types of electrical stimulators available, it is important to be aware of the characteristics of the electrical current applied to the human body. The waveform describes the configuration of the pulses of the electrical current. Very specific definitions have been assigned to wave-

forms, such as **alternating current (AC)** and **direct current (DC)**, to provide consistent terminology within physical medicine and to minimize confusion in communication with other professions. There are two major classifications of waveforms: monophasic and biphasic. DC and AC currents can be categorized as monophasic and biphasic, respectively, but DC and AC currents have no interruptions between pulses and continue indefinitely. **Monophasic currents** have uniquely positive and negative electrodes, while **biphasic currents** shift polarity continually, and each electrode has identical effects if the waveform is symmetrical. Polarity effects to the tissues are minimized or eliminated with a biphasic current (figure 7.2).

Both AC and DC currents can be hazardous when applied for clinical uses; therefore, the currents are modulated to produce safe, comfortable stimulators. Modulation of the waveform within the unit produces **pulsatile currents**, which have temporary interruptions between pulses. Pulsatile currents have various shapes, phase durations (usually short), and interpulse intervals (figure 7.3). The space that follows each pulse eliminates the normal inverse relationship between frequency and wavelength as with AC and all natural electromagnetic energy. This allows the clinician to independently control

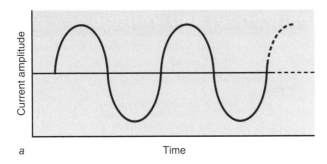

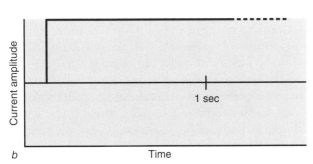

Figure 7.2 Continuous currents. Alternating current (AC): continuous sinusoidal, biphasic current with no interruption between pulses. *(a)* There is an inverse relationship between the phase duration and the pulse frequency. *(b)* Direct current (DC): monophasic current that flows in one direction for longer than 1 s.

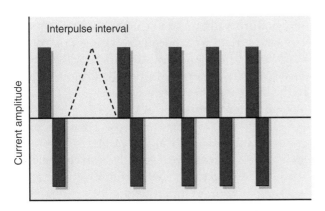

Figure 7.3 Relationship of frequency to pulse duration. A pulsatile current has interruptions called interpulse intervals between pulses that eliminate the relationship between pulse duration and frequency.

the number of pulses per second **(frequency)** and the phase duration of pulsatile currents (figure 7.4).

It is important to understand these waveforms and use proper terminology when discussing electrical stimulators. Consider the following true story: A member of the electrical engineering faculty at a college was referred for treatment by the team physician. This man had experienced an acute onset of mechanical low back pain while playing tennis. The

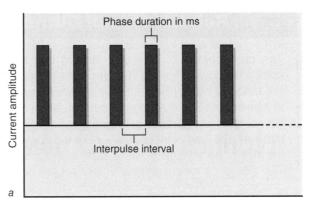

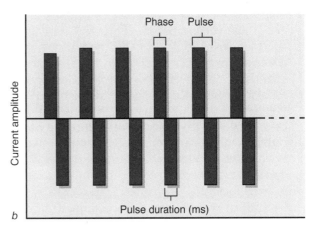

Figure 7.4 Pulsatile monophasic and biphasic currents. *(a)* Monophasic current flows in one direction only. One electrode is always positive (+) and the other is always negative (−). The interpulse interval allows independent control of phase duration and pulse frequency. *(b)* Pulsatile biphasic current flows in one direction, then the other. Neither electrode is exclusively positive (+) or negative (−) since they constantly switch. Each pulse (two phases) is separated by an interpulse interval, and there is independent control of pulse duration and frequency.

clinician elected to use TENS to treat the pain and muscle spasm. When the professor inquired what type of stimulation was used, he was told that the unit was a high-volt, pulsed galvanic stimulator. This patient informed the clinician that **galvanic** and DC are synonymous and that there was no such thing as pulsed, continuous current. He was, of course, correct. To be considered DC, the current must flow in one direction for at least 1 s, making it impossible to be pulsed (i.e., it cannot have more than one cycle in 1 s). The high-volt, pulsed galvanic stimulator was incorrectly named.

In addition to helping you use proper terminology, understanding the various electrical waveforms will help you use TENS in the clinic. Finally, and most importantly, understanding the basics of electricity and the physiological response to TENS will help you understand the differences between stimulators that produce different forms of pulsatile currents. The clinical effect and application of electrical stimulation are the focus of chapter 9.

PARAMETERS OF ELECTRICAL STIMULATION

When electricity is therapeutically applied to the body, certain effects are expected. A thermal effect is created when the frequency of the current is very high (over 100,000 Hz) and is associated with diathermies. A **physiochemical effect** occurs when there is a pH change in the tissues. Galvanic stimulation is required to alter the chemical composition under the electrodes and occurs because of the ionizing effects. And finally, a **physiological effect** occurs when the electrical stimulation causes the **depolarization** of a nerve and an action potential results. The physiological effect is desired with TENS and with neuromuscular electrical stimulation and will be the focus of this chapter. The specific effect is determined by the manipulations of the electrical current, the waveform, and the clinical parameters available on most machines. The parameters of electrical stimulation determine the effect of current on the body.

These are the characteristics of electrical current that will be considered:

- Amplitude
- Phase duration
- Frequency
- Rise time (rate of rise of the leading edge of the pulse)
- Duty cycle

Amplitude (Intensity)

The amplitude refers to the intensity or magnitude of the current. The **peak current** is the maximum amplitude of the current at any point during the pulse without regard to its duration. The peak current must be high enough to exceed threshold for the nerve or muscle fiber. Generally, large-diameter sensory and motor nerves (A-beta and A-alpha) have low thresholds, and smaller intensities of electrical current are needed to cause an action potential. The A-beta nerves are closer to the skin, so when the intensity on an electrical stimulator is turned up, a

sensory response precedes a motor response. A high peak current increases the depth of penetration of the electrical stimulation, which allows more fibers to be recruited. More nerves are stimulated with a higher amplitude, resulting in a stronger sensory or motor response.

Peak current is the measure from the isoelectric line (zero) to the maximum positive or negative point without regard to the duration of the pulse (figure 7.5).

Average current, however, refers to the amount of current supplied over a period of time, which takes into consideration both the peak amplitude and the phase duration. The average current may be described as the phase charge, and it is associated with the ability of the stimulator to produce physiochemical effects such as pH changes under each electrode, or the ability to perform denervated nerve stimulation or iontophoresis. These clinical uses require galvanic current that maximizes the phase charge. Depending on the waveform, it is possible to have a high peak but low average current. These features are characteristic of a high-voltage stimulator. The average current can damage tissue, and manufacturers limit the maximum amplitude on galvanic stimulators and minimize the phase duration on high-voltage stimulators for safety reasons. This is further discussed in chapter 8.

Peak current and root-mean-square values are used to describe the intensity of various waveforms. Peak intensity is measured from the isoelectric line to the highest point of the waveform.

Root mean square (RMS) is a means of determining phase charge or the effective area contained in the waveform that results in the physiochemical effects. It corresponds to an equivalent amount of direct current in the waveform and requires a complex calculus computation. The term "average current" is often used to describe the same effect. The RMS measure is preferred to the average current, especially as more complicated waveforms are used. The RMS is a more accurate

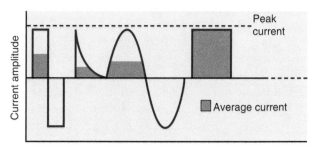

Figure 7.5 Peak current and average current.

measure of the effective current available with a specific waveform.

The RMS of a sinusoidal wave (alternating current) is 0.707 times the peak value. The average current of the same alternating current is 0.639 times the peak value.

Phase Duration

The duration of the individual phase of a current is the time it takes to leave the isoelectric (zero) line and return to the isoelectric line. If the current is biphasic, then there are two phase durations for each pulse. In monophasic currents, the phase duration and the pulse duration are the same. Tissues respond only to the phase duration, not the pulse duration. Biphasic currents do minimize the net charge by reversing the charge within each waveform (figure 7.6).

The phase duration must be long enough to overcome the capacitance of the targeted nerve and to cause an action potential. Each fiber type, depending on its characteristics of size and degree of myelination, has capacitance, that is, the ability to store charge before discharging. Large-diameter nerve fibers have low capacitance. They cannot store the charge, and an action potential results very quickly (within microseconds). Smaller nerve fibers and the muscle membrane itself have more capacitance and store the charge. In these tissues, there is minimal disturbance in the membrane potential with a short phase duration. When the current is applied, if the current does not flow in one direction long enough, there will not be an action potential (figure 7.7).

The strength–duration curve is important for describing the relationship of the amplitude (strength) of the electrical current to the duration (phase duration). These two parameters are linked in the phase charge.

Why is phase charge so important? As mentioned previously, nerve fibers act as capacitors and store an electrical charge. If the electrical charge delivered is sufficient to overcome the capacitance of a nerve fiber, it will depolarize (figure 7.8). If the electrical charge does not exceed the capacitance of a nerve fiber, the electrical charge will leak out of the fiber during the interpulse interval and the nerve will not depolarize. Likewise, if the amplitude is not high enough despite the duration, threshold will not be reached. Again, there will not be an action potential.

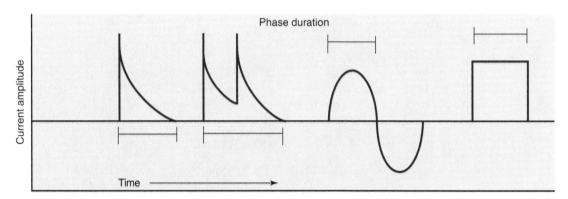

Figure 7.6 Phase duration: Length of time current flows in one direction before returning to the isoelectric line.

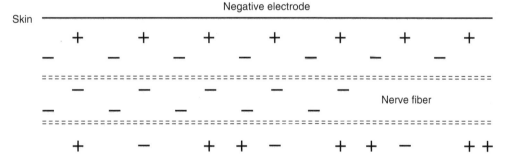

Figure 7.7 When the area surrounding a nerve becomes negatively charged by electrical current, the nerve fiber is no longer polarized in relation to the surroundings. When the nerve is depolarized, an action potential travels along the nerve to a synaptic junction.

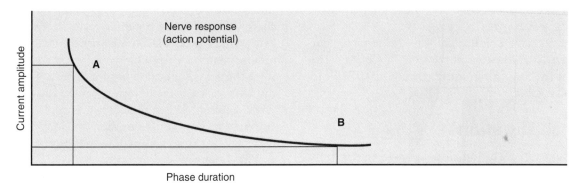

A = Short duration requires a higher amplitude for the nerve response

B = Longer duration allows a lower intensity for the same nerve response

Figure 7.8   Strength–duration curve.

Figure 7.8 depicts the capacitance of the nerve fiber types introduced in chapter 5 as well as the alpha motor neuron (A-alpha) and the sarcolemma of muscle cells. Using a monophasic square wave, figure 7.9 illustrates the concept of phase charge being increased to overcome the capacitance of each nerve fiber. Thus, in TENS application you can select the nerve fiber type or types to be depolarized.

If phase charge is so important, why is it not important to know the precise phase charge? If you adjust the phase duration and amplitude of TENS to cause a tingling sensation without muscle twitch, you have adjusted the phase charge to exceed the capacitance of A-beta afferent nerve fibers, but not A-alpha motor nerves. A muscle contraction indicates that the capacitance of the A-alpha motor nerves has also been exceeded. If TENS application results in a burning, needling sensation, you have exceeded the capacitance of A-delta afferents. Thus, by soliciting feedback from the individual and observing for muscle twitch, you can alter phase charge by adjusting amplitude and phase duration (figure 7.10).

Two concepts related to the adjustment of amplitude and phase duration are rheobase and chronaxie (figure 7.11). These terms are used primarily in electrodiagnostic evaluation of nerve regeneration. **Rheobase** is the minimum amplitude needed to depolarize a nerve fiber when the phase duration is infinite (DC current). If the peak amplitude of an electrical current fails to exceed rheobase, the nerve will not depolarize regardless of phase duration.

Chronaxie is the time or phase duration required to depolarize a nerve fiber when the peak current is twice rheobase. Chronaxie is thought to occur at the break in the capacitance curve. Stimulation parameters with an amplitude of twice rheobase and a phase duration slightly greater than chronaxie result in the greatest comfort for the recipient of TENS. Later this chapter provides guidelines for adjusting parameters to elicit the desired response with the greatest comfort.

Frequency

The frequency of the stimulation is the number of pulses generated per second (pps or Hz). The frequency affects the number of action potentials elicited during the stimulation. Although the same

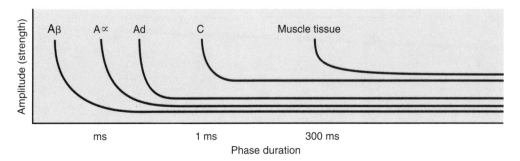

Figure 7.9   Strength–duration curves for various tissues. Because of the capacitance of the tissues, sensory nerves are the most easily excitable and can reach an action potential with a short phase duration. C fibers and the muscle membrane are difficult to excite and require much longer phase durations.

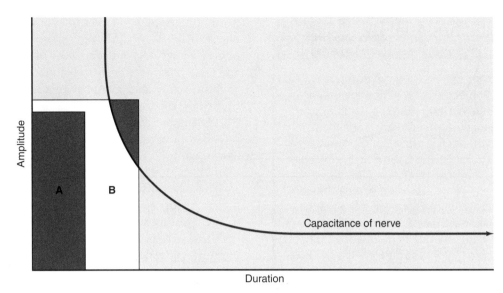

Figure 7.10 Capacitance is the ability of a nerve to store an electrical charge. The phase charge must exceed capacitance to depolarize the nerve. Pulse A lacks sufficient charge to overcome the capacitance of the nerve. However, by increasing amplitude and phase duration, you increase phase charge to overcome capacitance and cause depolarization.

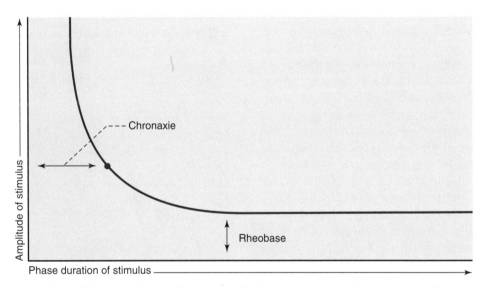

Figure 7.11 Rheobase is the minimum amplitude required to depolarize a nerve fiber, given an infinitely long phase duration. Chronaxie is the phase duration required to depolarize a nerve fiber when the amplitude is two times the rheobase.

number of fibers is recruited, a higher frequency causes them to fire at a more rapid pace, which ultimately increases the tension generated. Nerve membranes must repolarize, however, after discharging. There is an absolute refractory period during which the resting membrane potential is reinstated, and another action potential cannot be elicited during this time. The absolute refractory period is the rate-limiting factor in the number of impulses that can be generated by a nerve.

The classical delineations of current frequencies in the electromagnetic spectrum are low, medium, and high:

- Low frequency is 1,000 Hz (cycles per second) and below.
- Medium frequency is 1,000 to 100,000 Hz.
- High frequency is greater than 100,000 Hz.

Typically, low-frequency stimulators are used to produce the physiologic effect of action potential generation. When the frequency is raised beyond

Experimental Relationship of Intensity and Phase Duration

As an exercise, you may experiment with manipulation of the amplitude and duration of the electrical current. Note the minimal intensity needed to elicit a sensory response when the phase duration is preset to 50 μs. Increase the phase duration and again note the intensity at a minimal motor response. To achieve the same clinical effect, each of these parameters can be manipulated. However, if the machine does not allow a phase duration of greater than 1 ms, it will not be able to depolarize C fibers or the muscle membrane directly. Another type of stimulator is needed for these uses.

this range, the stimulation encroaches on the refractory period of the sensory nerve and actually causes inhibition by bombarding the membrane with continuous stimulation. This is called **Wedenski's inhibition**, or action potential failure, and clinically it can result in anesthesia between the electrodes.

Some confusion occurs with the terminology for the categories of stimulators when referring to frequency. The TENS applications refer to treatment frequencies as high (60–100 pps) and low (1–10 pps), but these stimulators may fall into the low- and medium-frequency stimulator (generator) categories.

Medium-frequency generators are used as TENS devices as well, but their current is modulated to produce a burst rate that the individual nerve fibers can respond to. For example, interferential current typically uses carrier frequencies of 4,000 to 5,000 Hz. However, two slightly different medium-frequency currents are crossed, or interfered, to create a net "beat" frequency. More about interferential therapy is discussed in chapter 8. Another example of manipulation of a medium-frequency current is with Russian stimulation. The carrier current of Russian stimulation is 2,500 Hz, and there is an intrinsic duty cycle of 10 ms on and 10 ms off. The result is "bursts" of stimulation at a rate of 50 per second.

High-frequency generators are used for thermal purposes and to elicit an electromagnetic field. High-frequency current is used with diathermies and has minimal sensory effects.

The frequency or pulse rate can be varied depending on the purpose of the application of the stimulation. When an AC current is used, there is an inverse relationship between the frequency and the wavelength

(phase duration), and either can be calculated when one is known. With pulsatile currents, the interpulse interval allows independent control of phase duration and pulse rate, so the potential variations are broader.

If the frequency does not affect the phase charge, then why is there a stronger sensation of stimulation when the pulse rate increases? Increasing the pulse rate adds more waveforms and ultimately more total charge within a given time (1 s), but the charge in each pulse is unaffected (figure 7.12).

When the pulse rate is increased with TENS, the higher frequencies cause the nerve fibers recruited to fire more rapidly, allowing summation of the stimulation to occur. The body cannot detect when one pulse ends and another begins, and a continuous sensory effect is noted when the pulse rate exceeds 20 pps (figure 7.13). When the frequency is increased, a **tetanic muscle contraction** may result. This usually occurs with a frequency of 35 to 50 Hz. Below this frequency, a twitch response occurs.

Rate of Rise of the Leading Edge of the Pulse

The rate of rise of the leading edge of the pulse, also known as pulse rise time, is a parameter that is

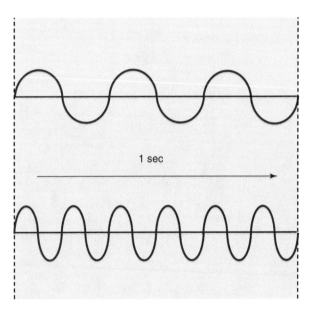

Figure 7.12 Alternating current has an inverse relationship of pulse duration and frequency. When the frequency is known (4,000 Hz or 5,000 Hz, for example), the pulse duration can be calculated: 1 s/4,000 Hz = 0.00025 s (250 μs) and 1 s/5,000 Hz = 0.0002 s (200 μs). Since the pulse duration is for both phases, the *phase* duration is half of the pulse duration. For example, 250 μs pulse duration = 125 μs phase duration.

Tetanic contraction

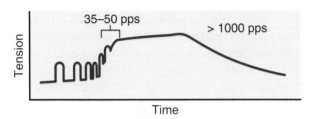

Figure 7.13 Temporal summation occurs when the frequency of stimulation increases and the sensory nerve and muscle contraction cannot differentiate between individual stimuli. The impulses add together.

incorporated into a waveform, but it will also affect the type of nerve targeted. The rate of rise refers to the time it takes to get from zero to maximal amplitude within each pulse. Fast rates of rise are necessary, especially with low-capacitance tissues such as large motor nerves. The low-capacitance membrane cannot store much charge and quickly accommodates to a stimulus. These nerves can dissipate the charge from a pulse with slow rates of rise, and the ion flux needed to alter the voltage to exceed threshold is never reached. Sensory nerves

Clinical Applications of Various Stimulation Frequencies

- Pain modulation techniques use different frequencies to elicit their desired responses.
  - Motor TENS uses frequencies of 2 to 10 Hz to elicit the neurohormonal response.
  - Sensory TENS uses frequencies from 60 to 120 Hz to elicit the enkephalinergic and gating effects.
- Neuromuscular stimulation for passive exercise uses modulated frequencies of 35 to 50 Hz that create a tetanic contraction.
- To increase blood flow or lymphatic drainage, a pulsing effect may be desired. A pulse rate of less than 10 pps causes twitching.

Phase charge determines which nerve fiber will depolarize during stimulation, and frequency determines how often the nerve fibers will depolarize.

that carry light touch, for example, have low capacitance and easily accommodate. This explains how a person is aware of clothing when it is first put on but then stops paying attention to the sensation at the skin; **accommodation** to this minimal stimulus has occurred. Generally, tissues with low capacitance accommodate to a stimulus easily, whereas high-capacitance tissues, because they store the charge, do not accommodate or dissipate the charge readily.

When you are determining whether there will be a physiological response within the tissues, the law of Dubois Reymond describes three important factors within each pulse of an electrical current that you must consider. First, the stimulus must be of adequate amplitude to reach the threshold level of excitatory tissues. Second, the rate of voltage change (rate of rise of the leading edge of the pulse) must be rapid enough that tissue accommodation cannot take place. Third, the length of stimulus or phase duration must be great enough to overcome the capacitance of the tissue to allow an action potential.

The rate of rise of the leading edge of the pulse is the preferred term to describe the onset of the stimulation, since rise time is often confused with ramp. Ramp time has to do with a gradual increase in the amplitude of subsequent pulses so that the intensity does not come on abruptly when a duty cycle is used (figure 7.14).

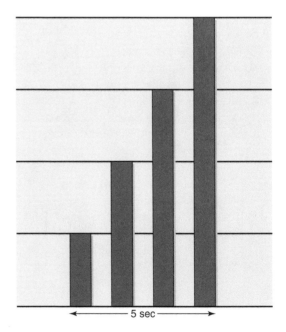

Figure 7.14 Ramping is a programmed increase in amplitude over several pulses (1–5 s).

Law of Dubois Reymond

The effectiveness of a current to target specific excitable tissues is dependent on three major factors:

1. Adequate intensity to reach threshold
2. Current onset fast enough to reduce accommodation
3. Duration long enough to exceed the capacitance of the tissue

Waveforms with an immediate onset of the pulse or fast rate of rise of the leading edge of the pulse (figure 7.15a) are used when the goal of stimulation is to excite the sensory nerve fibers. A long onset, such as with a sawtooth waveform (figure 7.15b), is used when sensory excitation is undesirable but a long phase duration is required to stimulate the muscle membrane directly. This treatment is used, for example, when a motor nerve has lost innervation but there is good sensation over the area, a common occurrence with Bell's palsy. A long phase duration is required to stimulate the denervated muscle, but the stimulation is noxious. A slow onset helps to minimize sensory excitation.

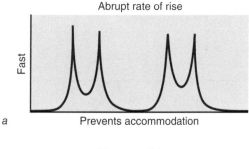

Abrupt rate of rise

Fast

a   Prevents accommodation

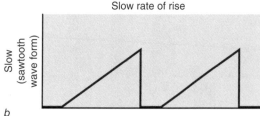

Slow rate of rise

Slow (sawtooth wave form)

b

Figure 7.15 *(a)* A fast rate of rise of the leading edge of the pulse minimizes the chance of exciting high-capacitance fibers. *(b)* A long rate of rise causes less stimulation of high-accommodation fibers while stimulating high-capacitance fibers.

Duty Cycle

The final parameter of electrical stimulation to discuss is the duty cycle. **Duty cycles** are either extrinsic (imposed by the clinician to interrupt the current periodically for several seconds) or intrinsic (used to modulate a current waveform). The extrinsic duty cycle, or "on–off" timing, creates a rest time that is variable on most units. An intrinsic duty cycle is used when pulses are packaged into small clusters. These duty cycles interrupt the current at specific intervals so that the manufacturer can produce time-modulated AC currents, otherwise known as burst mode. The carrier frequency is usually AC and is interrupted at regular intervals, often in the millisecond range. Interruptions are generally imperceptible, but they enable the clinician to take advantage of the characteristics of the carrier frequency to achieve deeper penetration or greater total current. The classic Russian stimulators use this method to modulate medium-frequency sinusoidal waves into bursts of 10 ms on and 10 ms off. Clinical use of Russian stimulation is discussed in chapter 9. The duty cycle reduces the high total current of the medium-frequency generators by introducing an "off" time in the current delivery, making this a safer modality (figure 7.16). The duty cycle also modulates the net frequency of medium-frequency generators to physiologically active frequencies (e.g., 2,500 Hz carrier frequency to 100 burst frequency).

The extrinsic duty cycle can be adjusted by the clinician to impose a rest period. This is often done when applying TENS to stimulate alpha motor nerves to cause muscle contraction. The duty cycle refers to the pattern of on–off sequencing. For example, you may want to stimulate the quadriceps muscles

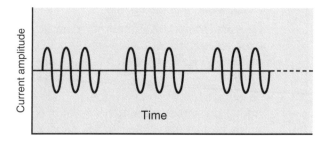

Current amplitude

Time

Figure 7.16 Time-modulated AC. An inherent duty cycle is imposed to create "bursts" of electricity. Each burst has a carrier frequency that is determined by the machine, and there are several bursts in 1 s. This example shows 3 bursts per second.

after knee injury or surgery because the patient has lost volitional control due to pain and swelling. The stimulation must be patterned to allow the muscles to recover between contractions. You might select a 12 s "on" time during which the quadriceps contract and a 12 s rest between contractions. The duty cycle would then be 12 s on and 12 s off, or 1:1. When maximal contractions are attempted with electrical stimulation, a 1:5 duty cycle is recommended to prevent fatigue.

ELECTRODE CONSIDERATIONS

To complete a circuit in electrical stimulation, at least one electrode from each output lead must be in contact with the athlete's skin. There will always be resistance to the current from the air–skin interface; to increase efficiency and consistency of the treatment, the clinician should minimize the resistance.

There are many types of electrodes available for electrical stimulation. Portable TENS units often have single-use or disposable electrodes that are self-adhesive. These electrodes are convenient, minimize the irritation of the skin that often occurs with tape adherents, and make the application simple. The electrodes may be remoistened with water when moved to a new location. The expense of these electrodes may prohibit their use when volume is heavy.

Most electrodes for commercial or clinical use are either metal backed or carbon rubber. Various sizes of electrodes are illustrated in figure 7.17. These require an interface such as moistened sponges or gauze. Gel may be used with the carbon rubber electrodes; however, this may reduce the longevity of the electrodes if they are not cleaned properly. Sponges are the most convenient, but gauze is more sanitary. The interface should be thoroughly wet, with no dry spots, but not dripping.

The electrodes should be firmly attached to the athlete using elastic straps. Weights may be used to secure the electrodes to the low back; however, the current density will change drastically if the electrodes move or become displaced during the treatment. This may cause discomfort to the athlete. The intensity should be adjusted after the electrodes have been secured, since any adjustment in the air–skin interface will affect the resistance and can potentially increase the current or amplitude dramatically. Electrodes should be flexible to conform to body parts such as the ankle or knee. To minimize electrode resistance,

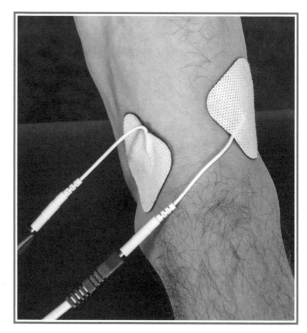

Figure 7.17   Small and large electrodes.

- use large electrodes,
- maintain even, firm contact with skin,
- use clean electrodes and sponges,
- keep the sponge interface well moistened, and
- remove excess hair and oil from skin.

Any lead can be **bifurcated**, or divided. It is imperative that each lead be used, since a common mistake in applying electrical stimulation is to use one bifurcated lead (two electrodes), which does not complete the circuit and therefore delivers no stimulation. Whenever bifurcated leads are used, current density becomes an issue. Each lead may be bifurcated as many times as needed (figure 7.18).

Current density depends on the size of the electrodes and the distance they are apart. There is an equal amount of current in each of the two essential leads. When unequal-sized electrodes are used, the current is more concentrated in the smaller electrode (figure 7.19). This causes a perception of increased intensity under the smaller electrode. When electrodes are very different in size, such as with a point stimulator, the patient may not be able to perceive current in the larger electrode. The larger electrode becomes the dispersive electrode since the current is dispersed over a broad area. When bifurcating leads, it is important to determine the total size of all electrodes that arise from each lead and to compare

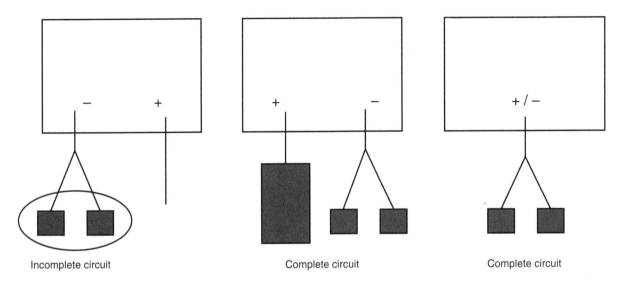

Figure 7.18 Monophasic versus biphasic stimulators. Make sure that there are at least two leads to complete the circuit to allow stimulation. The electrode configuration on the left does not complete the circuit.

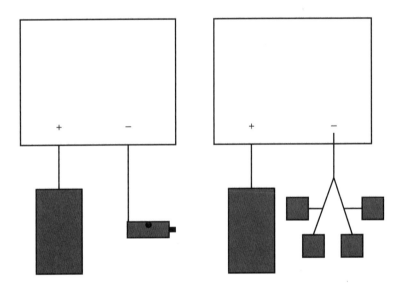

Figure 7.19 Current density concentrates current in the lead that has the smallest total surface area.

that total electrode surface area to the opposite lead surface area to determine if current density differences exist.

Current density can also refer to the concentration of current within the tissues. Current always flows in the path of least resistance. If the electrodes are placed very close together, the current is most dense or concentrated in the superficial tissues. If the electrodes are distant from each other, then the current can take a deeper path through the nerves and blood vessels, which have less resistance (figure 7.20).

Active and Dispersive Leads

All stimulators use either a monophasic or a biphasic current. By examining the stimulator, the clinician can determine the polarity. If the stimulator has a polarity switch, then the stimulator is monophasic, and the toggle will determine the polarity of the *active* lead. The active lead is demarcated on the unit as well. Most monophasic machines also have leads that arise from different locations on the stimulator, whereas most biphasic units have the two essential

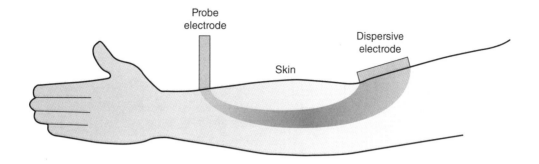

Figure 7.20 The small surface area of the probe electrode creates an area of high current density, resulting in perception of an intense electrical stimulus. The relatively large surface area of the dispersive electrode results in low current density and an excellent dispersion of the electrical stimulus.

leads arising from the same location or socket from the stimulator. In a biphasic machine, there is no physiological difference between the electrodes, and therefore it is not necessary to distinguish the leads (figure 7.21).

The dispersive electrode is needed to complete the circuit but is not relevant to the particular treatment. For example, it is not important to have sensory perception under the dispersive electrode, but electrical stimulation cannot be delivered without this pad in place.

Electrode Configurations

There are two general types of electrode configurations: monopolar and bipolar. Either type may be used with monophasic or biphasic currents. Quadripolar electrode configurations are often used with interferential current.

Monopolar Electrode Configuration

With a monopolar electrode configuration, two or more unequal-sized electrodes are used. One lead is

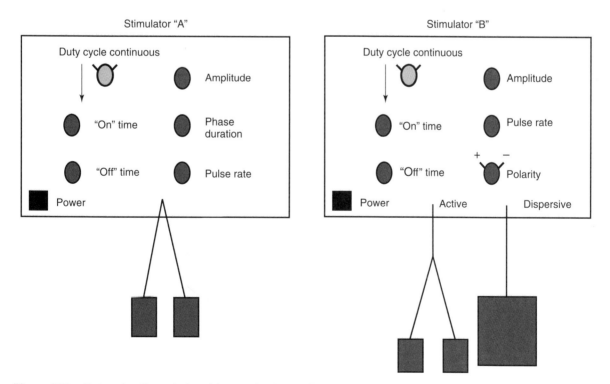

Figure 7.21 Determine the polarity of these stimulators. Stimulator A has no polarity switch, and both leads arise from the same location. Stimulator B has a polarity switch, and each lead is distinct.

designated as active and the other is designated as dispersive. The leads are placed at different locations, with the active lead at the target site and the dispersive lead placed away using a monopolar electrode configuration with a point stimulator. The small electrode with a high current density is desired at the treatment site, but it is more comfortable to use a larger electrode to complete the circuit. Often the patient does not perceive current from the dispersive site (figure 7.22). There are two primary reasons for using a monopolar electrode configuration. First, when electrodes are placed farther apart, the current penetration is deeper. As an example, with underwater stimulation there is less resistance in the water, so the current would preferentially go through the water instead of through the skin. When a monopolar configuration is used, the current has to travel through the body in order to reach the other electrode, which is at a site distant from the treatment location. Second, a monopolar electrode configuration is required when a polarity effect is desired. A monophasic current must be used to differentiate the polarity at the treatment site from the other lead.

The polarity is indicated by the active lead. Examples of this method are iontophoresis and situations in which one is creating an electrical field of a particular polarity for uses such as wound healing.

Bipolar Electrode Configuration

Bipolar electrode configurations can also be used with either monophasic or biphasic currents. In this case, equal-sized electrodes are used, with both placed over the treatment site (figure 7.23). This setup is the most commonly used method in TENS.

Quadripolar Electrode Configuration

The quadripolar electrode configuration is often used with interferential current. Two completely separate medium-frequency generators are used within the same unit, and the electrodes are placed to cross the currents. Ideally, *interference* is created where the two currents cross; however, since the body is not homogeneous, the current may vary. Many interferential stimulators have an adjustment that allows variation in the amplitude of one of the currents so that the location of the perceived

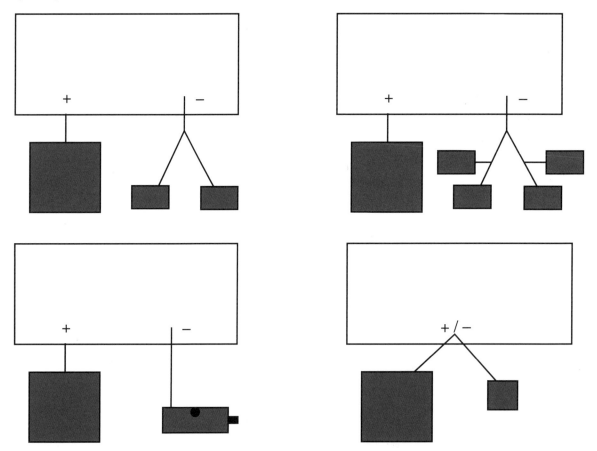

Figure 7.22   Monopolar electrode configuration. Note that either a monophasic or biphasic machine can be used. Each example uses different-sized electrodes.

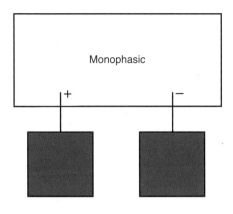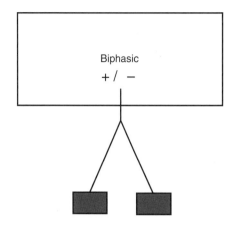

Figure 7.23 Bipolar electrode configuration. Similar-sized electrodes are used with either a monophasic or a biphasic machine.

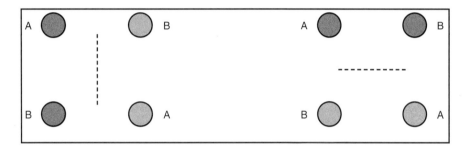

Figure 7.24 Quadripolar electrode configuration used with interferential current. The current is aligned so that it is concentrated between the electrodes to localize the stimulation depending on the pathology. A and B are the two channels.

current can be adjusted. Interferential current can also be placed on a flat surface such as the low back. The quadripolar arrangement implies a three-dimensional configuration of current; however, because the channels are not placed surrounding the tissues in this example, the current is aligned according to the alignment of the channels. Each channel has a red and a black lead. The concentration of the electrical field generated is in alignment with the same-color lead (figure 7.24).

Quadripolar electrode configuration is not the same as using two channels of TENS with four electrodes. Using two channels with TENS increases the number of stimulation points, which may be advantageous when one is treating a large surface area; however, the currents do not cross and cause interference.

SUMMARY

Electrotherapy is a broad topic that requires an understanding of the principles of electrical current and physiological responses before a discussion of clinical applications. Chapter 7 is a foundation for chapter 8, which addresses clinical uses of electrotherapy. The parameters of pulsatile current, used in all applications of transcutaneous electrical nerve stimulation (TENS), are defined. The link between stimulus parameters and capacitance of nerve and muscle tissue is illustrated in the strength–duration curve. The law of Dubois Reymond defines the stimulus characteristics essential for depolarization of nerve and muscle fibers. This chapter concludes with a discussion of electrode configurations used for administering electrotherapy. This discussion provides a transition into issues of clinical applications and decisions, which are addressed in chapter 8.

1. *Define volt, ampere, impedance, and resistance.*

Voltage is a measure of potential difference or electromotive force. One volt is required for 1 ampere of current to pass through 1 ohm of resistance. Electrical current, measured in amperes, is the flow of electrons. One ampere equals the flow of 1 C (6.25×10^{18} electrons) per second. Impedance is the sum of resistance, inductance, and capacitance. Resistance, measured in ohms, is the opposition to the flow of electrical current through a material.

2. *Describe the differences between alternating, direct, and pulsatile currents.*

There are two classifications of continuous currents: alternating (AC) and direct (DC). TENS units deliver electrical currents that are noncontinuous or pulsed. Pulsatile currents are classified as monophasic or biphasic.

3. *Define parameters of pulsatile current, including phase duration, amplitude, phase charge, and frequency.*

Pulsatile currents are characterized by pulses of electrical current interrupted by inter-pulse intervals. Phase duration refers to the length of time required to complete each phase of the waveform. Amplitude is the current or voltage (voltage equals the current if resistance is unchanged) in the electrical circuit. Phase charge, the number of electrons moved during each phase of an electrical pulse, is the primary determinant of which nerve fibers will be depolarized during TENS. Frequency is the number of pulses delivered per second.

4. *Describe the capacitance of nerve and muscle tissue and how it affects the strength–duration curve.*

Excitable tissue has a resting membrane potential and can carry an action potential. When electrical stimulation is applied, an action potential can be elicited in these types of tissues. Each tissue type has capacitance, which is the ability to store charge. If the capacitance is high, the electrical stimulation must have a higher phase charge to elicit an action potential. Means of increasing phase charge are to increase either the phase duration or the amplitude of the stimulation, or both. Thus the strength or intensity of the stimulation and the phase duration are related to create phase charge. The minimal amount of intensity or phase duration required to elicit a response depends on the capacitance of the targeted tissue.

5. *Understand the law of Dubois Reymond with respect to the application of electrical current.*

To create an action potential with electrical stimulation, three factors in the waveform are necessary. The intensity has to be greater than the threshold of the tissue; the phase duration must be long enough to overcome the capacitance of the tissue; and the rate of rise of the leading edge of the pulse has to be fast enough to prevent accommodation.

6. *Describe the types of electrode configurations used in applying electrical stimulation.*

Electrodes can be placed in a variety of configurations depending on the goal of the treatment. A monopolar electrode configuration uses two unequal-sized electrodes with the smaller, active electrode over the treatment site and the larger, dispersive electrode over a distant site. The electrode configuration is bipolar when two equal-sized electrodes are placed over the treatment site.

Clinical Application of Electrical Stimulation for Pain

OBJECTIVES

After reading this chapter, you will be able to

➊ understand the clinical uses for electrical stimulation in the rehabilitation process;

➋ analyze the waveform of the available device and determine whether the treatment goal can be met using that stimulator;

➌ incorporate theories of pain modulation with the principles of electrical stimulation to determine the amplitude, phase duration, and pulse frequency needed for a variety of clinical purposes;

➍ understand the use of microcurrent electrical stimulation; and

➎ identify contraindications for the application of electrotherapy.

A 30-year-old triathlete is referred to a sports medicine clinic for treatment of myofascial pain syndrome in the neck and shoulders. She has had recurring trouble with her neck and shoulder, mostly associated with prolonged training on her bicycle. Her pain became acutely worse 6 weeks after an accident in which the car she was driving was rear-ended. Her primary complaints are increased pain radiating into the right arm with cycling and with working at her desk for prolonged periods (she is a practicing corporate lawyer). She also reports occasional headaches associated with her neck and shoulder pain, which have become more frequent. X-rays were taken of her neck recently, and the orthopedic surgeon who referred her was unable to identify a structural cause for her pain. Examination reveals a fit, physically active woman with a forward-head, protracted-shoulder posture. There are multiple tender trigger points in her neck and shoulders. Upper extremity sensation, motion, and strength are normal. The middle and lower trapezius and serratus anterior are weaker than expected for her fitness level. A treatment plan is designed consisting of modalities for pain management, manual therapies, and exercises to strengthen the weak muscles and improve posture. She asks about using electrical stimulation for pain control and says that she received treatment in college from a certified athletic trainer for a back and hip injury sustained while running track.

Because of the patient's previous positive experience, electrotherapy is identified as the treatment of choice. Which type of electrotherapy is most appropriate to achieve the treatment goals? What are the optimal parameters of treatment? Is electrotherapy contraindicated? This chapter addresses these types of questions and provides the physical principles and physiological bases for the use of electrotherapy in sport rehabilitation.

Electrical stimulation units are often versatile in their parameters and often allow the clinician freedom to manipulate the phase duration, frequency, amplitude, and duty cycle. Although any type of electrical stimulation that crosses the skin to excite the nerve is considered **transcutaneous electrical nerve stimulation (TENS)**, some units are marketed for a specific clinical purpose, such as "muscle strengthening." A savvy clinician, knowing the capacitance and ability to excite target fibers, should be able to critically analyze the waveform and parameters offered to determine the cost versus benefit of a stimulator. The clinical uses of electrical stimulation are for pain, muscle stimulation through the alpha motor nerve, stimulation of denervated muscle, iontophoresis, and some subtle effects such as edema reduction and wound healing. For the purposes of this text, the stimulators are categorized according to their primary clinical function. There is mixed evidence for clinical uses for electrical stimulation with strong effects for TENS in certain cases such as osteoarthritis and low back pain. However, there is also research that does not support the use of TENS. Understanding how TENS can influence the physiology is imperative for appropriate clinical decision making.

The clinician should *not* use electrical stimulation if there are known myocardial problems or arrhythmias. TENS should not be used if there is a pacemaker or if pregnancy is suspected. Electrical stimulation should not be delivered through the chest or over the carotid sinus. Stimulation in the anterior neck elicits activity in the carotid sinus or may cause a contraction of the pharyngeal muscles. This can affect the blood pressure and pulse.

TRANSCUTANEOUS ELECTRICAL NERVE STIMULATION

Electrical stimulation for pain modulation is the primary reason for TENS. You should review the pain modulation theories presented in chapter 6, since the techniques described in this section will follow the guidelines associated with those theories. Specifically, the sensory, noxious, and rhythmical pain modulation theories should be reviewed. Understanding how TENS relieves pain requires integration of the pain control models and an understanding of nerve fiber capacitance. Examples of TENS units include biphasic low-voltage stimulators, portable TENS units, interferential units, and high-voltage stimulators.

Video 8.1 shows the setup of a multi-modality device.

One can achieve variations of TENS by adjusting the current parameters (figure 8.1). The proposed mechanisms of pain modulation appropriate for each type of electrical stimulation are discussed in this chapter. Because therapy with electrical stimulation treats the symptoms of an ailment and generally not the cause, proper evaluation of the etiology of the injury and rectification of the cause are important. Ideally, the pain modulation allows the athlete to perform therapeutic exercise, which will contribute to the alleviation of the problem.

Efficacy of TENS in the Reduction of Pain

A recent meta-analysis by Bjordal, Johnson, and Ljunggreen (2003) compared the effects of TENS with placebo controls. They identified 21 randomized controlled trials that examined postoperative analgesic use in patients who had undergone a variety of surgical procedures and concluded that TENS reduces postoperative pain compared to the placebo since patients had less analgesic demand during the first three days after surgery. Evidence-based research, however, remains mixed regarding whether TENS reduces pain with a variety of stimulation parameters. Several studies demonstrated that TENS was effective compared to sham treatment in relieving pain (Abelson et al. 1983; Hsueh et al. 1997; Jensen, Zesler, and Christensen 1991; Kumar and Marshall 1997; Moore and Shurman 1997; Møystad, Krogstad, and Larheim 1990; Smith, Lewith, and Machin 1983; Taylor, Hallett, and Flaherty 1981; Thorsteinsson et al. 1978; Vinterberg, Donde, and Andersen 1978). Other investigators found no analgesic effect with TENS (Grimmer 1992) or an effect on overall function (Feger et al. 2015). Databases have been created to identify randomized clinical trials to evaluate the use of TENS for both chronic pain and osteoarthritis. Most studies were

Goal: TENS pain control	Phase duration	Amplitude	Pulse frequency	Target nerve fiber
Sensory	<150 µs	Submotor	60-120 pps	A-beta
Motor	200-300 µs	Strong motor	<10 pps	A-delta
Noxious	>300 ms	Painful	High or low	C fiber
Neuromuscular stimulation	250 µs	Motor	50 pps	A-alpha
Iontophoresis	n/a (DC)	≤5 mamp	n/a (DC)	n/a
Stimulation of denervated muscle	n/a (DC)	≤5 mamp	n/a (DC)	Muscle membrane
Microcurrent	Variable	Subsensory	Variable	Sympathetic fibers

Figure 8.1   Examples of parameters used in the clinical application of electrical stimulation. The clinician can use a variety of machines to deliver the correct parameters.

eliminated from the evidence-based database because of poorly controlled or confounding variables.

Considerable variation in the site of stimulation and electrode placement was reported across the different studies. Some investigators reported that the electrodes were placed directly over the site of pain (Abelson et al. 1983; Hsueh et al. 1997; Mannheimer and Carlsson 1979; Taylor, Hallett, and Flaherty 1981; Vinterberg, Donde, and Andersen 1978). Others stimulated traditional acupuncture points (Ballegaard et al. 1985; Grimmer 1992; Jensen, Zesler, and Christensen 1991; Kumar and Marshall 1997; Lewis, Lewis, and Sturrock 1984; Lewis, Lewis, and Cumming 1994). Two reports did not specify the site of electrode placement in the study (Moore and Shurman 1997; Nash, Williams, and Machin 1990). Other investigators (Møystad, Krogstad, and Larheim 1990; Smith, Lewith, and Machin 1983; Thorsteinsson et al. 1978) applied TENS stimulation to acupuncture points and trigger points directly involved in the area of pain.

The variability in evidence linked to TENS is likely due to the range of parameters that are suggested for treatments. As our research in pain modulation mechanisms grows, we should align the treatment methodologies with the physiological effects that a treatment elicits. For example, in different approaches to pain modulation, each mechanism requires a certain type of stimulation. Sensory pain modulation requires a sensory response with A-beta fibers; rhythmical pain modulation requires rhythmical stimulation of A-delta fibers (intense); and noxious pain modulation requires the stimulation of pain fibers (C fibers). The parameter selection in the TENS device can be programmed to target those tissues. Future research should be consistent and report those parameters even when a manufacturer bundles the parameters together to make it easier for the clinician. Similarly, researchers should avoid the use of jargon when describing methods used to deliver the stimulation.

Considering the money that is spent on the treatment of pain, there is a significant need to further study the analgesic effects of TENS. Large, multisite randomized clinical trials are needed to evaluate the efficacy of TENS treatments and to validate clinical practice. TENS is thought to improve function through the central nervous system and peripheral mechanisms. Specific athletic injuries have been shown to respond favorably to TENS. These hypothesized mechanisms and applications are addressed here.

Mechanisms of Pain Modulation

The mechanisms of pain modulation for electrical stimulation parallel the pain modulation theories discussed in chapter 6.

Sensory TENS

Sensory TENS is also called high-rate or "conventional" TENS; it can be used for any painful condition, most commonly in the acute phase or postoperatively. The large-diameter, A-beta fibers are targeted with this treatment, and we know that those fibers are stimulated when the patient perceives a tingling sensation. The goal is to stay submotor because that ensures that only A-beta fibers are stimulated. If a muscle contraction occurs, there is a good chance that the smaller diameter (A-delta) fibers could be stimulated, potentially interfering with the gate theory. The stimulation is comfortable, and the intensity can be increased as long as it is comfortable and below the motor threshold.

To configure the stimulator to target the A-beta fibers for sensory TENS, think about the electrical principles presented in chapter 7. These fibers are large diameter and are found throughout the skin. They have low thresholds, and because of their diameter, they require a short phase duration and low intensity. Typically, these fibers can be stimulated with a phase duration as short as 50 μs, but it is generally around 100 μs. The intensity is then slowly increased until the stimulation is perceived. If the clinician has difficulty getting the appropriate response, the phase duration can be increased. Phase durations should remain less than 200 μs to make sure that A-delta fibers are avoided. Because we want to bombard the A-beta fibers with as much stimulation as possible, the clinician should choose a constant (continuous) stimulation at a high pulse rate (>100 pps) for an indefinite length of time. Most treatments are cut shorter to allow for other therapeutic interventions and rehabilitation; however, Pietrosimone and colleagues (2011) used continuous TENS on osteoarthritic knees both during rehabilitation and during daily activities to improve quadriceps function.

The treatment time can theoretically last up to 24 h. However, the athlete can be instructed to use the device for intermittent 20 to 30 min treatments to see whether the pain is diminishing. If pain is not reduced, then electrode placement should be adjusted. The clinician should emphasize that

TENS treatments do not replace rehabilitation progression. In the clinic, treatments generally are used in combination with ice or heat to reduce pain or spasm (figure 8.2). The treatment time for the TENS is consistent with the recommended time for thermotherapy, which ranges from 10 to 45 min depending on the depth of the target structure for the heat or cold therapy.

When the parameters of the stimulation are adjusted to target the large-diameter A-beta afferent nerve fibers, the release of enkephalins into the dorsal horn is triggered. Therefore, the pain relief generally lasts only as long as the stimulation. Any machine that allows stimulation of large-diameter sensory nerves (with short phase duration and high pulse rate) can be used for this treatment. Sensory TENS is commonly used to reduce pain after an injury or after surgery in combination with ice, elevation, and compression. Because the A-beta fibers accommodate to stimulation quickly, the intensity should be adjusted periodically. It is common to allow the patient to increase the stimulation during the treatment as long as the treatment remains below the motor threshold.

Many TENS units allow the clinician to use a "modulation" mode to decrease accommodation to the stimulation. This is most often used with sensory TENS, since the large-diameter nerve fibers that are targeted with this type of stimulation accommodate quickly. Some manufacturers modulate the amplitude, the pulse rate, or the phase duration, usually by varying the parameter by 20% above and below the preset value. Different parameters may be modulated, depending on the device (see figure 8.3). Some TENS units allow modulation of amplitude, phase duration, or pulse rate or "multimodulation," such that two or more parameters are modulated.

Rhythmical or Motor TENS

Rhythmical TENS may also be referred to as low-rate TENS. It has been equated with acupuncture in its mechanism of pain relief. This type of TENS is applied with a broad range of parameters in the literature, which may have resulted in variable responses. Some studies indicate that they used "acupuncture-like TENS," but the parameters do not fit into a category that would evoke the pain modulation theory previously described. It is very important to evaluate the parameters used with the appropriate goal when using TENS.

This mode of TENS incorporates the rhythmical pain modulation theory and commonly produces a strong, tolerable muscle contraction. Rhythmical TENS is more vigorous than sensory TENS and is used to treat subacute pain or trigger points. Rhythmical TENS should not be used on acute injuries; vigorous contractions may increase discomfort or cause bleeding.

Rhythmical stimulation is theorized to release endogenous opiates and inhibit pain through descending mechanisms and may provide relief for 1 to 3 h after a 30 min treatment. Pain relief may be delayed compared to that with sensory TENS, but it lasts longer. High- and low-frequency (sensory

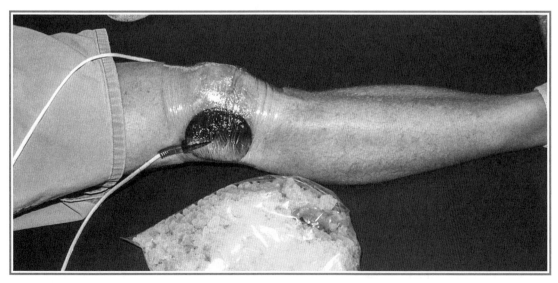

Figure 8.2 Sensory transcutaneous electrical nerve stimulation is often used with ice as a pain management technique with acute injuries. So that effective cooling may take place, make sure the electrodes do not insulate the area.

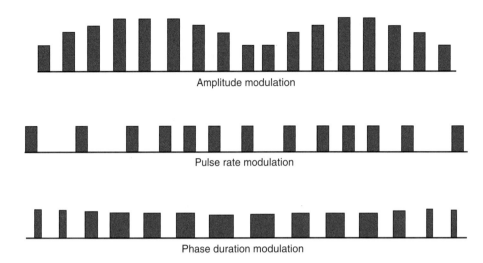

Figure 8.3   Modulation mode. Examples of modulation of the waveform include amplitude modulation, pulse rate modulation, and phase duration modulation. Modulation of the waveform helps to reduce accommodation.

and rhythmical) TENS has been compared from a neuroscience perspective by DeSantana et al. (2008). They provide evidence that low-frequency TENS also stimulates the large-diameter fibers and the subsequent analgesia via the spinal pathway. They also discuss an opioid stimulation from the more intense, rhythmical stimulation of low-rate TENS. Sluka and Walsh (2003) used microdialysis and high-performance liquid chromatography analysis in an animal model of joint inflammation to demonstrate that there is an increase in serotonin in the spinal cord during low-frequency, but not high-frequency, TENS.

Video 8.2 shows a demonstration of motor TENS.

To apply motor TENS, set the phase duration, pulse rate, and amplitude to the following specifications: The phase duration should be high, in a range of 200 to 300 µs, to target the A-delta (fast pain) nerve fiber. Because the motor nerve fibers are deep, elicitation of the A-delta fibers corresponds to a visible muscle contraction. The pulse rate should be low, with distinct, separate pulses in the range of 2 to 4 pps and generally less than 10 pps. The amplitude should cause the elicitation of strong, visible contractions but should not cause pain. A strong, tolerable muscle contraction indicates the stimulation of A-delta fibers. Treatment time generally lasts 20 to 30 min, although the pain relief may not occur for 30 to 120 min because of the descending

mechanism. A duty cycle is not necessary for motor TENS, and the continuous mode should be selected.

It is sometimes recommended that treatment be initiated with the sensory TENS technique to obtain the rapid onset of pain relief. As the pain subsides, the parameters can be adjusted to deliver motor TENS for prolonged pain relief. Again, this should be done only when the muscle contractions do not perpetuate the inflammatory response.

Noxious TENS

A noxious stimulus is applied to elicit pain relief through the diffuse noxious inhibitory control mechanism. This mode of TENS is commonly used with point stimulators because the amplitude should be at the maximum tolerable level to trigger descending serotonergic tracts to inhibit pain. Clearly this type of treatment is performed only when pain has exceeded its usefulness and a long-term interruption in pain is the goal. This type of treatment works well with persistent pain and with various myofascial disorders. The treatment may not be tolerated well in individuals with complex regional pain syndrome because of the sympathetic hyperactivity. Muscle spasms respond well to this type of treatment.

The small diameter of the probe creates a high current density to the target area without subjecting a broad area to the noxious stimulus. Units may incorporate an ohmmeter to identify points of lower skin resistance that correlate highly with trigger and acupuncture points. Body charts may help locate appropriate points for optimal pain relief.

The key to appropriate noxious TENS is to use a machine that allows the stimulation of C fibers. Very few machines allow a phase duration long enough to elicit a response of C fibers, since long phase durations have the potential to apply a great deal of current. The Neuroprobe or a galvanic stimulator can be used (figure 8.4). The recommended phase duration is between 10 and 20 ms. This is in contrast to what is possible with most TENS units, which have a maximum of 250 μs (milli- = 10^{-3}; micro- = 10^{-6}). Low-rate stimulation is commonly preferred to achieve the advantages of rhythmical pain modulation in conjunction with the treatment.

To apply noxious TENS, the parameters should be set to the following specifications. Again, the ability to stimulate C fibers may be prohibited in many stimulators to protect the athlete. The phase duration must be longer than 1 ms, 10^{-20} is recommended, and the amplitude should be as high as tolerable. The pulse rate may vary, but the clinician should choose either a high frequency or a low frequency. The high-frequency 100 to 150 pps prevents the discrimination of individual pulses and is classically used in noxious TENS. A low frequency of 2 to 7 pps, however, will elicit the benefits of motor TENS in conjunction with noxious TENS. If the stimulator parameters are capable of overcoming the capacitance of C fibers, then the A-delta fibers will be stimulated as well, providing an added benefit. Each point should be stimulated for 30 s, and generally 8 to 10 points are treated in a session.

Do not expect good results for TENS treatments if the athlete is taking narcotic analgesics. The electrical stimulation produces natural opioids that compete for the receptor sites occupied by the medication.

The pain modulation parameters are summarized in table 8.1.

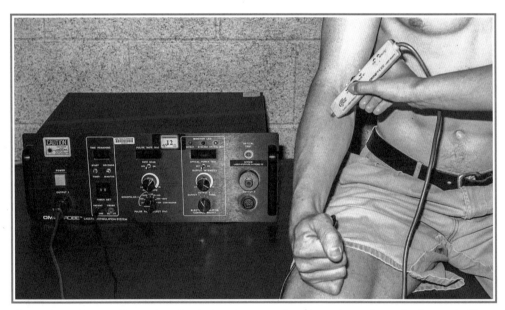

Figure 8.4 Neuroprobe point stimulation. A monopolar electrode configuration is used with the active electrode in the remote and the dispersive electrode in the patient's hand.

Table 8.1   Transcutaneous Electrical Nerve Stimulation Parameters

Type of TENS	Phase duration	Pulse frequency	Amplitude	Target nerve fiber
Sensory	<100 μs	>100 pps	Sensory, sub-motor	A-beta
Rhythmical	200–300 μs	2–4 pps	Strong muscle contraction	A-delta
Noxious	>1 ms	2–4 pps or 100–150 pps	Tolerable	C fiber

Types of TENS Units

Various types of machines can be used to deliver TENS in a clinical setting. Understanding the type of stimulator and how the treatment can be varied makes the clinician much more versatile. Companies that manufacture stimulators try to simplify the treatments by requiring the clinician to push one button to select the parameters. Computer chips are programmed appropriately. Although these machines simplify the delivery of stimulation, a clinician may not appreciate the nuances of parameter selection.

The following section describes different classes of electrical stimulators that are often used for TENS and pain modulation. These stimulators are biphasic low-voltage stimulators, portable TENS units, interferential units, and high-voltage stimulators.

Low-Voltage Stimulators

Low-voltage stimulators are all TENS units that do not belong to a special class. Many manufacturers produce stimulators in this category. They can have either monophasic or biphasic current and have variable waveforms. Usually they have specific controls for phase duration, intensity, frequency, and duty cycles. Most of these units have limitations on the phase duration for safety reasons, so they are not effective as noxious pain stimulators.

Portable TENS Units

Battery-operated portable TENS units allow a long duration of electrical stimulation (see figure 8.5). They can be lent or sold to an athlete or patient so

that TENS can be used throughout the day or night for pain management. Portable TENS units are often used for electrical stimulation treatments during travels with a team.

Video 8.3 discusses using a TENS device at home.

When using a portable TENS unit, complete a musculoskeletal evaluation to determine the source of pain and areas of associated pain. From the evaluation, determine sites for electrode placement, which may be around painful joints, on trigger or acupuncture points, at spinal nerve root levels or peripheral nerve trunks, or at a superficial point of the nerve supplying the painful area. Prepare the skin site by cleaning the area; electrodes should not be placed over abraded skin or open wounds. Secure electrodes at designated areas on the skin. Carbon-silicon-impregnated rubber electrodes require a conductive gel interface. Some pre-gelled electrodes contain an adherent. Thoroughly explain the treatment to the athlete.

Preset the phase duration and the pulse rate prior to application according to the type of TENS to be used. Gradually turn up the amplitude until the athlete feels a tingling sensation. Increase the amplitude until the stimulation is strong, but comfortable. Electrodes may have to be adjusted for better stimulation and pain relief. The athlete can be taught to adjust the amplitude independently but to keep the stimulation at the desired intensity (motor or submotor).

During treatment, the amplitude may be adjusted to maximize pain relief and to account for accommodation. The fast response to sensory TENS allows rapid evaluation of electrode placement and effectiveness. If the athlete is responding well to sensory TENS, other modes may be used. After 20 to 30 min, reevaluate the athlete for pain and inspect electrode sites for **hyperemia**.

The athlete may be instructed in home use. Sensory TENS can be used throughout the day, but the athlete should be taught to turn the stimulation off periodically and to monitor the duration of pain relief.

Interferential Stimulation Units

Interferential stimulation is another form of TENS used for pain relief, increased circulation, and muscle stimulation. We are categorizing interferential stim-

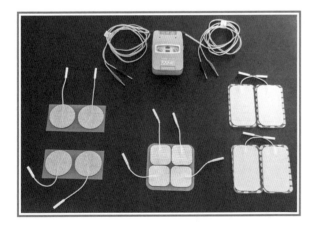

Figure 8.5 Portable transcutaneous electrical nerve stimulation units are available from many manufacturers. Most have two channels and allow the clinician to preadjust the rate, phase duration, and modulation.

ulation with TENS because it is primarily used for the modulation of pain. Interferential current simultaneously applies two medium-frequency currents to achieve deeper penetration of the stimulation. Medium- and high-frequency currents reduce the skin impedance that minimizes the penetration of low-frequency currents. Theoretically, a medium-frequency stimulation can be directed to a target tissue such as a joint. However, according to the pain modulation theories, sensory stimulation must evoke enkephalin intervention at the dorsal horn. Furthermore, because of bombardment of stimulation during the refractory period, medium-frequency currents must be modulated; otherwise there is minimal or no response in the tissues. Typical modulation techniques include the incorporation of an internal duty cycle as with Russian stimulation, or "interfering" the current to create a resultant "beat" frequency.

In order to modulate the medium frequency to a range that can create an action potential in the tissues, two slightly different medium-frequency (within the range of 1,000 to 10,000 Hz) sinusoidal wave currents are applied at the same time (figure 8.6). Typically, interferential units use a carrier frequency of 4,000 or 5,000 Hz. This results in a phase duration of 125 μs or 100 μs (1 s divided by 4,000 Hz = *pulse* duration). (Divide by 2 to get the

phase duration.) This phase duration is excellent for sensory pain modulation. The waveforms of the two carrier currents are superimposed on each other, which causes interference. Interference creates points of augmentation and attenuation of the phases where peaks and valleys are added together. The interference results in the modulation of a "beat" mode with a frequency that ranges from 1 to 100 beats per second, which is well within the conventional low-frequency range. The beat frequency is determined by the difference between the two carrier frequencies. For example, carrier frequencies of 4,000 and 4,150 have a beat frequency of 150 beats per second (bps); 2,500 and 2,550 have a beat frequency of 50 bps.

Video 8.4 demonstrates proper application of interferential current.

The medium-frequency currents used with interferential units can cause a cutaneous nerve inhibition, as with the action potential block mode of TENS. This action potential failure is known as Wedenski's inhibition, and it occurs because the stimulation is applied too quickly in relation to the refractory period of the nerve. At a frequency

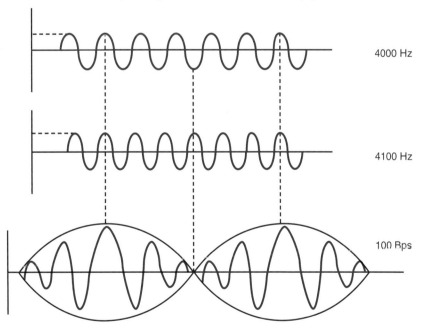

Figure 8.6 Interferential stimulation. Two different medium-frequency currents are superimposed so that there is augmentation and attenuation of the currents. The resultant frequency is the beat frequency and is the difference between the two carrier frequencies.

of 5,000 Hz, the membrane cannot stabilize, and the continuous function of the sodium-potassium pump causes an inhibitory effect. One can demonstrate Wedenski's inhibition by noting the anesthesia between the electrodes during medium-frequency stimulation. The patient should not be able to discriminate sharp or dull sensations between the electrodes during stimulation.

You can vary the frequency of the beats by changing one of the two carrier frequencies. The beat frequency, not the carrier frequencies, affects the tissues; changes in this parameter alter the stimulation responses. The number of muscle twitches increases as the beat frequency increases, until a tetanic contraction is attained. Some units have a feature that constantly changes the frequency of one of the carrier currents while the other remains constant. This mode is a "sweep frequency" that causes a rhythmic change throughout a range of frequencies. The purpose of the rhythmic mode is to reduce accommodation. Because the stimulation continuously changes, the body cannot adapt to it. The sweep frequency provides a more effective stimulation in this manner.

Some models include a rotating vector system that periodically changes the orientation of the electrical field 45° to further reduce accommodation. The efficacy of this modification has not been substantiated.

The beat frequency is selected according to the condition to be treated. A frequency of 60 to 100 bps is used for sensory TENS, 35 to 50 bps for muscle contraction, and 2 to 4 bps for motor TENS.

Four electrodes should be used for an interferential treatment, two for each carrier current in a quadripolar fashion. The electrodes of each current are placed diagonally over the treatment site (figure 8.7). The area to be treated should be surrounded by the electrodes if it is an extremity or joint. The electrodes should be placed all on one surface if the treatment area is large, such as the low back. Some interferential units also offer suction electrodes in which a mild vacuum is created under the electrode to allow it to stick to the body part. The electrodes are convenient to apply because they do not have to be strapped down and they stay in place throughout the treatment.

The passage of current through the tissues does not occur linearly between the electrodes but creates an electrical field. This field is purported to be shaped in a cloverleaf pattern situated three-dimensionally between the electrodes. If the conductivity of the tissues were uniform, this perfectly formed electrical field would occur with the maximal current concentration in the central region between the electrodes. However, differences in the tissue impedance affect the location of the electrical field and the degree of superposition of currents. Therefore, the concentration of current is not always centralized. To maximize the probability of properly placed electrodes and subsequent electrical fields, adjust the electrodes so that maximal intensity is perceived in the painful region.

Interferential stimulation can be used with other modalities. Although it is sometimes difficult with the suction electrodes, ice or heat can be used in conjunction with the stimulation. Treatment durations are dictated by the goal of treatment: pain relief, muscle reeducation, muscle spasm reduction, and so on. Interferential units have been shown to reduce pain and edema posttraumatically.

Contraindications to using interferential stimulators are the same as for any other form of TENS,

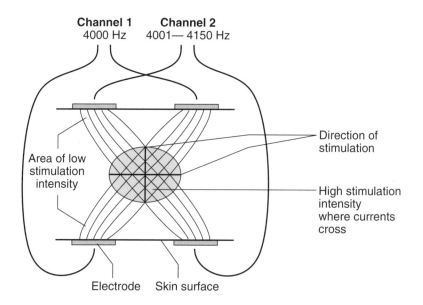

Figure 8.7 Stimulation produced with interferential current using four electrodes. The current is maximized between the electrodes, and the electrical field created is often depicted as a cloverleaf pattern.

Reprinted, by permission, from Dynatronics Corporation.

but interferential machines must be used cautiously in proximity to diathermy units. The electrical field generated can cause power surges in the electrical modalities.

Application

Turn on the power for the interferential machine before setting up electrodes. This prevents a power surge from transmitting to the patient when the machine comes on. Select the interferential mode if the unit has multiple stimulation options. There may be an option of selecting the carrier frequency. Generally your decision will be determined by your treatment goal. For example, if there are options of 2,500 Hz and 5,000 Hz, remember that the higher the frequency, generally the better the depth of penetration (according to the formula that affects impedance). However, a 2,500 Hz current has a phase duration of 200 μs (1/2,000 = 400 μs biphasic; therefore each phase is 200 μs). A current with 5,000 Hz has only a 100 μs phase duration. Therefore if a longer phase duration is desired, which may be the case with the use of **neuromuscular stimulation**, select the lower carrier frequency. Neuromuscular factors are presented in detail in chapter 9.

Select the treatment frequency. This also will be dictated by the treatment goal. Use the appropriate treatment frequencies for pain modulation or at tetany for neuromuscular stimulation. You may be able to select a frequency scan that modulates the frequency throughout a preset range to decrease accommodation. The treatment frequency is actually the difference between the two medium-frequency currents (e.g., 5,000 Hz and 5,100 Hz result in 100 bps).

Determine the duty cycle for the treatment. If the treatment is for pain, generally a continuous (no duty cycle) treatment is chosen. Neuromuscular treatments require a rest time, and both the on time and the off time should be selected as appropriate for the treatment.

Set up the electrodes. Moist sponges can be used to improve conductance. Two complete channels must be connected to the athlete. Ideally, the stimulation should cross between the electrodes. The electrodes should be firmly secured to the athlete.

Begin to increase the intensity of the stimulation, one circuit at a time. When the intensity of the second circuit is increased, the perception of stimulation may change. Increase each circuit a little at a time while getting feedback from the athlete about the location of maximal stimulation and the comfort level of the current. Amplitude should be adjusted only when the duty cycle is on rather than during the rest phase.

Some interferential units allow the clinician to "move" the current to allow better placement of the stimulation. This may be done with a joystick or a finger panel. This requires feedback from the athlete. Vector scan can be selected if the treatment site cannot be isolated. One circuit will intrinsically vary its amplitude, changing the location of maximal stimulation. This will reduce the time the treatment current is at the injury site, so a longer treatment duration is recommended. Check on the athlete for comfort during the treatment and make adjustments as necessary.

Premodulated Interferential

Premodulated interferential stimulation makes interferential stimulation easier to set up. Medium-frequency currents must be modified to a biologically active low frequency before they get to the body. The premise is that the two medium-frequency currents are crossed inside the machine so that only two electrodes or one channel is needed for the treatment. In actuality premod is a time-modulated AC, much like Russian stimulation. The medium frequency is delivered with interruptions at set times so that there are packages, or bursts, of medium-frequency current. The benefit is that the premod uses medium frequencies (>1,000 Hz), deeper penetration results from the reduced skin impedance of the higher frequency, and the stimulation is comfortable, likely from the Wedenski inhibition. Another clinical benefit is that the application requires only two electrodes, compared to the four required for the conventional interferential. This method is still an effective method of TENS application, since both sensory and motor pain modulation stimulation can be performed.

Application of Premodulated Interferential

Determine your treatment goal—for example, sensory pain modulation, muscle spasm reduction by fatigue, or neuromuscular. Select Premod on the unit. Adjust the treatment frequency and duty cycle based on the treatment goal.

Attach one channel (two electrodes) securely to the athlete and increase the intensity to the desired level, depending on the treatment goal.

High-Voltage Stimulators

High-voltage stimulators (HVS) are classified according to two distinct specifications: They must be able to transmit a voltage of at least 150 V, and they must use a twin-peaked monophasic current (see figure 8.8). The 150 V delineation is an arbitrarily set value that demarcates high- and low-voltage units. The major claims of this type of unit are that the high voltage allows deeper penetration of the energy and that the short phase duration of the twin peaks does not allow the capacitance of smaller sensory fibers (A-delta or C fibers) to be stimulated, resulting in greater comfort. Despite early concerns, these monophasic pulsatile waveforms do not cause ion flux. The phase duration is too short to drive the movement of charged particles. Therefore, TENS units with monophasic pulsatile waveforms do not cause skin irritation or the physiochemical responses seen with the application of DC current.

Since the stimulator is monophasic, there is a polarity difference in the electrodes, allowing the clinician to choose a positive or negative electrode for the treatment area. Again, since the phase duration is so short, there are minimal physiochemical changes under the electrodes. High-voltage units are used clinically for pain control, edema reduction, tissue healing, and muscle spasm reduction. Muscle reeducation or neuromuscular electrical stimulation (NMES) can be performed with high-voltage units if the stimulator allows a duty cycle.

The voltage amplitude available with most high-voltage machines ranges from 0 to 500 V. The amplitude, as with most electrical stimulators, is determined by patient comfort and the objective of the treatment (sensory or motor response). One

of the features of the high-voltage machine is that although the voltage is high, there is a low average current. It is therefore a very safe modality. The twin-peaked waveform allows the high peak voltage and low average current. The pulse decays almost immediately, and the second pulse begins before the first peak reaches the isoelectric line. The duration of both peaks together varies with each manufacturer, but it is generally between 50 and 120 μs. The phase duration is not adjustable, thus ensuring the safety of the unit.

Many claims have been made about the relevance of the polarity control of high-voltage units, although the low average current minimizes any ion flux or physiochemical response. However, during healing, the wound emits a charge potential depending on the stage of healing. It is believed that this potential is reinforced by application of a charge of like polarity, either positive or negative, from the stimulator. This process promotes a stronger physiological response and has been associated with **chemotaxis** of leukocytes, which may enhance healing and edema reduction. However, the electrophoretic effect with this type of unit is negligible, especially with short treatment durations. The net ion flux across the membrane is minimal and is self-limiting. The short phase durations cause only a minor shift in ion migration, and with the interpulse interval the membrane can neutralize any change in the normal ion status. Iontophoresis cannot be performed with this unit because no net ion flux occurs. Several studies have addressed the possibility of edema

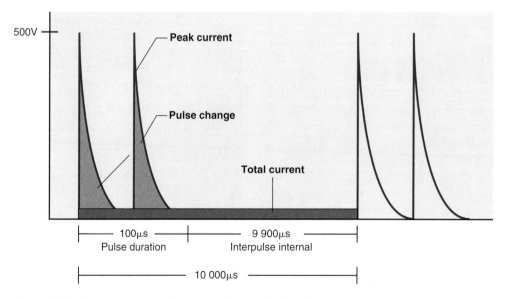

Figure 8.8 Twin-peak, monophasic waveform in high-voltage stimulators.

reduction with high-voltage stimulation in animal models (Dolan, Mychaskiw, and Mendel 2003) and humans (Goldman et al. 2003).

The frequency range offered by most high-voltage units is from 2 to 120 pps. The frequency adjustment allows the incorporation of either sensory or motor TENS principles when pain tolerance is the goal. The variation in frequencies also allows the clinician to optimize parameters for either muscle pumping or muscle reeducation. The phase duration cannot be changed and is so short that excitation of the smaller fibers for motor pain modulation or for a strong muscle contraction will be difficult to achieve.

Electrode placement for high voltage often uses the monopolar technique, although the bipolar can be used as well (see figure 8.9). The monopolar procedure uses one or more active electrodes and a larger dispersive electrode. The active electrodes are smaller and concentrate the current, and therefore the level of stimulation, over the treatment site. As the name implies, the dispersive electrode spreads the same amount of current over a larger surface area, causing minimal, if any, sensory perception under the electrode. The active electrodes are placed over the treatment site, and the dispersive electrode is placed on a site distant from the treatment area. Since the distance between electrodes is increased with the monopolar method, there is potentially a deeper penetration of the current.

The bipolar technique, which uses equal-sized electrodes over the same treatment area, can also be used with high voltage. The larger electrode is replaced by an equal-sized electrode, although the lead must be plugged into the dispersive socket in the unit; otherwise the circuit is not complete.

A key feature of the high-voltage unit is its ability to be used with appendage submersion treatments. Submersion is a preferred method of treatment for acute ankle injuries because it provides circumferential cooling and sensory TENS for irregular surfaces. Even though the extremity is in a dependent position, the submersion method allows active range of motion during the treatment. The active electrodes are placed in the cold water bath (13° to 18°C, 55° to 65°F), and a 20 to 30 min treatment is applied. The treatment is followed by other modalities and exercise as indicated for the condition. The treatment can be repeated several times throughout the day.

High-voltage stimulation with its monophasic current has the same applications as other TENS units—sensory and motor pain modulation and affecting blood flow and edema reduction. High-voltage stimulation has the same contraindications as all other TENS and should not be used through the chest, whenever there is a cardiac pacemaker, or during pregnancy. It should not be used over the carotid sinus in the neck because of the proximity of the baroreceptors.

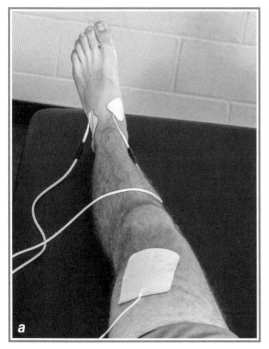 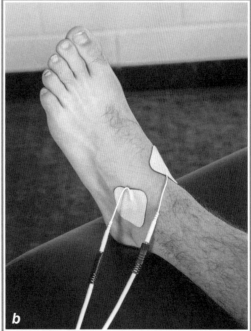

Figure 8.9 Setups using *(a)* a dispersive pad (monopolar) and *(b)* a small electrode (bipolar).

The evaluation should determine the goal of the HVS. The high-voltage unit does not have an adjustable phase duration; therefore, strong contraction as with motor TENS may not be possible. Check to see if your HVS has an adjustable duty cycle. If not, then the HVS cannot be used for NMES since there is no way to impose a rest time or duty cycle. The pulse frequency should be dependent on the goal of the treatment (sensory or motor TENS, muscle pumping or muscle contraction). If the HVS is to be used in a water bath, ensure that ground fault circuit interrupters are in good working order.

From the evaluation, determine whether a monopolar or bipolar electrode configuration is indicated and set up the electrodes. Make sure the dispersive pad is not causing trans-thoracic current.

Increase the amplitude to get the desired response (depending on the treatment goal—sensory or motor response). The HVS has a short phase duration, and the sensory nerves accommodate quickly to this stimulus. The amplitude may have to be increased periodically during the treatment. When the treatment time has ended, turn the amplitude back to zero and disconnect the electrodes. Evaluate the treatment response and inspect the skin. Return all electrodes and power down the stimulator.

IONTOPHORESIS

As discussed in chapter 7, there are two major classifications of waveforms: monophasic and biphasic. Biphasic waveforms have no polarity effects. Monophasic waveforms are polar since one electrode is positive and the other is negative. If the phase duration is short, as with an HVS, the polar effects are minimal and there are no physiochemical effects under either electrode.

Direct current, also known as galvanic current, has a long phase duration (at least 1 s), has strong polar effects, and is capable of changing the pH under the electrodes, creating a physiochemical effect. One electrode is always positive (the anode), and one electrode is always negative (cathode). Certain physiochemical effects occur in the tissues under each electrode (see figure 8.10, figure 8.11, and table 8.2).

Iontophoresis is the process in which ions in solution are transferred through the intact skin via an electrical potential. It is based on the electrical principle that like charges are repelled. Therefore, the ions in solution (of similar charge) migrate away from the electrical source into the body. Iontophoresis is a noninvasive method of introducing drugs locally (table 8.3). Iontophoresis has been shown to be effective in clinical trials (Gulick et al. 2000), but there are many negative and inconclusive reports (Runeson and Haker 2002; Smutok et al. 2002; Gudeman et al. 1997). Furthermore, you should check state practice acts before administering iontophoresis. Some states, such as Virginia, consider iontophoresis the application of a prescription medication. Therefore only physicians can apply

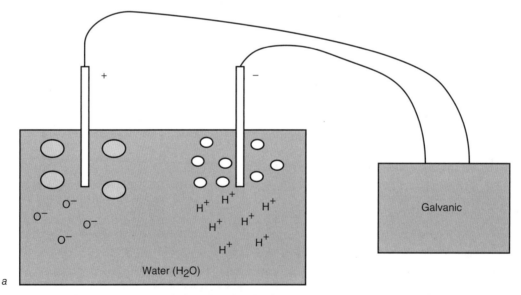

Figure 8.10 *(a)* Place each level of a galvanic stimulator into a container of water. Turn on the current and note the development of many small bubbles at the *negative* electrode (hydrogen ions) and the development of a few larger bubbles at the *positive* electrode (oxygen ions). *(continued)*

Table 8.2 Polarity Effects With Galvanic Stimulation

Positive	Negative
Attracts acids	Attracts alkali
Repels alkali	Repels acids
Hardens tissue	Softens tissue
Contracts tissue	Dilates tissue
Stops hemorrhage	Increases hemorrhage
Diminishes congestion	Increases congestion
Sedating	Stimulating
Relieves pain in acute conditions by reducing congestion	Reduces pain in chronic conditions because of softening effect
Scars formed are hard and firm	Scars are soft and pliable

Table 8.3 Pathology and Recommended Ions Used With Iontophoresis

Condition	Medication	Polarity
Pain and inflammation	Salicylate	−
	Hydrocortisone	+
	Lidocaine	+
	Dexamethasone	−
Calcium deposits	Acetic acid	−
Fungi	Copper	+
Adhesions	Chlorine	−
Edema	Magnesium sulfate	+
Spasms	Magnesium sulfate	+

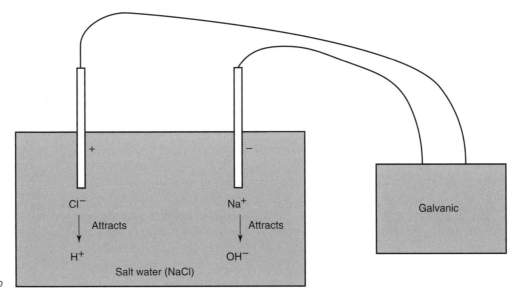

b

Figure 8.10 *(continued)* *(b)* Place each lead into a container of salt water. The salt water dissociates in water into Na^+ and Cl^- ions. The Cl^- is attracted to the positive electrode, which forms hydrochloric acid (HCl). The Na^+ is attracted to the negative electrode, which forms NaOH, a strong base. This is similar to what happens in the body.

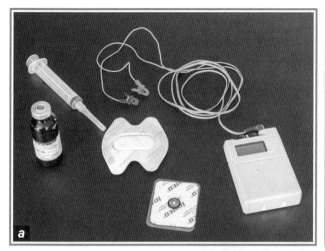
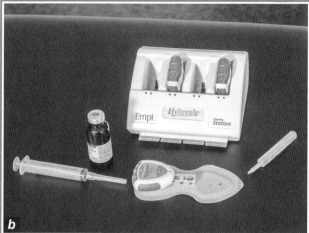
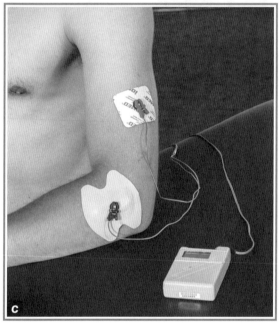
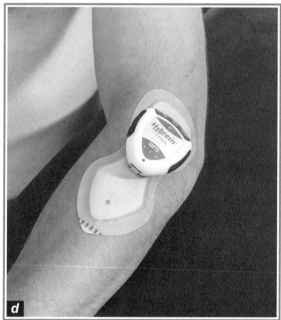

Figure 8.11   *(a)* and *(b)* Commercially available iontophoresis devices. *(c)* Application of battery operated unit with active electrode over lateral epicondyle and a dispersive electrode on the upper arm. *(d)* Application of a rechargeable battery unit with active and dispersive electrodes on the lateral elbow.

the device unless the treatment is delivered in an inpatient hospital setting. Pennsylvania requires a physician prescription for the medication, which the patient is responsible for obtaining. The treatment may be applied by an athletic trainer or physical therapist.

A DC generator is required for iontophoresis. Other monophasic stimulators have short phase durations, and the current does not flow long enough to cause physiochemical changes or a driving effect.

Commercially produced units make the application of iontophoresis very easy. The medication is placed into a specially made electrode and applied

at the treatment site. Some units have a feature to alter the duration of the treatment depending on the intensity of current used. The clinician sets the milliamp-minutes on this type of unit to keep dosage as consistent as possible.

The most common application of iontophoresis in sport rehabilitation is the use of dexamethasone to suppress inflammation, although there are no well-defined guidelines for such a treatment approach. The relationship between tissue repair and inflammation was emphasized in chapter 3, where it was pointed out that suppressing inflammation during tissue healing may be inappropriate.

In chronic inflammatory conditions, small amounts of **necrotic** tissue sometimes cause persistent pain that fails to respond to rest and other treatment interventions. For example, with age, the vascularity of tendon declines, which may compromise the body's ability to phagocytize necrotic tissues. In these circumstances there is empirical evidence that an injectable or iontophoresed steroidal anti-inflammatory medication can break a cycle of irritation and pain. These treatments can relieve symptoms for months or even permanently.

Lidocaine can be used to anesthetize a small area of skin and underlying tissues. The injection of lidocaine or other anesthetics into trigger points can be effective in managing myofascial pain syndromes. Iontophoresis offers a means of delivering the medication without needles. However, the treatment of multiple trigger points with iontophoresis would be extremely time-consuming.

At one time it was common to mix lidocaine and dexamethasone for iontophoresis to buffer the solution and thus minimize skin irritation. Iontophoresis must be conducted with water-soluble medications, but a direct current passing through water causes hydrolysis, lowering the pH of the drug solution. When lidocaine is used to buffer the free hydrogen ions, less change in pH occurs. Unfortunately, this practice also diminishes the delivery of dexamethasone into the tissues (figure 8.12). The use of buffered electrodes, which were marketed in the 1990s, minimizes the risk of skin irritation.

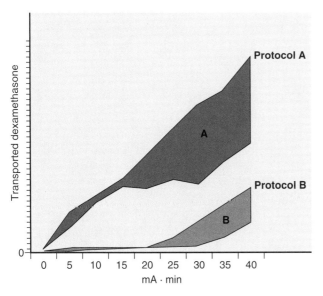

Figure 8.12 Dexamethasone delivery is enhanced by using a buffered electrode (protocol A) instead of a lidocaine-dexamethasone mixture (protocol B).

Effects of pH Buffering on Drug Delivery Iontophoresis

Iontophoresis must be conducted using water-soluble drugs. However, a direct current passing through an aqueous solution causes the hydrolysis of water, thus creating potentially harmful changes in the pH of the drug solution.

OH^- raises pH.

H^+ lowers pH.

Because the most commonly used drug in iontophoresis is the negatively charged dexamethasone sodium phosphate, a potential problem is the accumulation of hydroxide ions, which are also negatively charged. If allowed to accumulate, they will be driven into the skin along with the drug ions. Depending on the length of the treatment, this can result in alkaline burns at the skin surface. Fortunately, there are ways to prevent these potentially dangerous pH changes. The method most often used in delivering dexamethasone sodium phosphate involves mixing the drug with lidocaine hydrochloride. When the two substances are mixed and iontophoresis is performed, the following electrochemical reactions occur:

$$DexPO_4-2 + 2Na^+ + OH^- + H^+ \; LidoH^+ + Cl^-$$

Thus, there is no longer a need to mix lidocaine and dexamethasone.

An additional consideration with iontophoresis, which parallels concerns raised for phonophoresis, is the inability to precisely quantify the amount of medication delivered into the tissues. Continued investigation of the techniques is needed to identify effective treatment protocols.

Treatment Procedures

Since the purpose of iontophoresis is to introduce a medication, a physician should prescribe the treatment. Even topically applied steroids can have a systemic effect; therefore the administration of pharmaceutical agents should be monitored by a physician.

The electrical stimulators used in athletic training for iontophoresis deliver DC. The substance to be driven into the tissue must carry an electrical charge in solution. The solution is placed in a treatment electrode that is buffered to minimize skin irritation.

The maximum current delivered by the stimulator is 5 mA. Because DC is used, waveform duty cycle, frequency, phase duration, and ramp cannot be adjusted, and the only parameters of concern are polarity and dosage. The polarity of the treatment electrode should be the same as that of the ion to be driven into the tissue, because like charges repel. The unit of iontophoresis dosage is milliamperes multiplied by minutes (mA·min). With buffered electrodes, the maximum dosage is 80 mA·min. Theoretically, the higher the dosage, the greater the amount of medication driven into the tissues. The dosage is determined by the amplitude of current that produces a comfortable sensory stimulation multiplied by the length of the treatment. For example, if a 3 mA peak current produces a comfortable stimulation and the current is applied for 25 min, the dosage is 75 mA·min. DC current can cause skin irritation, and feedback from the recipient is essential for a safe treatment. Recent studies have investigated the manipulation of the current amplitude and time of stimulation on iontophoresis outcomes. The high amplitude with a short duration was similar to a low-amplitude, long-duration treatment (Saliba et al. 2011) and higher doses (80 mA·min) compared to lower doses (40 mA·min) had similar results (Glaviano et al. 2011). These results reiterate that the application of modalities help to stimulate tissues and that more is not necessarily better.

Safety

Safe application of iontophoresis requires proper equipment and clinical judgment. Iontophoresis carries all of the cautions and contraindications of TENS. In addition, medications to which the patient is allergic contraindicate iontophoresis. Even with modern electrodes designed for iontophoresis, skin irritation and chemical burns are possible. Instruct patients to report any sensation of burning, and if they do so, interrupt the treatment and inspect the skin. Ice should not be used before iontophoresis since it may diminish the patient's ability to perceive the sensory response to the stimulation. Stop treatment if you have any concern that burning may be occurring. Some people, especially fair-skinned people, are very sensitive and cannot be treated with iontophoresis.

Although homemade electrodes and DC generators have been used for iontophoresis, it is strongly recommended that you use commercial stimulators and electrodes designed specifically for iontophoresis to protect the patient as well as yourself. Proper equipment reduces the risk of skin injury substantially.

MICROCURRENT ELECTRICAL NERVE STIMULATOR FOR WOUND HEALING

Microcurrent is a form of electrotherapy in which the stimulus amplitude is in the microamperage (millionth of an ampere) range. Microcurrent stimulators have been referred to as microcurrent electrical nerve stimulators (MENS) and low-intensity stimulators (LIS). MENS is a poor name because the peak amplitude generated is usually below the rheobase of even A-beta afferent fibers. Thus, the electrical current does not result in nerve depolarization. Moreover, the theoretical basis underlying the application of microcurrent does not involve nerve fiber depolarization.

A substantial body of evidence shows that electrical stimulation has physiological effects that are not related to nerve fiber depolarization. Electrical stimulation has been shown to speed repair in slow-healing surface wounds such as decubitus ulcers in humans (Barron, Jacobson, and Tidd 1985; Houghton et al. 2003). Enhanced repair in deeper tissue has been reported in animal models with the use of indwelling electrodes (Akai et al. 1988; Nessler and Mass 1987; Litke and Dahners 1994; Owoeye et al. 1987). Exciting work on the effects of microcurrent on edema formation in the acute inflammatory phase is ongoing; however, this work is limited to animal models.

There is also great interest in the use of pulsed ultrasound and pulsed electromagnetic fields to facilitate the healing of nonunion and slow-healing fractures. The effects of these stimulators are discussed in chapter 9.

Although the effects and potential benefits of microcurrent stimulation warrant continued investigation, the work completed so far has limitations. There is no evidence that using electrical stimulation facilitates the normal repair response in healthy humans. Whether microcurrent should be used to treat musculoskeletal injuries sustained by physically active people has yet to be determined.

Table 8.4 Indications and Contraindications for Electrotherapy

	Indications	Contraindications
TENS neuromuscular stimulation	Pain control Restore neuromuscular control Retard atrophy	Electrode placement over carotid artery Cardiac pacemaker (unless approved by MD; monitoring may be necessary) Pregnancy
Iontophoresis	With dexamethasone: chronic inflammation With lidocaine: local anesthesia	Electrode placement over carotid artery Cardiac pacemaker (unless approved by MD; monitoring may be necessary) Pregnancy Medications to which individual is allergic or hypersensitive
Stimulation of denervated tissues	Lower motor neuron lesion	Same as for TENS
Microcurrent	Slow-healing wounds Inflammatory conditions	Same as for TENS

There is some testimonial evidence of the benefits of microcurrent in the treatment of these injuries; however, controlled investigations using delayed-onset muscle soreness as a model for musculoskeletal injury suggest that microcurrent may relieve pain but does not speed recovery (Denegar et al. 1992). Some reports even question the pain-relieving effects of microcurrent (Lerner and Kirsch 1981; Weber et al. 1994). The subsensory effects of microcurrent may influence the peripheral mechanisms of the inflammatory and pain processes.

Where does the evidence leave the certified athletic trainer who must decide whether to apply microcurrent? At this time, the only application of microcurrent shown to be effective is in the treatment of slow-healing skin lesions, a condition that a certified athletic trainer is not prepared to treat. The prospects for other uses of microcurrent will depend on future research findings. Clearly, electricity can alter tissue responses. However, research based on animal models and the use of indwelling electrodes does not provide answers about using surface electrode stimulation in humans to facilitate deep tissue repair or alter capillary membrane permeability to minimize swelling.

Microcurrent stimulation is safe, although the cautions identified for TENS should be observed. The major challenge is developing a theoretical basis and substantiating the clinical efficacy of microcurrent in the treatment of musculoskeletal injuries. Throughout your career you should continue to review the research literature and critically assess whether there is enough evidence to warrant the application of any modality, including microcurrent stimulation. Table 8.4 summarizes the indications and contraindications for the forms of electrotherapy discussed in this chapter.

SUMMARY

This chapter addresses the clinical uses of electrical stimulation for pain and inflammation. The relationship between the waveform, stimulus parameters, and treatment goals is presented to help the clinician apply electrotherapy effectively while appreciating that in some cases differing units and waveforms yield the same physiological responses. For clinical purposes, the relationship between stimulus parameters and theories of pain modulation introduced in chapter 6 is discussed in detail, as are the parameters necessary for effective NMES. Applications of galvanic (direct) current for iontophoresis and microcurrent electrical stimulation are also presented. Safety and the identification of contraindications to the application of electrotherapy are emphasized.

1. *Understand the clinical uses for electrical stimulation in the rehabilitation process.*

Electrical stimulation has many clinical uses, including pain modulation, neuromuscular facilitation, and wound healing. An athletic trainer can use various commercial stimulators to complement the rehabilitation process. Electrical stimulation helps to reduce pain, making therapeutic exercise and daily activities more comfortable. The stimulation can also be modified to encourage muscle reeducation. When the muscle activity is facilitated, active exercise can be directed to assist the return to function.

2. *Analyze the waveform of the available device and determine whether the treatment goal can be met using that stimulator.*

There are many stimulators on the market. Many new machines offer programmed treatment parameters, making treatment selection as easy as pushing a button. However, the athletic trainer should understand the functions of the preprogrammed treatments with respect to waveform, amplitude, phase duration, and frequency. Understanding how the electrical configuration can be changed to target different tissue types is essential in understanding therapeutic modalities. The athletic trainer should be able to differentiate waveforms, types of stimulators, and methods of application used in electrical stimulation treatment.

3. *Incorporate theories of pain modulation with the principles of electrical stimulation to determine the amplitude, phase duration, and pulse frequency needed for a variety of clinical purposes.*

Theories of pain modulation were reviewed in chapter 6. Electrical stimulation can be varied to target different nerve fiber types to maximize the analgesia addressed by each of the theories of pain modulation: sensory, noxious, and motor. The phase duration, amplitude, and frequency can be adjusted to target the A-beta, C, and A-delta fibers to apply these theories clinically.

4. *Understand the use of microcurrent electrical stimulation.*

Microcurrent electrical stimulation uses subsensory stimulation to promote wound healing. There are various suggestions regarding the waveforms, phase duration, frequency, and amplitude to maximize the results.

5. *Identify contraindications for the application of electrotherapy.*

Electrical stimulation should not be used during pregnancy, on a patient with a cardiac pacemaker, or over the carotid sinus in the neck. Caution should be exercised with the use of stimulators with high phase charges such as galvanic stimulators. Additionally, the electrical stimulation should not be placed so that it goes through the chest.

Arthrogenic Muscle Inhibition and Clinical Applications of Electrical Stimulation and Biofeedback

OBJECTIVES

After reading this chapter, you will be able to

❶ identify the three components of neuromuscular control;

❷ differentiate between neuromuscular control deficits and muscle atrophy as causes of muscular weakness;

❸ discuss the effects of swelling, pain, and altered mechanoreceptor input on neuromuscular control and arthrogenic muscle inhibition at the knee, ankle, hip, and shoulder;

❹ describe the clinical uses for neuromuscular electrical stimulation, including Russian stimulation, in the rehabilitation process;

❺ describe the uses of a galvanic stimulator;

❻ define *biofeedback*;

❼ describe the application of EMG biofeedback in the treatment of impaired neuromuscular control;

❽ describe the instrumentation and signal processing related to EMG biofeedback;

❾ describe the use of biofeedback in relaxation training; and

❿ identify contraindications for the application of electrotherapy.

A downhill ski racer has had multiple knee injuries with subsequent surgical procedures. She presents to the clinic with moderate pain on the medial joint line and has some quadriceps weakness. There is no apparent effusion, but she has some early osteoarthritic changes due to the traumatic injuries that she has sustained. A thorough evaluation reveals quadriceps dysfunction on the involved limb with a central activation ratio of 85%, and reduced hip and knee flexion moments compared to the contralateral limb. How can we modify the neuromuscular factors of joint injury? She trains specifically with an ACL prevention program in addition to core and overall strength training, but would adjunctive therapy with electrical stimulation enhance her outcome?

This case study illustrates that injury, pain, swelling, and joint instability can impair neuromuscular control. Clinicians caring for patients with musculoskeletal injuries must be able to detect and address deficits in neuromuscular control through a progressive rehabilitation plan. Deficits in strength and power (rate of force development) limit function, slow progression to sport-specific retraining, and likely increase the risk of recurrent and new injuries upon return to competition.

Part II of this text introduced the inflammatory response and tissue repair processes, acute pain, and lasting pain. This chapter combines an introduction to neuromuscular control and **arthrogenic muscle inhibition** with the use of neuromuscular electrical nerve stimulation (NMES) and electromyographic (EMG) biofeedback for the treatment of strength impairments. The concepts of biofeedback are expanded to address control over muscle relaxation. Neuromuscular control is a broad concept that incorporates the integration of sensory input and motor recruitment in performing physical tasks. Neuromuscular control can be compromised following injury. When the ability to recruit strong, coordinated muscle contraction is compromised by joint injury, the problem is called arthrogenic (caused by a joint) muscle inhibition, or AMI. This chapter identifies the causes of impaired neuromuscular control and more specifically AMI following injury, and it introduces basic concepts of neuromuscular reeducation. Techniques to restore neuromuscular control through neuromuscular electrical stimulation and biofeedback are then presented.

Six components of a progressive rehabilitation program were identified in chapter 1 (see figure 1.5). Therapeutic modalities are commonly applied to control pain and interrupt the pain–spasm cycle. Pain control and appropriate postinjury care to minimize swelling will help restore range of motion. The next priority in rehabilitation is to return neuromuscular control, the last component of the rehabilitation program affected by modality application (figure 9.1).

INTEGRATION OF COMPONENTS OF NEUROMUSCULAR CONTROL INTO A REHABILITATION PLAN

Restoration of control over volitional contractions, reflex reactions, and complex functional movements was identified in chapter 1 as part of a progressive rehabilitation plan of care. These components encompass the continuum of neuromuscular control. By recognizing that neuromuscular control consists of three components, clinicians can integrate activities to restore neuromuscular control

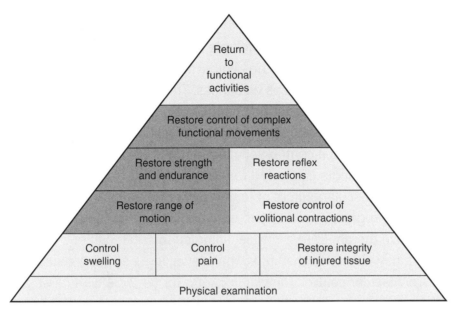

Figure 9.1 Hierarchy of rehabilitation goals.

Reprinted, by permission, from J. Hertel and C.R. Denegar, 1998, "A rehabilitation paradigm for restoring neuromuscular control following athletics injury," *Athletic Therapy Today* 3(5): 13.

throughout the plan of care (figure 9.2). AMI of the peroneal muscles is observed in the loss of ability to balance on the affected leg or in the loss of ability to hop and gain single-leg balance. This loss of balance performance is sometimes attributed to impaired proprioception. However, proprioception is really the afferent component of neuromuscular control. Furthermore, in tasks such as balancing, the person's ability to recruit skeletal muscle to maintain stance is based on sensory input from mechanoreceptors, Golgi tendon organs, and muscle spindles. Thus, these assessments really measure neuromuscular control rather than parse out true proprioception.

The final component of neuromuscular control relates to complex functional movements. When one becomes proficient in athletics, complex integration of afferent input is required to precisely control movement through efferent pathways. Conscious effort is absent once the movement begins. For example, when learning to play golf, the player is consciously aware of each movement. As the player becomes proficient, he or she executes the swing without conscious control. However, injury can disrupt the ability to perform well-practiced functional movement patterns. The person who cannot perform a straight leg raise will also demonstrate abnormal stair climbing patterns and running gait, indicating disrupted neuromuscular control of functional and sport-specific movements. Sport-specific movements also require that muscle develop force

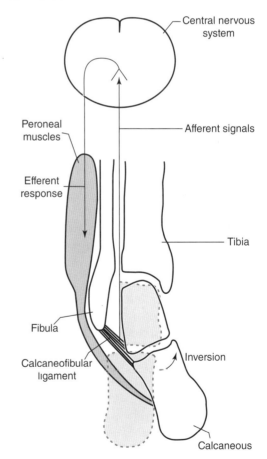

Figure 9.2 Reflex circuits.

Reprinted, by permission, from Human Kinetics, 2000, *Progressive rehabilitation of lower extremity sport injury* (Champaign, IL: Human Kinetics), 52.

Neuromuscular Control and Muscle Atrophy

Muscles generate force when motor nerves send impulses to the muscle fibers they innervate. The more muscle fibers stimulated to contract, the more force is generated. The cross section of muscles also influences the amount of force they can generate. When muscle is not used for a period of time, the cross section diminishes, or atrophies, which is a relatively slow process. When the ability to recruit muscle fiber contraction in a coordinated manner is impaired, neuromuscular control has been lost, a process that can occur quickly.

Thus, a loss of neuromuscular control should not be confused with muscle atrophy. Several weeks of muscle disuse, such as immobilization in a cast, will result in atrophy as well as loss of neuromuscular control. Fortunately, the importance of early motion after musculoskeletal injury is widely recognized, and prolonged immobilization is used only when absolutely necessary.

rapidly. Thus there is more to restoring neuromuscular control than improving the force developed by muscle. If the rate of force development is slowed, the athlete or worker may be unable to dynamically stabilize and protect a joint from injury.

WHY IS NEUROMUSCULAR CONTROL LOST?

The case study at the beginning of this chapter provides a clinical example of lost neuromuscular control due to knee injuries, which is defined as AMI. Inhibition of quadriceps function after knee injury is commonly encountered in clinical practice. The relationship between knee injury and neuromuscular control of the quadriceps has received considerable attention in medical literature. However, much more study is needed for us to fully understand the impact of musculoskeletal injury on neuromuscular control and refine therapeutic approaches to restoring it.

Clinical observations and scientific investigations suggest that more than one factor contributes to decreased neuromuscular control after musculoskeletal injury. This chapter explores the impact of swelling, pain, and altered mechanoreceptor input on the ability to consciously perform volitional muscle contractions. Mechanoreceptor input is often altered when the ligaments and the capsule protecting a joint are sprained and the joint becomes unstable. As discussed in chapter 5, pain and swelling are associated with acute inflammation. Furthermore, as discussed in chapter 6, pain may occur in the absence of inflammation. In any case, these factors contribute individually and collectively to impaired neuromuscular control.

Activities to restore pattern-generated movements and reflexive muscle contractions usually do not involve therapeutic modalities. However, volitional control over isolated muscles, such as that which occurs when a straight leg raise is used to recruit the quadriceps, or when controlled functional motions such as bending and stair climbing are initiated, can be restored by the application of therapeutic modalities. Furthermore, conscious control of muscle must be restored before reflex patterns and more complex movement patterns can be retrained. Thus, rehabilitation often requires identifying and correcting deficits in volitional control over skeletal muscles.

Swelling

Swelling within the joint capsule of the knee decreases quadriceps function. Clinicians often observe this phenomenon after knee injury, and researchers have studied it. By infusing saline solution into the knee, researchers have been able to inhibit quadriceps function as measured through electromyography (EMG) (Kennedy, Alexander, and Hayes 1982; Spencer, Hayes, and Alexander 1984). Vastus medialis activity can be inhibited by as little as 30 ml of fluid. This small increase in fluid volume would appear as very mild effusion on clinical exam. Larger increases in volume affect the function of the other quadriceps muscles. A 200 ml increase can severely limit the ability to perform a straight leg raise even in the absence of knee injury. Neuromuscular inhibition appears to persist as long as joint capsule volume remains elevated.

The reason joint effusion inhibits quadriceps femoris function is not fully understood. However, much of the knee joint capsule is innervated by articular branches of the femoral nerve (figure 9.3). In particular, the articular branch of the femoral nerve to the vastus medialis supplies a large portion of the anteromedial joint capsule. Swelling within the cap-

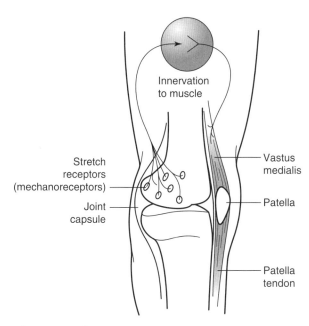

Figure 9.3 Swelling within the capsule may stimulate stretch receptors, which in turn trigger reflex inhibition of the motor neuron pool.

Innervation to muscle

Stretch receptors (mechanoreceptors)

Joint capsule

Vastus medialis

Patella

Patella tendon

sule may stimulate stretch receptors, which in turn trigger reflex inhibition of the motor neuron pool. The suprapatellar pouch accommodates increases in joint fluid volume more than do other parts of the joint capsule. The tendency of fluid to accumulate in this area of the knee may partially explain why the vastus medialis is most affected by swelling within the knee joint.

Tsang (2001) found that the infusion of saline into the joint capsule of the ankle impaired postural control and inhibited recruitment of the peroneal musculature. His results suggested that the phenomenon of swelling-induced loss of neuromuscular control is not isolated to the knee joint. The impact of extracapsular swelling on measures of neuromuscular control has not been examined in a laboratory model and warrants investigation.

Pain

Pain also appears to affect neuromuscular control. Athletes who injure a lower extremity often limp to protect damaged tissue and minimize pain. The altered movement patterns represent changes in neuromuscular control. Could the observed gait deviation be due to swelling and altered mechanoreceptor input? Perhaps, but careful observation suggests that pain contributes to deficits in neuromuscular control. Athletes with little or no swelling

and no history of trauma may exhibit decreased neuromuscular control.

For example, some individuals with patellofemoral pain (PFP) experience little or no swelling. The connective tissues housing mechanoreceptors have not been damaged, nor are these receptors stimulated due to swelling. However, if you ask the person with PFP to tighten the quadriceps muscle and you palpate the vastus medialis, it will feel softer than the fully tightened quadriceps of the uninjured leg (figure 9.4) because the person cannot effectively recruit the vastus medialis. Similarly, AMI is observed in patients with osteoarthritis in their knees. Many have no history of trauma that would damage sensory receptors. Even in the absence of measurable effusion, these patients report pain and demonstrate AMI.

Observations such as these support the notion that pain uniquely contributes to the loss of neuromuscular control. Unfortunately, it is difficult to isolate the impact of joint pain on neuromuscular control in research. Ethical and methodological considerations do not permit researchers to induce joint pain in the way that swelling can be safely induced to study AMI. However, there is evidence that pain-relieving modalities (focal cold application or transcutaneous electrical nerve stimulation) disinhibit the quadriceps in patients with knee osteoarthritis

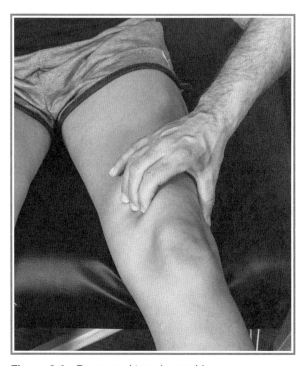

Figure 9.4 Decreased tone in quadriceps.

(Pietrosimone et al. 2009). Thus, research and clinical observations provide evidence that pain, even in the absence of swelling and joint instability, can alter neuromuscular control.

Despite the limited research evidence, clinical observation offers insights into successful clinical practice. The first such insight relates to the discussion of PFP. When knee pain inhibits the function of the vastus medialis, patellar mobility increases. With greater patellar mobility, there is more irritation of the joint tissues and more pain. Thus, a cycle is created that gradually turns into patellofemoral pain syndrome. With sufficient irritation, swelling will also develop, further compromising neuromuscular control and exacerbating the cycle.

This phenomenon explains why some athletes who present with the signs and symptoms of patellofemoral pain syndrome have no history of knee injury. Other factors (such as changes in training routine) and biomechanical problems (such as subtalar hyperpronation and genu varus) clearly are contributors. However, these factors do not explain the loss of neuromuscular control of the quadriceps. Thus, it appears that pain decreases neuromuscular control.

The role of pain in the loss of neuromuscular control is an important consideration during therapeutic exercise. When active exercise is painful, normal neuromuscular patterning is disrupted. Painful exercise inhibits muscle groups, perpetuates abnormal motor control, and slows recovery from injury. With the exception of passive stretching of muscle and connective tissue, therapeutic exercise must remain pain free if neuromuscular control is to be reestablished and maintained.

Altered Input

The proprioceptors in the skin, muscles, tendons, and joints provide the central nervous system (CNS) with a constant flow of **somatosensory information**. The CNS responds by generating appropriate motor commands to allow the body to move safely through a changing environment.

Instability at the knee results in AMI. A systematic review by Hart et al. (2010) revealed evidence of AMI in anterior cruciate ligament (ACL)–deficient as well as reconstructed knees. Researchers studying quadriceps musculature in patients with ACL-deficient knees found 10% to 30% decreases in pain-free isokinetic force production despite minor atrophy and little morphological change (Lorentzon et al. 1993). The inhibition of the quadriceps muscles is accompanied by facilitation of the hamstring muscles (Solomonow et al. 1987). While these changes in recruitment may serve to minimize anterior translation of the tibia, the loss of quadriceps function affects movement quality and may leave the knee vulnerable to reinjury upon return to sport and recreational activities. A previous injury to the ACL is a recognized risk for a new injury or reinjury.

Similarly, a history of an ankle sprain is a strong risk factor for ankle injury. The role of AMI has yet to be fully explored. When the ankle is inverted toward the limits of the range of motion, afferent input is generated in three ways: The mechanoreceptors within the ligaments and joint capsule alert the CNS to the precarious position of the ankle; muscle spindles within the muscles that evert the ankle (peroneus longus and brevis) signal that the muscle is rapidly stretching; and skin receptors signal the distortion and stretch of the skin over the lateral ankle. The CNS processes these afferent signals and responds by activating the motor pathways that cause the everters to contract and by inhibiting motor activity in the antagonistic muscles to counteract the sudden inversion of the ankle. Thus, the proprioceptors sense the potential for ankle joint injury, and the CNS responds through a dorsal horn synaptic reflex loop to prevent joint injury.

The sensory input from mechanoreceptors can trigger muscle contractions through the spinal reflex loops. Moreover, the continuous flow of sensory input from mechanoreceptors is essential to the performance of coordinated movements. Mechanoreceptors are most active at the anatomical limits of the physiological range of motion. Damage to ligaments and joint capsules alters mechanoreceptor input in the damaged tissue and subsequently affects neuromuscular control. Swelling that limits full range of motion also alters mechanoreceptor activity. These changes in the pattern of sensory input from mechanoreceptors decrease neuromuscular control.

The evidence suggests that changes in neuromuscular control persist after pain and swelling have resolved. Much of our understanding of the impact of swelling and pain on neuromuscular control has come from the study of knee injury. However, changes in kinesthetic awareness and slowed reflex contractions have been observed after injury to other joints.

Ankle Injuries

It is clear that neuromuscular control is lost after sprains of the lateral ligaments of the ankle. Researchers have reported deficits in position sense (Freeman 1965) and balance in single-leg stance (Gross 1987) and postural control (Docherty et al. 2006). In addition, the response of the peroneal muscles is slowed after ankle sprain (Lofvenberg et al. 1995). One of the goals of treatment after an ankle sprain is to restore neuromuscular control of the muscles surrounding the ankle. This is accomplished through a return to pain-free weight bearing as early as possible, depending on the severity of the injury, and a progressive program of balance and coordination exercises (Hale, Hertel, and Olmsted-Kramer 2007) (figure 9.5). Balance and neuromuscular retraining improves function in patients with chronic ankle instability (McKeon et al. 2008; Lee and Lin 2008). Research into the effects of balance training on the incidence of reinjury is ongoing (Janssen et al. 2011). Given the high incidence of reinjury and the increasing recognition of a link between ankle injury and osteoarthritis, we need to continue our efforts to understand ankle injury and AMI and to prevent reinjury.

Hip Injuries and Arthritis

The influence of hip injury, femoral-acetabular impingement, and osteoarthritis on neuromuscular control has received relatively little research attention. Clinical observation suggests that some patients with hip pain and arthritis demonstrate inhibition of the powerful gluteus maximus muscle. Freeman, Mascia, and McGill (2013) reported that patients undergoing **MRI arthrograms** due to hip-related conditions experienced inhibition of the gluteus maximus during functional tasks, including supine bridge exercises. These data suggest that the gluteal muscles respond to hip pain and swelling in a manner similar to quadriceps AMI in the presence of knee pain and swelling. Given the prevalence of hip osteoarthritis and the role of the gluteal muscles in

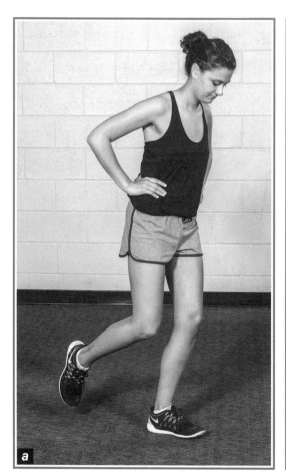
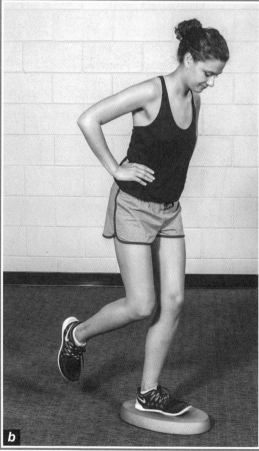

Figure 9.5   An example of balance and coordination exercises: *(a)* single-leg balance and *(b)* single-leg balance on foam.

such tasks as rising from a chair and climbing steps, as well as protection from falling, further investigation into the treatment of hip-related AMI is needed.

Shoulder Injuries and the Low Back

Pain, disruption in ligamentous stability, and swelling appear to inhibit the rotator cuff, especially in the supraspinatus and perhaps the scapular stabilizers. The stabilizing function of these two muscle groups is essential for normal, pain-free shoulder function. For many years, people with rotator cuff tendinitis and glenohumeral impingement were treated with rotator cuff strengthening exercises. Some improved rapidly, whereas others improved very slowly. Closer examination of those who failed to respond to rotator cuff strengthening revealed that many demonstrated impaired neuromuscular control of the rotator cuff, the scapular stabilizers, or both (figure 9.6).

Injury to the ligaments and capsule of the glenohumeral joint compromises the sense of shoulder positioning and movement detection. Clinically these injuries compromise the athlete's ability to keep the shoulder out of positions likely to cause dislocation and further injury.

Training with visual and EMG biofeedback addresses neuromuscular control deficits and speeds recovery. Pain, instability, and swelling appear to affect the shoulder muscles in much the same manner as occurs with the quadriceps after knee injury. Strengthening alone does not relieve shoulder

pain or promote recovery after shoulder dislocation. The injured person must relearn proper control of the glenohumeral and scapular stabilizers—in other words, reestablish neuromuscular control.

The impact of swelling, pain, and instability in other joints on neuromuscular control warrants further study. Certainly, there is a component of neuromuscular retraining after any injury; however, it may be more easily accomplished in some parts of the body than in others. One area receiving greater attention is the low back, where pain may alter the neuromuscular function of paraspinal muscles. This loss of neuromuscular control is a significant challenge in treating a physically active person with a history of back injury and pain.

ROLE OF THERAPEUTIC MODALITIES IN RESTORING NEUROMUSCULAR CONTROL

Neuromuscular electrical stimulation and EMG biofeedback are the modalities most commonly used to help patients regain volitional control of muscle contraction. There are no direct modality applications for retraining protective reflex responses or control of complex movements. However, several therapeutic modalities may be used to permit pain-free exercises aimed at restoring these components

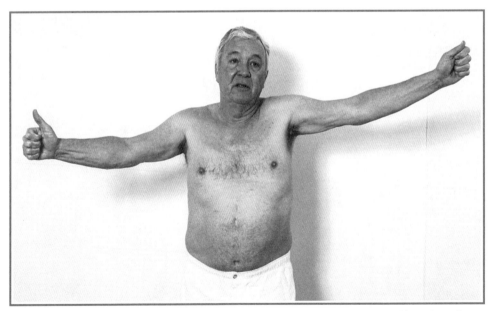

Figure 9.6 Shoulder hiking in an effort to abduct the arm is a common manifestation of impaired neuromuscular control.

of neuromuscular control. When rehabilitation is viewed as a hierarchy of goals and modalities are used to achieve specific goals, the relationship between modality application and efforts to restore neuromuscular control becomes evident.

Muscle function is initiated with electrical impulses from the alpha motor nerve. Muscular function is associated with the nervous system on multiple levels. Information from the sensory system—from the skin, fascia, muscle, and joints—can have profound effects on the function of the muscular system. Likewise, cognitive and higher centers affect the muscle in both inhibitory and excitatory fashion. People with neuromuscular diseases or who have had brain injuries have lower levels of inhibition that ultimately reduce voluntary control and produce spasticity. We need inhibition of muscle tone for normal muscle function. However, following an injury, our efforts are often directed to minimizing inhibition so that pre-injury strength returns.

Because of the electrical control of muscle, a contraction can be induced with electrical stimulation. When the motor nerve is intact, the stimulation will be via the alpha motor nerve. This phenomenon is an example of the law of Dubois Reymond. The alpha motor nerve is a large-diameter (low capacitance) fiber and is easily stimulated. These nerves are generally deeper than the sensory nerves that supply the skin; therefore the patient will perceive the sensation first, and then as the intensity is increased, a muscle contraction will be produced. Generally, longer phase durations (>250 μs) are used to stimulate the muscle in this manner despite the low threshold. If the nerve is not present, then stimulation may occur at the motor endplate. The muscle cells have a resting threshold similar to nerves, but the capacitance is very high. A phase duration of at least 300 ms is required to stimulate the muscle directly. Only galvanic (DC) stimulators are configured to have such long phase durations.

Both types of muscle stimulation will be addressed in this chapter. Most commonly, neuromuscular electrical stimulation is used for muscle reeducation and to promote or enhance muscle function. This type of stimulation can be used on patients with spinal cord injury since the peripheral nerve is intact (it is just not connected to the brain). Various methods are used in rehabilitation or to replace a nonfunctional muscle. Electrical stimulation for **denervated** muscle will also be discussed.

MUSCLE REEDUCATION

Electrical stimulation can be used clinically to help to retrain the neuromuscular function that is lost due to AMI after injury or surgery. The muscles "shut down" in order to protect the joint, but this inhibition must be overcome to allow controlled rehabilitation. One mechanism to help retrain the muscle function is with neuromuscular electrical stimulation. The treatment is still TENS by definition, but the goal of the treatment is to elicit a strong muscle contraction through stimulation of the alpha motor nerve. The injured person is taught to contract the muscle with the stimulation to overcome the natural inhibition. This use of electrical stimulation is termed neuromuscular electrical stimulation or NMES because the goal is to retrain the neuromuscular component to achieve an improved ability to produce muscle force.

NMES was originally developed to increase the strength of muscles in trained athletes. Kots (1977) claimed that NMES combined with intense training resulted in greater strength gains than training alone. However, there is little evidence that NMES is any more beneficial than volitional isometric contractions in building strength. In fact, because isometric strength gains are position specific, NMES is less effective than resistance through the normal range of motion in a healthy person.

NMES can also be applied to slow disuse atrophy in innervated muscle. At one time NMES was most commonly used to prevent disuse atrophy in postoperative care following anterior cruciate ligament reconstruction. When intra-articular graft placement procedures were developed, fixation of the graft was difficult, and patients were placed in plaster casts for up to 6 weeks following surgery. It was found that NMES limited disuse atrophy during cast immobilization. However, improved graft fixation now allows for range of motion and active quadriceps and hamstring contractions to be initiated soon after surgery, minimizing the need for long-term NMES. Today, prolonged cast immobilization is reserved for unstable fractures. NMES is contraindicated in these cases because active muscle contractions can alter the alignment of the fracture site and delay healing.

Evidence-based medicine shows that NMES assists muscular function when neuromuscular inhibition is present following injury or surgery (Snyder-Mackler et al. 1991, 1995; Ward and Robertson 1998; Arna Risberg, Lewek, and Snyder-Mackler

2004; Currier et al. 1993; Kim et al. 2010). Some data are inconclusive (Lieber, Silva, and Daniel 1996), and NMES is not as helpful when applied on normal subjects who can exercise independently.

Somewhat different from NMES is patterned electrical neuromuscular stimulation (PENS). PENS is a form of electrical stimulation that is based on electromyography activity during functional tasks recorded in healthy individuals. The purpose of PENS is to replicate the typical firing pattern through reeducation from precisely timed electrical stimulation. PENS is currently used for neuromuscular reeducation or with sport-specific activities that clinicians can use later in the rehabilitation plan. Some examples of the sport-specific activities PENS can be used with are walking, running, jumping, skating, and kicking.

Neuromuscular reeducation with PENS uses previous EMG activity in healthy persons to help re-create the proper firing patterns after injury. One novel component of PENS is the use of a triphasic pattern between agonist and antagonist muscle groups. During muscle contractions, the agonist muscle will initially fire, followed by the antagonist muscle, and lastly a small amount of activity will be fired from the agonist muscle again (Brown and Gilleard 1991; Hallett, Shahani, and Young 1975). For example, the biceps will fire to initiate elbow flexion, followed by activity of the triceps (the antagonist) to decrease the rate of elbow flexion, and then a small amount of activity is found again in the biceps to allow for exact corrections to the end position (Cooke and Brown 1990).

PENS has been applied to a variety of pathological conditions with positive results. Researchers have found that the use of PENS in conjunction with rehabilitation produced decreased pain and improved function in individuals with knee osteoarthritis (Burch et al. 2008) and other chronic conditions (Palermo, 1987; Palermo, Picone, and Freeberg 1991). Gulick et al. (2011) found that 6 weeks of jump training with PENS improved vertical jump height by 9.7% in healthy college athletes.

Muscle Strengthening Versus Force Capacity Enhancement

In order for a muscle to become stronger, a load must be placed on the muscle and adaptation must occur. Strength is measured by an increased ability to do work, usually by the ability to lift weights or produce more force. For strength to increase merely through electrical stimulation, the stimulation must be as great as a similar overload imposed in the form of exercise. Currier, Lehman, and Lightfoot (1979) report that a force equal to 40% to 60% of the maximal voluntary force must be imposed with electrical stimulation for strengthening to occur. For example, if the athlete can lift 20 lb with the biceps volitionally, to strengthen the muscle electrically the stimulation should be strong enough to lift 8 to 12 lb. This level of electrical stimulation is rarely tolerable, and in normal situations it is easier to exercise rather than use electrical stimulation for muscle strengthening.

In an injured population, electrical stimulation can assist neuromuscular function. If there is inhibition of a muscle from effusion or prolonged immobilization, electrical stimulation can be used to help teach the athlete to contract the muscle. In this manner, the force capacity or ability of the muscle to contract is enhanced, but the muscle is not truly strengthened. Electrical muscle stimulation always occurs through the motor nerve rather than by depolarizing the muscle membrane directly whenever the peripheral nerve is intact. Therefore, although muscle contraction is the goal, the technique is termed neuromuscular electrical stimulation, or NMES.

NMES can be used in sports medicine for muscle reeducation following injury or surgery, the reduction of disuse atrophy with immobilization, or augmentation of the function of an impaired muscle (functional electrical stimulation). For example, NMES may be used to assist dorsiflexion with foot drop. NMES may also be used for focal stimulation of a weakness (e.g., stimulation of paraspinals on the convex side of scoliosis).

Endogenous Versus Exogenous Muscle Contractions

The all-or-nothing principle affects the type of muscle contraction that is elicited with NMES (exogenous contractions), and this creates a difference from physiological contractions (endogenous contractions). According to the law of Dubois Reymond, if the amplitude of the stimulation exceeds threshold, the phase duration exceeds capacitance, and the rate of rise of the leading edge is fast enough to prevent accommodation, there will be an action potential. When electrical stimulation is applied to target alpha motor nerves, the entire motor unit associated with the stimulated nerve will respond.

The large-diameter motor nerves are preferentially stimulated because they have a lower capacitance. Large-diameter motor nerves correspond to fast-twitch (glycolytic) fibers. These muscle fibers fatigue quickly because of the energy system used to produce a contraction. This is in contrast to a normal physiological contraction; in such contractions, slow-twitch fibers are recruited first, and if the task requires a greater force, the fast-twitch fibers will be called upon as needed.

Furthermore, because of the all-or-nothing principle, the contraction will be maintained as long as the stimulation is applied. There is no inhibition if the contraction becomes too strong; therefore the body cannot protect itself against an intense contraction. An electrically stimulated contraction is also synchronous, meaning that the individual motor units cannot "rest" as with an endogenous contraction. These factors contribute to the increased fatigue associated with NMES. The differences between physiological and electrical muscle contractions are summarized in table 9.1.

Fatigue and Neuromuscular Electrical Stimulation

Electrically produced contractions cause greater fatigue than physiological contractions, primarily because of the energy system used in the fast-twitch fibers. In order to reduce fatigue with electrical stimulation, a duty cycle or *rest time* must be imposed. Generally, a 1:5 on-to-off time is required to allow enough time to regenerate the local energy utilized for the contraction. The phosphocreatine energy system is depleted rapidly (in 10–15 s) and requires 30 s to 1 min to replace. The rest time allows quality contractions to be produced throughout the treatment. With the use of NMES for muscle reeducation or to promote quality muscle function, generally a 10 s contraction is followed by a 40 to 50 s rest time. As the athlete accommodates to the overload (after 1 to 2 weeks of training), the rest time can be reduced to 30 s. If the force of the contraction is very low, as might occur in the early phase of treatment, shorter rest times might be appropriate. Because of muscle fatigue, the duty cycle is probably the most important feature of a neuromuscular stimulator. Interestingly, PENS does not produce the fatigue that NMES does. Thus, PENS can be used for a longer period of time and prior to activity.

Parameters of Neuromuscular Electrical Stimulation

The electrical stimulator's parameters of phase duration, pulse frequency, amplitude, and duty cycle can be adjusted to optimize the NMES treatment.

The phase duration with NMES should be high enough to overcome the capacitance of motor nerve fibers. Although the capacitance of these motor fibers is low, these fibers are deep, and a high phase duration is recommended (250 to 300 μs) so that there is increased recruitment of many motor units.

The goal is to produce a tetanic contraction; therefore the pulse rate should be 35 to 50 pps. Usually 50 pps is used. Higher frequencies (over 100 pps) do not cause a stronger contraction, and they promote early fatigue.

Table 9.1   Differences Between Physiological and Electrical Muscle Contractions

	Physiological	Electrical
Order of recruitment	Slow-twitch fibers are excited first. Fast-twitch fibers are excited if increased force is required, preserving energy.	Larger-diameter, fast-twitch fibers are recruited first because they have a lower capacitance. Slow-twitch fibers are recruited if the stimulation is increased.
Synchrony of firing	There is asynchronous firing to promote a continuous contraction. This reduces the potential for fatigue of any one motor unit.	There is synchronous firing, depending on the frequency of the stimulation. The contraction continues until the stimulation is off.
Inhibition	If the stimulation is strong, the Golgi tendon organ (GTO) will cause inhibition, which relaxes the muscle to prevent too strong a contraction.	The GTO is excited, but inhibition of the alpha motor neuron is overcome because of direct stimulation of the peripheral nerve.
Fatigue	There is minimal fatigue because of the order of recruitment and asynchrony of firing of motor units.	The muscle fatigues rapidly from the fast-twitch fiber recruitment, which uses the phosphocreatine energy system, and from the synchronous nature of the firing.

Video 9.1 shows the progression of NMES with volitional effort.

The amplitude with NMES depends on the goal of the treatment. If the purpose is to teach the athlete to contract the muscle, then the intensity should produce a strong, tolerable contraction. The athlete should perform a voluntary contraction with the electrical contraction whenever possible to enhance the force produced. If the goal is strengthening the muscle, then the amplitude should be 40% to 60% of the maximal volitional force.

Video 9.2 demonstrates NMES stimulation protocol for the quadriceps using the Russian stimulator.

As described previously, the duty cycle is probably the most important parameter in NMES treatment since the electrically produced contractions cause more fatigue than endogenous contractions. The duty cycle should be 1:5 (10 s on and 50 s off) in the initial treatments, and as the athlete adapts to the stimulation the duty cycle can be reduced to 1:3. The "on" time does not include the ramp time, so if a long ramp time is desired, increase the "on" time. For example, if the on time is 10 s, but there is a 3 s ramp, then the maximal intensity is on for only 7 s. Increase the on time in this case to 13 s so that there is a maximal contraction for the full 10 s.

Types of Neuromuscular Stimulators

Any machine can be used as long as there is a duty cycle control. Ideally, the unit should be able to produce a strong tetanus contraction. Commonly the *Russian stimulator* is used; this machine has unique parameters that were popularized by Kots, a Russian researcher who presented impressive results on muscle strengthening with electrical stimulation in 1977. The Russian stimulation parameters are preset and cannot be adjusted to vary the treatment.

PENS has a variety of parameters, including but not limited to its triphasic pattern and upper and lower extremity sport-specific activities. These activities allow the clinician to select an optimal electrical stimulation for reeducation directed at the athlete's return to play. PENS is an asymmetrical low-volt pulsed current. It uses a pulse rate of 50 Hz and phase duration of 70 μs. This pulse rate still allows for a tetanic contraction of the muscle, but when paired with a shorter phase duration, the amount of discomfort is considerably less than with traditional NMES. This short phase duration also allows the athlete to complete the sport-specific activity in conjunction with the stimulation. The PENS uses a triphasic pattern between agonist and antagonist muscle groups. A 200 ms stimulus train is applied to the agonist, followed by a 200 ms stimulus to the antagonist, and finally a 120 ms stimulus train to the agonist. A 40 ms overlap occurs between the agonist and antagonist. This parameter has been selected from previous EMG findings, and the clinician cannot change it (figure 9.7).

Application of Neuromuscular Stimulation

The following is an example of a stimulation protocol for the quadriceps muscle.

Explain the treatment protocol to the athlete, who is encouraged to increase the current intensity for as strong a contraction as can be tolerated. Also encourage the athlete to perform a volitional contraction in conjunction with the stimulation.

Place one electrode over the femoral nerve in the femoral triangle and the other over the distal quadriceps proximal to the patella. The athlete should be positioned in a device such as an Orthotron that

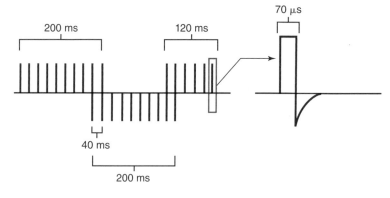

Figure 9.7 Triphasic pattern of the PENS treatment.

Russian Stimulation Parameters

(Time-Modulated Medium-Frequency AC Stimulation)

- Sinusoidal AC current with a carrier frequency of 2,500 Hz (200 μs phase duration)
- Bursted or time-modulated AC with a 10 ms "on" time and 10 ms "off" time, which ultimately results in a 50 burst per minute frequency
- Duty cycle preset at 10 s on and 50 s off (with a 2 to 3 s ramp)

adds isometric resistance to the contraction and limits the complete excursion of the limb. Terminal extension should be avoided to prevent joint "jamming" and soft tissue damage (figure 9.8). The optimal knee angle to obtain maximal quadriceps muscle force using NMES is at 60° of knee flexion.

Treatment parameters may vary according to the type of unit used. The phase duration is often preset; otherwise select 200 to 300 μs. The pulse frequency is also often preset, but if it is adjustable, select 40 to 50 Hz (30 to 40 Hz postoperatively) for tetany. The amplitude should be adjusted and increased to tolerance of a maximal contraction. Make sure that the amplitude is adjusted only when the stimulation is on rather than during the rest phase. The duty cycle should be set at 15 s on and 50 s off (this is preset on some units; otherwise use a 1:5 on-to-off ratio). Select the ramp time at 2 to 3 s.

The treatment duration may vary according to the type of neuromuscular stimulator being used and the goal of the treatment. For example, only 10 to 15 contractions are required when maximally tolerated contractions are elicited. However, when the patient is being "taught" to contract a muscle following a surgical procedure, more submaximal contractions can be performed. With the use of home portable units, the treatment can be repeated up to three times a day for up to 1 h, although overfatigue of the muscle groups should be discouraged. Generally these units do not elicit a maximal contraction.

The patient should be placed in a position to allow the best contraction of the muscle. If there is a deficit in the muscle function in part of the range, such as with an extension lag of the knee, then the muscle should be strengthened in the weak aspect of the range (figure 9.9).

If reciprocal stimulation of agonist–antagonist muscle groups is desired, then the joint should be positioned so that both muscle groups can benefit. This is generally in the midrange of the joint motion.

When one is trying to increase the force generated by the muscle with augmentation of electrical stimulation, the end range of the joint should be blocked. This is to minimize potential injury to the joint, since the inhibition caused normally by the Golgi tendon organ cannot take place as long as the stimulation is on. Blocking terminal extension also prevents hyperextension of the joint.

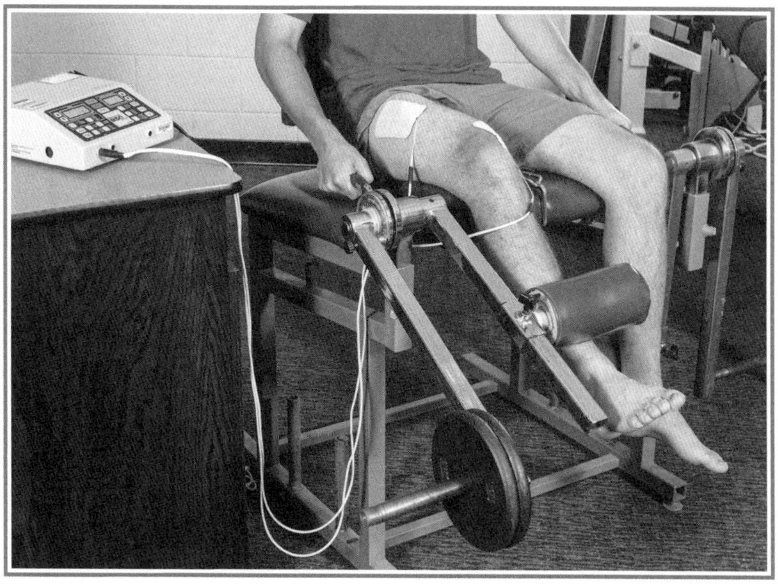

Figure 9.8 Neuromuscular electrical stimulation for enhancing force capacity. Block terminal extension to protect the joint. Use a concomitant maximal volitional contraction.

Electrical Stimulation for the Treatment of Arthrogenic Muscle Inhibition

Arthrogenic muscle inhibition (AMI) is a clinical condition characterized by a decreased ability to activate an uninjured muscle surrounding an injured joint (Hopkins and Ingersoll 2000). Evidence suggests that both spinal and supraspinal inhibitory

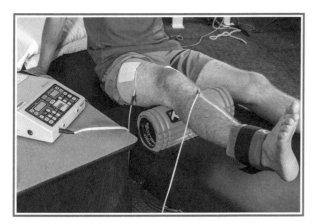

Figure 9.9 Neuromuscular electrical stimulation for muscle reeducation. Use the electrical stimulation to teach the athlete how to contract the muscle after an injury or surgery. Active exercise with the stimulation is encouraged.

mechanisms play a role in decreasing the excitability of motor neurons within a muscle, thus decreasing the muscle's overall function (Palmieri, Ingersoll, and Hoffman 2004). Although this has been hypothesized as a protective mechanism aimed at decreasing forces that act around a joint immediately after injury, AMI may be a limiting factor in restoring optimal neuromuscular control during rehabilitation.

Previous research has supported the use of conventional modalities such as TENS, cryotherapy, and NMES in restoring muscle activation after joint injury (Palmieri-Smith, Thomas, and Wojtys 2008). NMES applied to the inhibited muscle works under the premise that the electrical stimulation in conjunction with voluntary exercise will recruit motor neurons that are being reflexively inhibited. Conversely, **disinhibitory TENS** and cryotherapy should be applied directly to the injured joint (Hopkins et al. 2002); they are hypothesized to increase excitatory afferent stimulation of the spinal cord, which decreases the relative amount of inhibitory activity, causing a reflex activation of the inhibited motor neurons. Therapeutic exercise should be performed after a cryotherapy intervention and may be best performed in conjunction with a disinhibitory TENS treatment of the inhibited joint (Pietrosimone et al. 2011). Although research is currently being conducted to determine the most effective way to use these modalities to disinhibit the motor neuron pool, it should be noted that AMI is a serious clinical condition that may be treated by strategically placed conventional modalities.

Direct Stimulation of Denervated Muscle

When the conduction of impulses to muscle by **alpha motor neurons** is disrupted, the person loses control of the affected muscle. Alpha motor neurons conduct impulses from the spinal cord to the muscle and are known as lower motor neurons, in contrast to the motor neurons of the spinal cord that are called upper motor neurons. When the nerve to the muscle is not functioning, the muscle is denervated, or without innervation.

Denervation can be caused by injury or disease, but you will most likely encounter denervated muscle secondary to trauma. Severe knee sprains and dislocations can injure the peroneal nerve where it passes behind the head of the fibula, denervating muscles in the anterior tibial or lateral compartments of the leg. Injury to the brachial plexus can denervate the deltoid and other muscles of the arm.

Unlike upper motor neurons of the spinal cord, injury to which results in permanent paralysis, alpha motor nerves can regenerate, and active control of the muscle can be restored. This reinnervation process is very slow and does not always occur.

However, because reinnervation is possible, clinicians have tried to maintain the muscle with electrically stimulated contractions. The efficacy of electrical stimulation of denervated muscle has not been established. Electrical stimulation does not bring about reinnervation; however, a regularly stimulated muscle may recover force-generating capacity sooner if reinnervation occurs.

Although lower and upper motor neuron lesions are uncommon in an athletic environment, it is important to understand the difference between these types of lesions. It is also important to understand that with lower motor neuron injury, the parameters of stimulation required for NMES will not elicit a contraction because the capacitance of muscle is much greater than that of the alpha motor nerve. Therefore, when NMES fails to elicit a contraction of the target muscle, one must suspect a lower motor neuron injury. If this diagnosis is confirmed, a low-frequency AC or DC current must be applied to overcome the capacitance of the muscle. The stimulation of denervated muscle carries the same contraindications as TENS.

The stimulation is uncomfortable because of the depolarization of small-diameter afferent nerves. Work closely with the directing physician in treating people with lower motor neuron lesions, and obtain the necessary equipment should stimulation of denervated muscle be requested.

BIOFEEDBACK

Neuromuscular control incorporates the efferent neural output to skeletal muscles with the afferent neural input received by the central nervous system. Coordinated, purposeful movement requires precise feedback from the periphery to allow for refined control over muscle contractions and ultimately, movement of the body through space.

This paradigm includes three levels of neuromuscular control: volitional muscle contractions, reflex responses, and control of more complex, coordinated movement. The focus of this chapter is on volitional control and the treatments that can help to restore volitional control. Unlike NMES, biofeedback is used to monitor the electrical activity of muscle rather than induce a contraction. The general concepts of biofeedback will be presented followed by a more detailed description of EMG biofeedback. EMG biofeedback can help physically active people regain control of volitional muscle contractions and transition to functional activities. Several examples of clinical strategies to promote control of volitional contractions and more complex movements are provided to illustrate functional progression.

VOLITIONAL CONTROL AND BIOFEEDBACK

Biofeedback is the use of instrumentation to bring physiological events to conscious awareness. Electromyographic biofeedback permits awareness of neural recruitment of muscles by transducing the electrical activity during muscular contractions into audio or visual signals. Biofeedback devices can also measure heart rate and galvanic skin response (sweating) during relaxation training. Visual feedback during therapeutic exercise can be enhanced with mirrors. Sometimes a combination of feedback devices is used in neuromuscular reeducation following musculoskeletal injury.

Although EMG biofeedback is used more commonly to increase tension and force production by a muscle or groups of muscles, it can also be used with other types of biofeedback to help athletes learn to control tension and stress responses. An introduction to this aspect of enhancing neuromuscular control is provided at the end of this chapter.

Why Is Biofeedback Effective?

Biofeedback is really a teaching aid. Effective learning requires precise and timely information about the quality of performance. This is true in the cognitive, psychomotor, and affective domains. Feedback must be timely so that we can assess our performance and identify ways to improve. As a student, you know that tests returned months after you take them lose their value as learning tools because your focus has shifted to other coursework and new information.

The feedback provided must also be as precise as possible, as illustrated by the process of learning golf. Everyone in sports medicine should try to learn golf because proficiency in this game requires considerable coordination, and the learning process is a study in neuromuscular education. Step up to the tee, swing the club, and see what happens. Unless you are truly gifted, your first swing will result in the ball's rolling forward or slicing wickedly, or perhaps in no contact at all. You are not sure what went wrong, only that the outcome was flawed. Slowly you improve through trial and error. To speed the acquisition of the basic skills, find a good golf coach and watch the improvement. Effective coaching provides precise information about the reasons for poor shots. Swing speed, swing plane, head and hand position, and other factors can be quickly assessed and improved. Thus, precision of feedback is as important as timeliness.

We have discussed the reasons for impaired neuromuscular control. At this point we hope you appreciate the certified athletic trainer's role in restoring volitional control of both simple and complex motor tasks. Here we introduce biofeedback in relaxation training, but before we proceed, we must review the instrumentation, especially that used for EMG biofeedback.

Instrumentation

If EMG biofeedback is to provide useful information, the electrical activity of the muscle must be recorded and transformed into visual and auditory signals. This process begins with the detection of electrical activity by electrodes. In clinical practice, surface electrodes are used. In some research applications, the electrodes consist of fine wires inserted into the muscle. The indwelling electrodes provide very specific information from a portion of a muscle but are not appropriate for clinical use. Surface electrodes provide less specific information, but the convenience of these electrodes and their ability to quantify the activity of muscles and muscle groups make them ideal for sport rehabilitation.

There are several configurations of surface electrodes. All consist of two active leads and a ground. The self-adhesive electrode with a single three-pole attachment is illustrated in figure 9.10. These electrodes are easy to apply, stay in place, and are inexpensive.

Once the raw electrical signal is detected at the electrode, it is conducted to the electrical circuitry within the EMG biofeedback unit. Within the unit, the raw EMG signal received through the electrodes is filtered, amplified, rectified, integrated (figure 9.11) and transduced into visual and audio output that is proportional to the amount of electrical activity in the muscle. Advances in technology allow for signal processing with much smaller components, permitting greater portability of the unit and expanding the applications of EMG biofeedback in rehabilitation.

Filtering removes "noise" from high- and low-frequency sources. Electrical activity of muscles falls into the 80 to 250 Hz range. It is important that electrical activity below and above this range be filtered before the signal is processed. For example, the electrical current that runs the lights and equipment in athletic training rooms and clinics is 60 Hz, so without effective filtering, turning on an ultrasound or a TENS unit could cause signal fluctuation.

Effective signal processing requires that the raw EMG signal be amplified. Actual electrical activity in muscle falls in the microvolt range, so a signal amplifier is used to amplify the signal into the millivolt range.

When a signal is rectified, all deflections from the isoelectric line are made positive or negative. Signal integration involves sampling the rectified signal and fitting a curve through the sampled points. This process essentially smoothes the signal, allowing for the area under the curve to be quantified (integrated). The integrated electrical signal is then used to power lights, sound, or a signal meter to provide immediate and highly specific feedback about the amount of electrical activity within the target muscle.

Other forms of biofeedback operate in a similar manner. Heart rate monitors detect the electrical activity of heart muscle contractions. Changes in the conductivity of the skin (galvanic skin response) can provide feedback about the body's response to stress. Feedback is provided through measurement of changes in the conductivity of an almost imperceptible electrical current and conversion of the electrical signal into visual and auditory feedback.

Skin temperature can also provide valuable feedback. Surface temperature monitoring does not require electrical signal processing, but it does

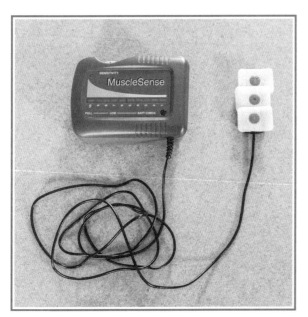

Figure 9.10   An electromyography electrode.

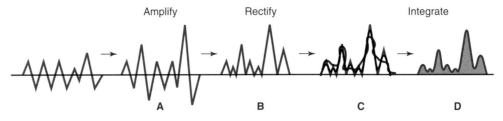

Figure 9.11   Electromyographic signal processing. Electrical signal detected at an electrode is *(a)* amplified and *(b)* rectified. *(c)* The signal is then integrated by taking samples at specific time intervals (e.g., every 0.1 s for a sampling rate of 100 Hz). *(d)* The sampling points are connected, and the electrical activity is quantified by calculating the area under the curve.

require thermometers that can be attached to the skin and very sensitive temperature gauges.

RESTORING CONTROL OF VOLITIONAL CONTRACTION

Restoring control over isolated, volitional muscle contraction is often an early goal of rehabilitation, especially after knee injuries and surgeries. If you examine an injured physically active person the day before arthroscopic knee surgery, you will probably find that all of the quadriceps muscles contract strongly during active quadriceps setting and straight leg exercises. Reexamine the knee the day after surgery, and a decrease in active control of the vastus medialis is often evident with these activities. The effect is more dramatic after arthrotomy. Kirnap et al. (2005) reported that EMG biofeedback facilitates the recovery of quadriceps function after arthroscopic partial meniscectomy.

The response to EMG biofeedback occurs because the affected muscles have not atrophied. Rather, the patient has lost the ability to contract the muscles fully because of neural inhibition. As in learning to play golf, precise and immediate feedback speeds neuromuscular reeducation. Electromyography provides positive feedback when the appropriate neural pathways are activated, eliminating much trial and error in this early stage of rehabilitation (figure 9.12).

There are also limited data (Draper and Ballard 1991) suggesting that EMG biofeedback is as effective or more effective than neuromuscular stimulation in recovery of quadriceps function after anterior cruciate ligament reconstruction. Surgical techniques and rehabilitation strategies have advanced since these data were published. These results, however, suggest that EMG biofeedback, which may be better tolerated by patients, is a viable treatment option. In cases where patients cannot generate a muscle contraction despite the use of biofeedback and their best effort, neuromuscular stimulation (NMES) can be applied to induce a muscle contraction. Using an electrical current to contract a target muscle (usually

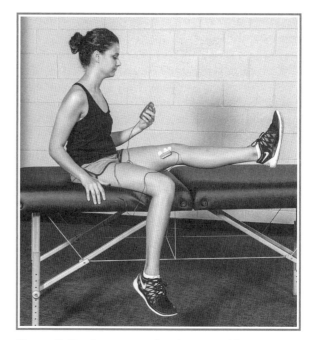

Figure 9.12   A person performing a quadriceps set with biofeedback.

the quadriceps after knee injury or surgery; figure 9.13) generates afferent input. The object of NMES in these situations is to restart the motor efferent–proprioceptive feedback loop by inducing muscle contraction. Be aware, however, that strong electrically stimulated contractions are poorly tolerated.

Using a stimulus with the phase duration and frequency described in chapter 8, apply a 10 to 15 s "on" time with a 4 to 5 s ramp and a 10 to 15 s "off" time. Longer recovery between contractions is not necessary because of the submaximal nature

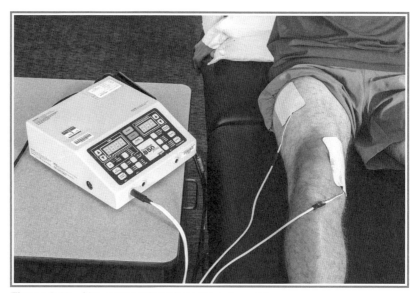

Figure 9.13   Neuromuscular stimulation of quadriceps.

of the muscle contractions; in addition, longer off time promotes boredom. In 10 min the injured person will experience 20 to 30 muscle contractions. The person should be encouraged to contract the affected muscle volitionally during the stimulation. Some people are very timid at first and must be encouraged to adjust the amplitude of the stimulus during the treatment. Allowing the person to control the strength of the stimulus reduces apprehension and makes the treatment more effective.

Once the injured person can contract the affected muscle volitionally, EMG biofeedback can be used to enhance neuromuscular control. You can use NMES and EMG biofeedback in a single treatment session depending on how quickly the person responds to NMES and how much exercise he or she can tolerate.

Neuromuscular inhibition is not limited to postoperative applications. Many physically active people with patellofemoral pain syndrome also demonstrate inhibition of the vastus medialis. Yip and Ng (2006) reported somewhat greater improvements in patients with patellofemoral pain whose exercise program was supplemented with EMG biofeedback training. Furthermore, many people with shoulder pain due to glenohumeral impingement, instability, and rotator cuff lesions fail to properly stabilize the scapula or activate the rotator cuff during shoulder flexion and abduction. Shoulder pain appears to inhibit neuromuscular control in these muscles, leading to altered movement patterns, losses in motion, and greater losses of shoulder function. Electromyographic biofeedback, mirrors (figure 9.14), and, occasionally,

shoulder taping can restore neuromuscular control throughout the shoulder range of motion.

REFLEX RESPONSES

Although the application of NMES and EMG biofeedback can be extended from simple open-chain exercises such as straight leg raises to more complex movements such as a step-up, the speed of the motion does not mimic that of normal function. Reflex responses, however, may be impaired due to damage to the peripheral receptors, pain, or swelling. A program of progressively greater challenges to reflex responses can improve performance and reduce the rate of reinjury. For example, balance training on disks and wobble boards has been reported to decrease the sense of instability in athletes with chronic ankle instability (Tropp, Ekstrand, and Gillquist 1984), decrease postural sway (suggesting greater control of balance) (Gauffin, Tropp, and Odendrick 1988; Mattacola and Lloyd 1997; Bernier and Perrin 1998), and decrease the incidence of recurrent ankle sprain (Wester et al. 1996; Holme et al. 1999). Mattacola and Dwyer (2002) identified intermediate and advanced rehabilitative exercises for the treatment of ankle injuries. Similar exercise progressions have been suggested in the rehabilitation of the injured knee (Drouin et al. 2003).

Myers and Lephart (2000) described the impairment of proprioception and neuromuscular control following capsuloligamentous injury at the shoulder. Several open- and closed-chain exercises directed at enhancing neuromuscular control over

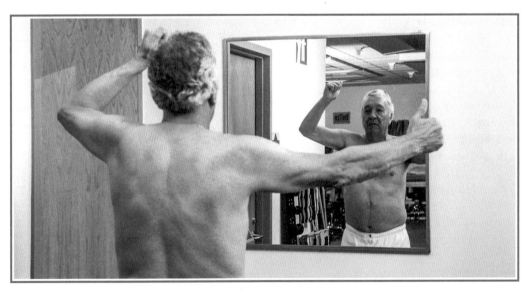

Figure 9.14   Shoulder hiking with abduction of the arm.

the scapulothoracic are depicted by Paine and Voight (1993). The importance of identifying and treating deficits in reflex control in the shoulder complex following injury through a progressive exercise regimen cannot be overemphasized. Ultimately the exercise program advances to exercises that integrate controlled motion throughout the kinetic chain, especially in work with "throwing athletes," including racket sport players and golfers. McMullen and Uhl (2000) provided a thorough review of the theoretical basis for and progression of kinetic chain exercises for shoulder rehabilitation, as well as several illustrations of specific exercises.

Progression from reflex retraining to sport-specific functional activities is the final transition in the neuromuscular control progression. At this point the rehabilitative activities become more sport specific and individualized. Clearly the demands of sports such as gymnastics and soccer differ markedly. Take, for example, the rehabilitation of a gymnast and a soccer player following a lateral ankle sprain. The gymnast might be required to perform on a beam, complete a floor routine, or "stick" a landing after vaulting or completing a bar routine—all very demanding tasks. The soccer player, however, might have to play on wet, slippery surfaces and must redevelop touch with the ball. Knowledge of the demands of the athlete's sport is essential in completing the rehabilitation progression.

FUNCTIONAL PROGRESSION

Sport, work, and daily tasks require coordinated, complex motions rather than isolated control of a single muscle or muscle group. Performing quadriceps setting and straight leg raises has little carryover to walking, climbing stairs, running, cutting, and jumping. The rapid, coordinated recruitment of all the muscles needed to complete relatively complex motor tasks is not generated through conscious control of each muscle. Rather, complex motor tasks are executed from a motor pattern.

Again using the golf swing as an example, we can see that many muscles must contract at precisely the right moment to hit the ball well. If one were to concentrate on controlling only one muscle, let alone several muscles, performance of the swing would suffer badly. Yet the accomplished golfer can consistently hit good shots. Why? The accomplished golfer can execute a complex movement generated from higher centers and continuously adjust

through afferent feedback. Injury, pain, swelling, and instability inhibit the execution of the coordinated, complex movement. Thus, rehabilitation cannot end with restoration of volitional control over muscles or proprioceptive training. Once the early goals of rehabilitation are met, a functional progression of increasingly complex tasks must be introduced. Functional or sport-specific rehabilitation and work hardening are advanced stages of rehabilitation in which coordinated, complex movements are refined and the stamina and strength needed to return to sport and work are built.

The treatment of patellofemoral pain syndrome (PFPS) provides an example of the use of EMG biofeedback in an exercise progression. The initial assessment of an injured person with PFPS often reveals inhibited recruitment of the vastus medialis, which is more affected by knee pain and swelling than the other quadriceps muscles. Selective inhibition of the vastus medialis worsens PFPS in some people because the imbalance between the forces generated by the vastus medialis and lateralis results in lateral glide of the patella. This, in turn, is believed to irritate the patellofemoral joint, resulting in more pain, swelling, and neuromuscular inhibition and perpetuating the condition.

Early treatment of PFPS should focus on relieving pain and swelling. As these treatment goals are accomplished, EMG biofeedback during open-chain exercises such as quadriceps setting and straight leg raises will restore volitional control over the vastus medialis. Although volitional control in open-chain activities is an important goal, the lower extremity rarely functions in an open chain. Thus, the therapeutic exercise program must be progressed to closed-chain and to work- and sport-specific activities: namely, pattern-generated movements.

Early restoration of neuromuscular control is most effective when activity is isolated to a particular muscle or muscle group such as the quadriceps. Open-chain exercises allow athletes to isolate their effort on a single muscle group and then proceed to closed-chain exercises in a progressive exercise program. Failure to establish volitional control in the open chain before beginning closed-chain exercises often reinforces substitute motor patterns. Some people can perform a leg press after anterior cruciate ligament reconstruction yet struggle to move an 8 lb (3.5kg) plate in an open-chain 90° to 60° quadriceps contraction because they substitute gluteal and hamstring force generation for the quadriceps function they lack. Thus, it is important to assess and retrain volitional control in an open chain before progressing to more functional, closed-chain movements.

After more complex movements are initiated, EMG biofeedback provides valuable information about muscle recruitment. If we continue to use PFPS as an example, once the athlete has gained control over the vastus medialis in the open chain, EMG biofeedback can be used during activities such as step-ups, lunges, quarter squats, and balance exercises (figure 9.15). Electromyographic biofeedback is also useful when you are instructing athletes to use machines for resistance exercises, including leg extensions and leg presses (figure 9.16), and for gait training. The EMG biofeedback permits you and the injured person to monitor the quality of motor recruitment in these more advanced and functional exercises. Once the appropriate motor pattern has been established, EMG biofeedback is no longer needed. At this stage more complex balance and landing tasks should be introduced. As skills are mastered, sport- and work-specific exercises and drills are initiated in preparation for unrestricted participation.

Proper execution of exercises is essential for success. Practicing faulty or substitute motor patterns will ingrain the pattern and slow recovery or even exacerbate the injury. This process is very important for people who will complete a home-based or independent exercise program during their rehabilitation.

The use of EMG biofeedback is not limited to rehabilitation of the lower extremity. Biofeedback is useful for people with back pain who struggle to gain control over the abdominal musculature during pelvic tilts, abdominal curls, and standing pelvic tilts. Ultrasound imaging (USI) is a relatively new technique that clinicians use to actually visualize the local stabilizing musculature. The transversus abdominis (TrA) or the lumbar multifidis can easily be visualized with USI while the patient is taught core strengthening exercises (Partner et al. 2014) For the TrA, the patient is taught to do an abdominal drawing in maneuver (ADIM) to minimize the contraction of the global movers and to maximize control of the TrA (figure 9.17). As the patient becomes more proficient with the ADIM, additional stresses such as an unstable surface or more challenging exercise can be added.

Electromyographic biofeedback is useful in treating many types of shoulder dysfunction. Impingement syndrome, rotator cuff tendinopathy, and glenohumeral ligament laxity are similar in that tissues in the subacromial space become inflamed. The resulting pain appears to cause neuromuscular

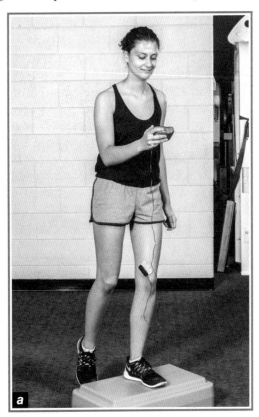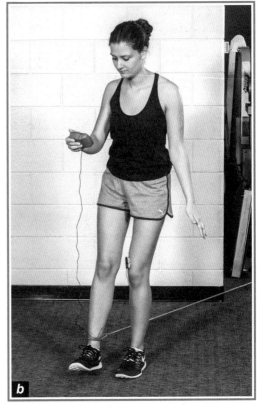

Figure 9.15   *(a)* Biofeedback during step-ups and *(b)* tubing-resisted kickers.

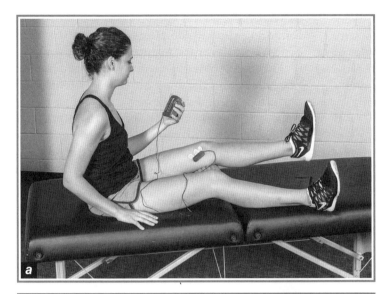

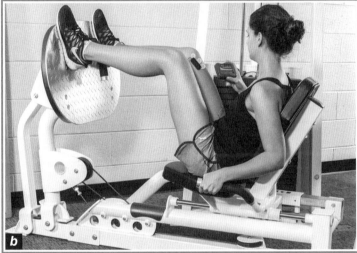

Figure 9.16 *(a)* Biofeedback during short arc leg extension and *(b)* leg press.

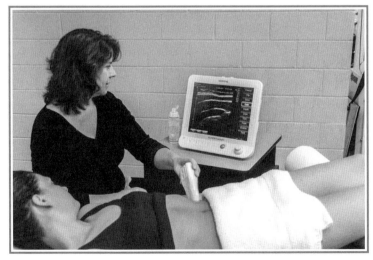

Figure 9.17 Biofeedback at the abdominal site during ADIM.

inhibition of the rotator cuff muscles, especially supraspinatus and to a lesser degree infraspinatus.

The use of EMG biofeedback during exercises that isolate these rotator cuff muscles, such as scaption, empty can, and active external rotation, speeds neuromuscular rehabilitation. An effective method is to use the biofeedback on the lower trapezius muscle to encourage proper scapular stabilization during the exercises (figure 9.18). Using a mirror to provide visual feedback enhances the ability to relearn the appropriate neuromuscular pattern. This technique is helpful when the injured person demonstrates a "shoulder-hiking" pattern with glenohumeral abduction. This substitution pattern, which develops to avoid a painful arc during glenohumeral abduction and flexion, can be difficult to suppress without visual, and sometimes EMG, biofeedback.

The role of the scapula in shoulder dysfunction has received much attention in the past 15 years. Many physically active people with impingement syndrome demonstrate weakness in the scapular stabilizers, especially the middle and lower trapezius and the serratus anterior. People with myofascial pain patterns involving the neck and upper back often present with similar dysfunction. Most of these people also have poor postural awareness. Thus, improved scapular stabilization is a common treatment goal. Once again, EMG biofeedback can speed neuromuscular reeducation and recovery. Visual feedback through the use of mirrors or videotaping can also facilitate recovery of postural and neuromuscular control.

As with the treatment of knee injuries, EMG biofeedback for the shoulder can be used as the therapeutic exercise program becomes more work and sport specific. This is especially true when scapular stabilization is being developed. Electromyographic biofeedback helps the person relearn how to "set" the scapula both before and while throwing (figures 9.19*a* and 9.19*b*) and lifting.

Gaming devices such as the Nintendo Wii and the Microsoft Kinect can also be used to promote biofeedback and encourage methods of neuromuscular function. Specific games can be used in conjunction with traditional balance exercises to add variety to exercise programs and to challenge the patient to improve lower extremity stabilization (Sims, et al. 2013).

LEARNING RELAXATION

This chapter is devoted to the topic of restoring neuromuscular control, and we introduce EMG

biofeedback as a part of that process. However, increasing neuromuscular activity is only one of many possible treatment goals for biofeedback. Many people who suffer from myofascial pain find that their symptoms are exacerbated when they are fatigued or under stress. Unfortunately, many people seem unable to relax. Biofeedback from EMG, galvanic skin response, heart rate, and skin temperature can be used in relaxation training.

Multiple forms of feedback are often used because people vary in their responses to stress. Some people

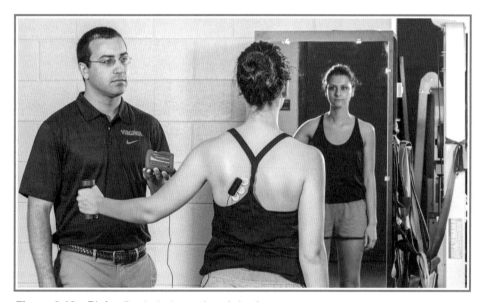

Figure 9.18   Biofeedback during active abduction.

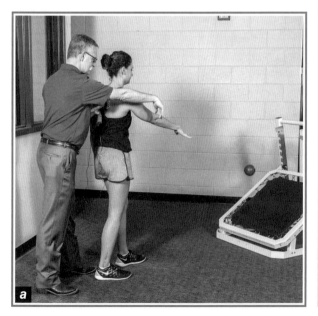 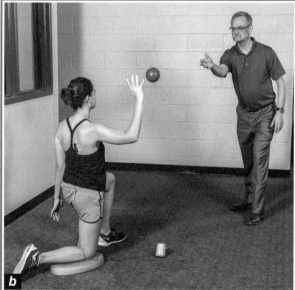

Figure 9.19   EMG during shoulder complex stabilization exercises: *(a)* Stabilization during the cocking phase. *(b)* Stabilization during arm deceleration.

experience an increase in neuromuscular activity in response to stress. Others may experience a galvanic skin response or a drop in temperature. By identifying thoughts or events that increase stress and developing strategies to decrease it, physically active people can improve their ability to relax and break the cycle of stress, pain, and spasm.

These strategies can also be used to help athletes return to competition after injury. Psychological preparation to return to sport following injury has been receiving increased attention; physical rehabilitation alone is not enough to enable a person to return to the environment where the injury occurred. Biofeedback can help the athlete, and the sports medicine team, to assess the stress response to returning to competition. Videotape of competition, biofeedback, and thought stopping can be very effective in managing this stress response.

Physicians, physical therapists, and athletic trainers typically have not devoted much attention to the psychological aspects of rehabilitation. Clinical psychologists and sport psychologists can be invaluable in the management of persistent pain and the individual's psychological response, respectively. All clinicians involved with caring for a patient should recognize the potential value of stress management and biofeedback in a rehabilitation plan of care.

SUMMARY

This chapter returns to the subject of neuromuscular control in the rehabilitation plan of care, specifically with electrical stimulation interventions (NMES and PENS) as well as biofeedback. The electrical stimulation artificially produces a muscle contraction that can facilitate muscle reeducation, while biofeedback brings physiological processes to conscious aware-

---

Biofeedback and Relaxation

Biofeedback Techniques

Muscle tension

Galvanic skin response

Temperature

Heart rate

Often, several forms of biofeedback are used simultaneously to identify how individuals respond to stress and to train them in relaxation.

Relaxation Techniques

Thought stopping

Visual imagery

Breathing exercises

Isolated muscle contraction and relaxation

Specialized preparation in relaxation training is needed to effectively use these techniques. Do not attempt intervention with these techniques without appropriate training or with individuals whose psychological or psychiatric dysfunction is beyond your scope of practice.

---

ness. In the rehabilitation of musculoskeletal injuries, electromyographic (EMG) biofeedback can help patients in regaining control over muscle to restore force production or facilitate relaxation. These interventions for treating impaired neuromuscular control are reviewed, and specific parameters related to the treatments are described.

1. *Identify the three components of neuromuscular control.*

   Neuromuscular control can be divided into three components: (1) conscious, volitional control over isolated muscle contraction; (2) protective reflex patterns; and (3) control over complex, functional movements.

2. *Differentiate between neuromuscular control deficits and muscle atrophy as causes of muscular weakness.*

   Muscles generate force when motor nerves send impulses to the muscle fibers they innervate. The more muscle fibers stimulated to contract, the more force is generated. The cross section of muscles also influences the amount of force a muscle can generate. When muscle is not used for a period of time, the cross section diminishes, or atrophies, which is a relatively slow process. When the ability to recruit muscle fiber contraction in a coordinated manner is impaired, neuromuscular control has been lost; this can occur quite rapidly.

3. *Discuss the effects of swelling, pain, and altered mechanoreceptor input on neuromuscular control and arthrogenic muscle inhibition at the knee, ankle, hip, and shoulder.*

   Laboratory research and clinical observation reveal that pain, swelling, and instability that alter mechanoreceptor input can independently impair neuromuscular control. These elements are often present in the clinical care of musculoskeletal injuries. Managing pain and reducing swelling set the stage for recovery of neuromuscular control. Progressive exercise is important in regaining the ability to generate large, controlled muscle force rapidly, but neuromuscular electrical stimulation or biofeedback can be valuable in the care of patients who struggle to make progress.

4. *Describe the clinical uses for neuromuscular electrical stimulation, including Russian stimulation, in the rehabilitation process.*

   Muscle inhibition is common after an injury or a surgical procedure. NMES can facilitate muscle contraction and thus help reeducate the muscle. NMES is most effective when used in combination with active exercise.

5. *Describe the uses of a galvanic stimulator.*

   Galvanic current is the same as direct current (DC). This unique current in physical medicine is a monophasic current with a phase duration of at least 1 s. It has the highest phase charge or average current of any stimulator. Its primary uses are for iontophoresis to transcutaneously deliver medication and for stimulation of denervated muscles. Muscles that have lost the peripheral nerve can maintain some contractility while the nerve is regenerating. The stimulation does not promote nerve growth.

6. *Define* biofeedback.

   Biofeedback is the use of instrumentation to bring physiological events to conscious awareness. Electromyographic (EMG) biofeedback permits awareness of neural recruitment of muscles by transducing the electrical activity during muscular contractions into audio or visual signals.

7. *Describe the application of EMG biofeedback in the treatment of impaired neuromuscular control.*

An EMG biofeedback device monitors the electrical activity of muscle through electrodes applied to the skin. The patient is asked to contract the targeted muscle, such as the vastus medialis. The biofeedback unit is adjusted to indicate successful recruitment of the target muscle through audio or visual feedback. As neuromuscular control improves, greater recruitment of the target muscle is required to induce positive feedback, and more complex activities are added to the therapeutic exercise regimen.

8. *Describe the instrumentation and signal processing related to EMG biofeedback.*

When a raw electrical signal is detected at the electrode, it is conducted to the electrical circuitry in the EMG biofeedback unit. Within the unit, the raw EMG signal is filtered, amplified, rectified, integrated, and transduced into visual and audio output that is proportional to the amount of electrical activity in the muscle. Filtering removes "noise" from high- and low-frequency sources. Electrical activity of muscles ranges from 80 to 250 Hz. Electrical activity below and above this range is filtered before the signal is processed. Effective signal processing requires that the raw EMG signal be amplified. Actual electrical activity in muscle falls in the microvolt range. The signal is amplified into the millivolt range by a signal amplifier. When a signal is rectified, all deflections from the isoelectric line are made positive or negative. Signal integration involves sampling the rectified signal and fitting a curve through the sampled points. This process essentially smoothes the signal, allowing the area under the curve to be quantified (integrated). The integrated electrical signal is then used to power lights, sound, or a signal meter to provide immediate and highly specific feedback about the amount of electrical activity within the target muscle.

9. *Describe the use of biofeedback in relaxation training.*

Biofeedback can be used to teach relaxation and management of tension and stress. Biofeedback can be used to make a person aware of muscle tension (EMG biofeedback), heart rate, sweating, galvanic skin response, and temperature—areas that reflect the stress response in most people. By identifying thoughts or events that increase the physiological response to psychological stress, and strategies to decrease this response, athletes can improve their ability to relax and break the cycle of stress, pain, and spasm.

10. *Identify contraindications for the application of electrotherapy.*

NMES carries all of the contraindications and precautions of TENS application for pain control. Additionally, NMES should not be applied in any case where active motion (e.g., early stages of fracture healing) is contraindicated. Since EMG biofeedback does not conduct energy to the body, there are no specific contraindications, but EMG biofeedback should not be used to restore the force-generating capacity of muscle until active range of motion is indicated.

Cold and Superficial Heat Therapies

The application of cold through ice packs, water baths, and other means is common in the treatment of musculoskeletal injuries. Similarly, the application of superficial heat also can relieve pain and reduce muscle spasm. In part IV, these treatments are described with attention to understanding the physiological responses and potential for therapeutic benefit. The best available evidence to guide clinical decisions about the application of cold and superficial heat is reviewed. Contraindications for treatment and strategies to assure patient safety are provided in chapter 11.

Principles of Cold and Superficial Heat

OBJECTIVES

After reading this chapter, you will be able to

1. describe the four energy transfer mechanisms used by therapeutic modalities;

2. describe the thermal changes that occur with local cold and superficial heat application;

3. discuss the effects of local cooling and superficial heat on blood flow, muscle, and the nervous system;

4. discuss the evidence on the treatment outcomes of local cold and superficial heat application;

5. describe the application of cold in a program of cryokinetics; and

6. describe contrast therapy.

In your high school athletic training facility, two different individuals are referred to you for care. The first is a 17-year-old female volleyball player (outside hitter) who reports twisting her right ankle about 5 minutes prior. She ambulates with the assistance of her teammates and reports experiencing pain (5/10) in the area of the anterior talofibular ligament and calcaneal fibular ligament. She also presents with mild swelling and edema in the same area. The remainder of your examination is unremarkable with a negative Ottawa Ankle examination. The other patient is the department secretary, who is 60 years old and physically active. She has no significant health complications but is experiencing neck pain after slipping at the grocery store the day prior. She presents with pain (4/10) in the bilateral soft tissue areas of C5-T1. She denies any loss of consciousness or impact to the head during the incident but has begun to experience mild headaches. She presents with no other signs of trauma or neurological involvement and you do not suspect any vertebral fracture.

Is cryotherapy or superficial heat indicated in the treatment of either individual? What physiological effects occur as a result of temperature change in local tissues? How does energy transfer occur between the various forms of cold and superficial heat modalities? This chapter examines current evidence of efficacy for cold and superficial heat.

Cold and superficial heat are probably the most commonly applied therapeutic modalities. These modalities are those thermal agents that alter tissue temperature by conducting heat (energy) to or away from the body. The purpose of altering tissue temperature is to elicit a physiological response leading to an application effect or treatment outcome. The application of a cold agent decreases the temperature of the target tissue, such as skin and deeper tissues. It is worth noting that the decrease in tissue temperature occurs as a result of heat being removed from the body rather than cold being added. Cold agents are the only therapeutic modalities that exert a physiological effect based on this mechanism. In contrast, the application of heat modalities increases target tissue temperatures. More specifically, superficial heat modalities increase the temperature of superficial tissues and joints. An increase of temperature in deeper tissues (including muscle) with superficial heat modalities is limited

and likely has little clinical meaning. Heating of deeper tissues (including muscle and tendon) is better accomplished with other modalities such as ultrasound and diathermy; these are discussed in later chapters. This chapter focuses on modalities that cool tissue or warm superficial tissue.

Despite the simplicity and widespread use of cold and superficial heat, the evidence of clinical benefit is somewhat limited, and the results of clinical trials are often contradictory. Therefore it is important for clinicians to establish desired application effects when selecting modalities. Furthermore, while the mechanisms that bring about the desired effects appear rationally sound, they may not be fully elucidated in the literature. Although thermal agents are applied to help people recover from injury, clinicians must remember they can also cause injury or harm to the patient. Thus, this chapter presents fundamental concepts of energy transfer, the physiological responses to thermal modalities, and the indications and contraindications for cryotherapy and superficial heat. A review of clinical trials investigating the treatment outcomes of cold and superficial heat is also provided.

ENERGY TRANSFER

Thermal energy can be transferred to or from the body by four mechanisms: **conduction**, **convection**, **radiation**, and **conversion**. In addition, these mechanisms are affected by various principles of physics covered in chapter 1 (inverse square law, cosine law, temperature gradient).

Conduction is the transfer of heat through the direct contact between two objects, a hotter and a cooler area (Michlovitz 1990). When heat or cold is applied directly to the skin, the amount of temperature change depends primarily on the temperature difference between the two surfaces (gradient) and the length of time the two surfaces are in contact. Surface cooling begins immediately; however, the deeper the tissue, the longer the cooling process takes. When a larger surface area is heated or cooled, temperature at the center of the area being treated changes somewhat more rapidly than when smaller areas are treated.

Convection is the transfer of heat by the movement of air (gas) or liquid between regions of unequal temperature. For example, a convection oven circulates heated air around the food that is being cooked. In a therapy clinic, a whirlpool or a fluidotherapy unit can be used to heat or cool via convection. As with conduction, the rate and extent of temperature change are determined primarily by differences in temperature between the medium and the tissue (gradient), the length of exposure, and the size of the area treated.

Radiation is energy that is emitted from surfaces with temperatures above absolute zero (Michlovitz 1990); therefore the body emits radiant energy. However, the body can also absorb radiant energy, and radiant energy can increase the temperature of superficial tissues. The obvious example of radiation is sunbathing. At one time infrared or baker's lamps were commonly used for superficial heating in athletic training and physical therapy. Although less common today, these modalities are quite useful for warming large areas. The amount of heating caused by radiant energy relates primarily to the output of the infrared bulb, the distance between the bulb and the skin, and the length of exposure.

The relationship between the heating effect and the distance between the bulb and the skin is stated as the inverse square law (chapter 1).

Conversion implies that energy is changed from one form to another, so this concept does not relate to the application of cold and superficial heat. However, it does relate to two modalities discussed later and is included here for completeness. Ultrasound machines deliver acoustic (sound) energy to tissues where it is reflected and absorbed. When sound energy is absorbed into the tissues, it is converted to thermal energy. A similar phenomenon occurs when the tissues are exposed to continuous electromagnetic energy as with diathermy. These two modalities increase tissue temperature through the conversion of energy within the body.

CRYOTHERAPY

Cryotherapy is the application of a cold agent for therapeutic purposes. When therapeutic exercise is performed during or immediately after cold application, the combination of cold and exercise is referred to as **cryokinetics**, literally cold and motion. Cryotherapy has been used in the treatment of acute musculoskeletal injuries and during rehabilitation for many years. These treatments are generally inexpensive and easy to apply. Despite the widespread use and empirical acceptance of cryotherapy, the extent to which patients benefit from cold application warrants further investigation. The lack of understanding and the need for research are reflected in the lack of evidence-based recommendations for the frequency, length of treatment, and duration (number of days) of treatment needed to improve the outcomes of care. The lack of consensus on optimal parameters was noted by Bleakley, McDonough, and MacAuley (2004). These uncertainties are reflected in this chapter and more broadly in discussion of the clinical use of cold therapies.

Temperature Decreases and Physiological Responses

Localized cooling results in a number of physiological responses at the superficial and deeper levels, including changes to blood flow, nerve conduction, and muscle function. It has been suggested that the extent of cooling, and thus the physiological responses, is affected by the amount of adipose tissue present (Lowdon and Moore 1975; Johnson et al. 1979). Adipose tissue acts as an insulator and prevents the loss of energy from deeper tissues in the presence of lower surface temperatures. Grant (1964) and McMaster, Little, and Waugh (1978) suggested the amount of adipose tissue present would influence the time required for temperature decrease; thinner people require less time for temperature decrease in comparison to those with more adipose tissue. In summary, the magnitude of change in surface temperature is not a good indicator of changes in intramuscular temperature and will vary between patients.

Superficial Tissue Cooling and Rewarming

When an ice pack is applied or a limb is immersed in an ice bath, the superficial tissues (i.e., skin, afferent sensory fibers, nociceptive fibers) cool rapidly. After a few minutes, the rate of cooling (temperature gradient) slows and finally levels off at a few degrees above the temperature of the ice pack or ice bath (Knight 1995). If a compression wrap is applied over the ice pack, greater decreases in skin temperature are observed (Knight 1995).

When the cold is removed, a similar pattern of rewarming occurs. There is an initial rapid rise in temperature (which is of lesser magnitude than the sudden drop that occurs with cold application), followed by a more gradual return to preapplication temperature. During this period, the skin temperature can remain below preapplication levels for over 1 h following 30 min of cold pack application. More rapid rewarming occurs when cooling is followed by physical activity (cryokinetics).

Deeper Tissue Cooling and Rewarming

In general, deeper tissues cool more slowly and to a lesser extent than superficial tissues. Measures of gastrocnemius muscle tissue temperature at a depth of 2.3 cm revealed slow cooling during a 22 min ice pack application (Hartviksen 1962). However, temperatures continued to drop for several minutes following the removal of ice packs in subjects at rest, and cooling plateaued at approximately 28°C.

The research evidence suggests that changes in intra-articular temperature follow a pattern similar to that observed in muscle (Haimovici 1982; Oosterveld et al. 1992). However, there is a greater temperature decrease in the joint than in the surrounding muscle (Wakin, Porter, and Krusen 1951). When the joint is held at rest, temperatures continue to drop after cold is removed (Bocobo et al. 1991; McMaster, Little, and Waugh 1978). Cold water immersion results in greater cooling of the intra-articular space than an ice pack (Bocobo et al. 1991) because a greater surface area of the joint is exposed to cold.

After cold application, deep tissues maintained at rest rewarm very slowly, and the rewarming of muscle and intra-articular spaces has been reported to exceed 2 1/2 hours (Knight 1995; Knight et al. 1980). The research into rewarming has implications for applications in various clinical settings. For example, in the treatment of a person who will remain at rest following knee surgery, ice can be applied to control pain and swelling. Based on the research findings, a 20 to 30 min ice pack application will cool tissues, creating the desired physiological effect, for 2 h or more. In addition, reapplication of cold during the rewarming period will result in further decreases in tissue temperatures. This is important when considering contraindications with cold modalities. Although there are not enough data to recommend a specific cooling–rewarming ratio, Knight (1995) recommended a rewarming period of at least twice the cooling period with application of ice directly to the skin. This is still sound advice.

When the patient is active after cryotherapy, rewarming occurs much more quickly. Physical activity rapidly increases core body temperature along with muscle and joint temperatures. Thus, deep tissue temperatures return to normal much more rapidly when cryotherapy is followed by exercise. Interestingly, recent data suggest that effective cooling of muscle can occur when someone walks around with ice applied over the working muscle (Compton et al. 2008). These results have implications in daily practice because athletes and patients are often pressed for time and are unable or unwilling to rest during ice application. Further investigations are needed to establish the efficacy of "to-go" cold therapy protocols.

Impact on Blood Flow

Localized cooling creates a number of physiological responses, including decreased blood flow in the skin. The skin is the largest thermoregulatory organ and is capable of mediating temperature changes by controlling its vascularity. When the skin is cooled, superficial vasoconstriction occurs primarily through reflex mechanisms as arteriole sphincters are directly stimulated by the cold. In addition, a decrease in local histamine and prostaglandin (vasodilators) contributes to vasoconstriction. Fluid viscosity (thickness of a liquid) also is increased, resulting in less blood flowing in the local area. Maximum decrease in local blood flow is reported to occur at approximately 57°F (13.9°C). A point to keep in mind for later discussion is that constriction or decrease in the diameter of lymphatic vessels occurs at approximately 59°F (15°C).

Changes in blood flow through deeper tissues occurs due to decreased metabolic activity. Perfusion is decreased at rest and increased during exercise. Various researchers have examined whether a local application of ice affects muscle perfusion, and recent evidence shows that blood flow in a skeletal muscle is not changed with cryotherapy (Selkow et al. 2012). Therefore, ice may have a positive effect on pain and other factors, but it would not limit the delivery of oxygen to the tissues. Hypothetically, if a large area is cooled as with whole body cooling or cold submersion, there may be deeper vascular changes. As cooling lowers the metabolic activity and oxygen demand of local cells, less blood flow is routed to the area.

The cold-induced effects of vasoconstriction, increased fluid viscosity, and decreased blood flow must be examined within the context of the injury environment. For example, the combined effects of vasoconstriction and increased fluid viscosity may be of significance in response to an acute injury involving blood loss. However, these same effects may not be important when treating a musculoskeletal injury, as blood loss has already been managed by the actions of the clotting cascade. In contrast, cooling may slow neutrophil migration acutely and reduce lymphatic drainage as the acute inflammatory response subsides.

Impact on Neural Tissue

Cold application affects the nervous system, especially sensory, nociceptive, and motor nerves. Cooling of nerve fibers slows the conduction of neural impulses. An example is seen in local numbness that occurs after cold application. After several minutes of cold application, sensation is diminished because the impulses of sensory nerves cannot be transmitted from the periphery to the sensory cortex. When the same mechanism occurs to active nociceptive nerves, the result is decreased perception of pain, pain modulation. Patients have described a progression of sensations during cold application. Initially, intense cold is perceived. This is followed by an aching pain,

which gives way to sensations of pins and needles or warmth and finally numbness. Although not everyone will experience these sensations, this general description suggests that cold initially stimulates cold and pain receptors. Nevertheless, the numbness or analgesia experienced during cryotherapy results in the first goal of rehabilitation: pain relief.

Muscle function is controlled by motor nerves within the nervous system. In this section, we will examine muscle spasm and function separately. In addition to relieving pain and thus breaking the pain–spasm cycle, cold also reduces muscle spasm by directly affecting the muscle spindle.

When injury occurs, the body responds through reflex contraction of surrounding muscles. These involuntary contractions or spasms splint the injured area and prevent further injury. However, spasm occludes blood flow and exacerbates the pain–spasm cycle. **Muscle spindles** sense the stretch of a muscle. The spindles are innervated by gamma efferent fibers, which allow the spindle to adjust to changes in muscle length. Thus, muscle spindles respond to the protective spasms during injury by intensifying contractions.

Cold application appears to decrease spasm through direct and reflex mechanisms. When cooled, the muscle spindles are less sensitive; thus, the muscle relaxes and spasm is relieved. However, decreases in muscle spasm begin to occur before the muscle cools significantly, suggesting that a reflex response to cold also occurs. Certainly, the antispasmotic effects of cryotherapy are an important consideration when one is selecting a therapeutic modality to treat musculoskeletal injuries.

A normal component of muscle function is force production. Knight (1995) summarized the findings of several investigators and concluded that maximum isometric and isotonic strength and rate of force development are reduced when the muscle tissue is cooled below 15°C to 18°C. While the mechanism for this response is not completely understood, it is conceivable that a reduction in efferent motor nerve conduction and neural impulses and neurotransmitter signaling may be involved.

Impact on Proprioception and Sensation

Although cooling slows nerve conduction velocity and relieves pain and muscle spasm, the effects on proprioception, postural stability, and sensation are less evident. Studies on the effect of cryotherapy on balance, proprioception, postural stability, and function have presented conflicting conclusions. Ice bath immersion of the ankle and lower leg appears to temporarily reduce postural stability and balance (Gerig 1990; Rivers et al. 1995; Steinagel et al. 1996), while ice pack application to the ankle and knee has been reported not to affect postural stability and balance (McDonough et al. 1996; Thieme et al. 1996). Open kinetic chain repositioning is not changed after cold water immersion (LaRiviere and Osternig 1994; Hopper, Whittington, and Davies 1997). Cold application (15 min, 10°C ice bath) was not found to affect control of force production or two-point discrimination in the hand, although pressure sensitivity was reduced (Rubley et al. 2003). A similar treatment was found not to affect the haptic system responsible for nonvisual perception, such as when an implement is held in the hand (West 1998). Cryotherapy applied to the shoulder has been reported not to affect shoulder joint position sense (Dover and Powers 2004) and to impair proprioception and throwing accuracy (Wassinger et al. 2007).

There is also conflicting information on the effect of cold on cutaneous sensation. Cooling of the forearm and hand appears to alter cutaneous sensation in the fingers and thumb (Provins and Morton 1960; Rubley et al. 2003). However, cooling of the foot does not affect cutaneous sensation on the plantar surface. The differences in these findings are probably due to the greater sensitivity of the hand. Rewarming of the hand appears warranted before performance of fine motor tasks. Cataldi et al. (2013) examined the sensory effect of cryotherapy and noted that the maximal cutaneous effect from an ice bag occurred within less than 15 min of application. Ice massage required the shortest duration (8 min), while cold immersion took up to 20 min for cutaneous sensory changes to occur.

Performance of maximal-effort jumping and agility tasks may also be affected by tissue cooling, although once again the results of studies are conflicting. Some investigators (Cross, Wilson, and Perrin 1995; Greicar et al. 1996) reported that cold adversely affects jumping and agility, whereas others (Evans et al. 1996; Shuler et al. 1996) found no performance differences after cryotherapy.

The previously mentioned research may appear confusing, and you may question when to apply cold in light of the potential to affect functional performance. However, when cold is used to treat musculoskeletal injury, these issues are usually of minimal concern. Persons treated with cryotherapy are rarely capable of maximal-effort, functional exercise or activity. For the few who are capable of such exercise but need to apply cold for pain management, a period of rewarming with safe, rhythmic exercises is advised (Pritchard and Saliba 2014). One must question, however, whether throwing, jumping, and agility exercises are appropriate for injured people who need cryotherapy for pain management.

Cryotherapy and Acute Inflammation

Tissue injury results in an inflammatory response that was discussed in detail in chapter 4. The acronym PRICE reflects the recommendation for treatment in response to acute injury. **P** - protection, **R** - rest, **I** - ice, **C** - compression, and **E** - elevation are the five elements of care. Protection through splinting, casting, and the use of assistive devices such as crutches can lessen pain and the risk of additional tissue injury. Rest overlaps with protection and implies reducing activity, especially activity that is pain provoking. Compression and elevation are introduced to minimize swelling. Why is cold or ice application recommended?

Ice has been proposed to lessen inflammation, minimize secondary tissue injury, and relieve pain. First consider the issue of inflammation. As demonstrated in chapter 4, inflammation is not simply a pain-provoking physiological response to tissue damage, but it is also the process through which tissue is repaired. Thus, complete interruption of the inflammatory process prevents repair. If cold application truly affected the inflammatory process, then tissue repair and functional recovery would be delayed, rather than facilitated (Butterfield, Best, and Merrick 2006). Inflammation results in pain. Cold application can relieve pain, but the application of cold can be painful. The analgesic response to cold application in patients suffering from acute musculoskeletal injuries has, to our knowledge, never been truly quantified. Many reading this book can probably recall a situation when cold application did relieve the pain associated with an injury but also recall a situation when the exposure to cold was frankly painful. The foundation for this paradox is addressed in chapter 5. Some nociceptors are cold sensitive, thus cold application is pain provoking. However, in the presence of pain resulting from injury, cold can slow nerve conduction, especially in the pain carrying, unmyelinated C-afferent fibers. Thus, cold can reduce the conduction of pain signals reaching the dorsal horn of the spinal cord and ultimately the sensory cortex.

It has also been proposed that cold decreases secondary tissue injury or cell death. Knight (1995) suggested that secondary injury is due to **hypoxia** at a cellular level. He theorized that during an acute inflammatory response, disruption of capillaries and congestion due to edema decrease the oxygenation of healthy cells close to the tissue damage. Hypoxia leads to further cell death. Thus, after musculo-skeletal injury there is a period of additional tissue damage, or secondary injury, due to hypoxia. Certainly cooling of tissue lowers the metabolic activity and reduces oxygen demand. When oxygen demand is reduced through cooling, cells can survive a period of hypoxia. Because more cells survive, there is less total tissue damage, a more rapid resolution of the signs and symptoms of acute inflammation, and a more rapid recovery.

Despite our limited understanding of secondary cell death and tissue repair processes, the application of cold is a widely accepted and practiced treatment (Merrick 2002, 2003). Some may view the issue of secondary tissue injury and cell death as academic, having little clinical relevance. However, given that the clinician cannot influence primary tissue injury (cell death occurring immediately after trauma) and that no intervention has been proven to speed tissue repair, further investigation into the phenomenon of secondary tissue injury and the influence of cryotherapy on neutrophil and macrophage activity is clearly needed. A better understanding of these issues may identify the most effective use of cold applications. Further investigation may also lead to additional therapeutic adjuncts that the health care provider can use to help injured patients.

Cryotherapy and Therapeutic Exercises

Knight (1995) described the application of cold before or during exercise and coined the term cryo-kinetics ("cold and motion"). Cryokinetics involves cold application, usually consisting of cold water immersion, cold whirlpool, or ice massage, and active exercise. Cold is applied until analgesia is achieved (10-15 min). Once the painful area is numbed, a careful progression of exercises is initiated. When the numbing effects of the cold wear off, cold is reapplied. Several repetitions of cold application and exercise can be performed.

Cryokinetics can speed functional recovery. Loss of function is a consequence of pain and swelling. The loss of function is the result of increased "tone" or spasm in muscle and a loss of the ability to recruit muscle to generate force. The increase in tone and loss of force generation through volitional muscle contraction occur in reciprocal muscle groups. For example, following a knee injury, an increase in tone or spasm of hamstring muscles and a loss of the ability to contract the quadriceps will occur. Similarly, low back pain is associated with spasm of the paraspinal (extensor) muscles and inhibition of transversus abdominis and multifidus. Cold application can break the cycle of pain and muscle spasm before therapeutic exercise. As discussed in chapter 9, the loss of the ability to recruit muscle to generate force is termed arthrogenic muscle inhibition (AMI). While more is known about AMI involving the knee and quadriceps muscle, pain and swelling at the hip and ankle have also been studied. Cryotherapy can disinhibit the quadriceps in those with knee swelling and likely can facilitate functional improvement in patients with knee pain and/or arthritis as well as conditions affecting the ankle, hip, and other joints (Rice, McNair, and Dalbeth 2009; Hopkins et al. 2002).

Sound clinical judgment must be used in initiating cryokinetics. With relatively minor injuries, such as a grade I lateral ankle sprain with injury isolated to the anterior talofibular ligament, cryokinetics can be initiated 1 to 2 days after injury. Activities such as walking and jogging do not stress the ligament. Thus, the injured person can return to activity when his or her function allows, provided that the ankle is protected from forced inversion. However, if the ankle injury is more severe and involves, for example, injury to the syndesmosis (articulation between the distal tibia and fibula), walking and jogging must be delayed until the damaged ligaments heal. These activities greatly stress the syndesmotic ligaments and would delay healing and result in an unstable ankle.

In general, cold decreases sensation and relieves pain but does not provide anesthesia. If exercise during cryotherapy is painful, it should be discontinued. You can reapply the cold and resume exercises after numbness has returned, or you can end the exercise session. Likewise, if the injured person becomes too aggressive with a therapeutic regimen, pain, spasm, and swelling will increase the following day, and rehabilitation will be slowed for 1 to 3 days while the newly inflamed tissue recovers. Two good rules in any rehabilitation exercise program are as follows: (1) pain that alters normal movement patterns indicates that the person is not ready to perform the exercise, and (2) the person should be able to do tomorrow what was done today. Clinical experience will refine your ability to judge the appropriateness of an exercise for each individual, but these rules are commonsense guidelines for the progression of therapeutic exercise, especially cryokinetics.

Cryotherapy in the Treatment of Persistent Pain

Cryotherapy may also be effective in managing some persistent pain problems. For individuals with myofascial pain syndrome, characterized by very sensitive trigger points, cryotherapy offers a safe, cost-effective home treatment. Travel and Simons (1983) described the use of ethyl chloride spray and stretch in treating myofascial pain. Ice massage using brief stroking can produce similar responses. Brief, intense cold to sensitive points may decrease pain by stimulating descending spinal pathways described in chapter 5. A more prolonged ice massage decreases the sensitivity of free nerve endings and slows the conduction velocity of afferent fibers. The numbing effect of the ice breaks local pain–spasm cycles, relieving the symptoms of myofascial pain. Cryokinetics may also be useful in the management of myofascial pain and, as noted, patients suffering AMI. Therapeutic exercises to restore motion, improve posture, and reestablish pain-free, functional movement patterns are often better tolerated after cryotherapy.

Cold is not indicated in the treatment of all persistent pain problems. Complex regional pain syndrome may be exacerbated by cryotherapy; the intense stimulus of the cold can result in excruciating pain and worsen the problem.

Does Cold Application Improve Treatment Outcomes?

In chapter 3, issues of treatment outcome and evidence-based practice were introduced. This chapter has introduced application techniques, reviewed why cold is used in clinical practice, and discussed an evolving theoretical basis for therapeutic cold application. Despite the widespread use of cold as a therapeutic agent for many years, the effectiveness of treatment needs to be assessed. Does cold application speed or enhance recovery from injury or surgery? And how strong is the evidence? Interestingly, the number of published reports that provide evidence for the effects of cold application is not large. Belanger (2002) listed fewer than 15 references to clinical trials involving cold application for musculoskeletal conditions (ankle sprain and knee surgery) of interest here.

Bleakley, McDonough, and MacAuley (2004) completed a systematic review of randomized controlled trials related to cold therapy. Their summary suggests that cryotherapy is better than superficial heating or contrast in the treatment of acute ankle injuries. Treatment with cryotherapy is reported to increase range of motion and reach distance in subacute ankle sprain, but a single application of ice and compression is unlikely to be of benefit. In contrast, cold following arthroscopic knee procedures, combined with exercise, was reported to reduce pain and facilitate weight bearing when compared to performing exercise alone. There was, however, little evidence to support cold therapy after anterior cruciate ligament reconstruction.

Van den Bekerom et al. (2012) focused on the recommendation for rest, ice, compression, and elevation (RICE) in the treatment of acute ankle sprains in adults. Their conclusions were no more compelling than those of Bleakley, McDonough, and MacAuley (2004). van den Bekerom wrote "Insufficient evidence is available from randomized controlled trials to determine the relative effectiveness of RICE therapy for acute ankle sprains in adults. Treatment decisions must be made on an individual basis, carefully weighing the relative benefits and risks of each option, and must be based on expert opinions and national guidelines."

The reviews by Bleakley et al. and van den Bekerom incorporated research conducted over many years. In examining some of this work, Daniel, Stone, and Arendt (1994) reported no benefit of cold wrap adjusted to as low as 45°F (7°C) on pain, medication use, or other outcome measures after arthroscopically assisted anterior cruciate ligament reconstruction. Dervin, Taylor, and Keene (1998); Edwards, Rimmer, and Keene (1996); and Konrath et al. (1996) reported similar results using a continuous flow of cool water through Cryocuff cooling pads and ice packs. Ohkoshi et al. (1999); Cohn, Draeger, and Jackson (1989); and Barber, McGuire, and Click (1998) reported, however, that cooling reduced reports of pain and analgesic use after surgery. Lessard et al. (1997) reported similar findings after arthroscopic knee surgery. These conflicting findings highlight concerns over the insulating effects of postoperative dressings and the need for investigators to be very specific when describing treatment protocols.

Cold application may be of benefit in some patients preoperatively. Mora et al. (2002) reported that pulsatile cold/compression applications decreased swelling in patients awaiting surgical management of displaced ankle fractures when compared to patients treated solely with splinting and bed rest. There is also agreement (Levy and Marmar 1993; Leutz and Harris 1995) that cold therapy lessens blood loss after total knee arthroplasty, but these groups of investigators differed about whether any additional benefits are realized with cold application. Levy and Marmar found small differences in pain report and medication use in patients receiving cold therapy, while Leutz and Harris reported no additional benefit. Hubbard, Aronson, and Denegar (2004) completed a systematic review of the effects of cold treatments on return to work or sport. The focus on functional return yielded only four clinical trials. They concluded that cryotherapy may promote more rapid functional recovery and return to participation. The magnitude of effect of cold application could not be estimated from the data retrieved. Sloan, Hain, and Pownall (1989) reported that immediate cold therapy patients treated in an emergency department with compression and nonsteroidal anti-inflammatory medication plus early cold application were not significantly better at 7-day follow-up than those treated with medication and compression only. Thus, repeated applications are likely needed to achieve the more rapid return to work and sport identified by Hubbard, Aronson, and Denegar, but an optimal treatment protocol has not been established.

These reviews of treatment outcomes demonstrate the need for additional study. Many clinicians routinely apply cold therapy or other modalities based on what they were taught and the practice habits they have developed. At this time we conclude that when patients are free of contraindications, cold can be safely applied. It is likely to reduce pain, it may influence secondary tissue injury, and it may speed recovery after ankle sprains and knee surgery. The evidence for expedited recovery, however, is not compelling.

SUPERFICIAL HEAT

Superficial heat is the application of heat energy to the body for therapeutic purposes. Superficial heat is commonly used in the treatment of musculoskeletal injuries during rehabilitation to decrease pain and muscle spasm. As with cryotherapy, despite their being empirically accepted, the extent to which patients benefit from superficial heat modalities warrants further investigation. This lack of understanding is reflected in the limited availability of evidence-based recommendations for treatment applications that will improve the outcomes of care. These uncertainties are reflected in this chapter and more broadly in current discussions about the clinical use of superficial heat therapies. The rest of this chapter addresses physiological effects and evidence of the effectiveness of superficial heat.

Temperature Increases and Physiological Responses

As previously mentioned, adipose tissue (fatty layer of tissue beneath the dermis) insulates the deeper tissues; therefore, modalities that heat the skin are classified as superficial heating modalities. Much as with cold, the primary clinical benefits of superficial heat are pain control and relief of muscle spasm. However, the mechanisms responsible for these physiological responses are not well understood.

These modalities can increase intra-articular temperature but have little or no effect on the temperature of deeper tissues such as muscle (Draper et al. 1998; Holcomb 2003). Therefore, cellular metabolism or muscle blood flow in deeper tissues is also minimally affected. Despite the limited effects on deep tissue temperature, superficial heat modalities are commonly used to attain a number of physiological responses at the superficial levels, including changes to blood flow, neurological tissue, and muscle function.

Depth of Tissue Heating

Superficial heating increases the skin temperature several degrees. The intra-articular temperature of superficial and small joints such as the knee (Oosterveld et al. 1992; Oosterveld and Rasker 1994) and interphalangeals can be increased to therapeutically beneficial levels. The temperature of deeper tissues such as large muscles and deep joints (e.g., hip) rises insignificantly. Draper et al. (1998) reported a 3.8 °C temperature rise at 1 cm depth but only a 0.74 °C rise at 3 cm after a 15 min hot pack application. Holcomb (2003) reported no change in temperature at 3.75 cm at the same hot pack temperature and application time used by Draper. Thus superficial heat placed over the hamstrings or the glenohumeral joint of a muscular person will not raise the temperature of those tissues enough to have a therapeutic benefit.

Impact on Blood Flow

Superficial heating increases blood flow in local tissues by means of different mechanisms: vasodilation of capillaries and decreased fluid viscosity. In the superficial tissues, the increase in blood flow occurs mainly through reflex mechanisms as smooth muscles in arteries relax in response to the increased temperature. A spinal-level reflex that increases the release of bradykinin (a vasodilator) adds to the increased blood flow. There is also an increase in permeability of the local tissues (including lymphatic vessels). Fluid viscosity (the thickness of a liquid) is decreased, resulting in greater blood flow in the local area. The maximum increase in local blood flow is reported to occur up to 60 minutes after application.

As with cryotherapy, the induced effects of capillary dilation and decreased fluid viscosity in superficial tissues must be examined within the context of the tissue environment. For example, the combined effects of vasodilation and decreased fluid viscosity may be detrimental during the acute inflammatory response to injury. However, these same effects may permit a greater ease of motion in patients with arthritis.

Impact on Neural Tissue

The physical sensation of the superficial heat modality as it is applied to the body, such as a heat pack placed on the gastrocnemius, activates larger-diameter (A-beta) neural fibers. A sustained activation of these fibers may result in pain modulation via the ascending pain modulation model, the gate response. However, this response is not unique to superficial heat modalities; therefore it is unlikely that the complete pain modulation response occurs through the gating mechanism.

The sensation of heat is carried by small-diameter neural fibers (A-delta and C fibers). Thus it is possible that a descending pain modulation mechanism is involved. Input into the central nervous system via small-diameter afferent fibers may stimulate descending pain control mechanisms. Clinical observation suggests that this theory may have merit. Superficial heat applied for 20 to 30 min often has a calming, sedating effect.

Others have suggested the analgesia experienced with superficial heat may be the result of a decrease in "congestion," thereby lessening mechanical pressure on nociceptive fibers as well as "washing out" neurochemicals responsible for nociceptive activation. Nevertheless, the mechanisms behind the calming, analgesic effects of superficial heat are not well understood; however, the answers may lie in the advances in neuroscience described in chapter 6.

The mechanism behind the antispasmodic effect of superficial heating is equally speculative. One explanation is that by relieving pain, superficial heating breaks the pain–spasm cycle. However, other factors may be involved. When heat is applied, the sensitivity of muscle spindles decreases, even though the temperature of the spindle is not affected. Thus, superficial heating may alter muscle spindle activity through a spinal reflex mechanism. Although speculative, this is the best explanation for the decrease in spindle sensitivity and the relief of spasm associated with superficial heating.

Impact on Proprioception and Sensation

It is suggested that the increase in temperature results in an increased nerve conduction velocity in sensory and motor fibers. However, this is not sufficiently supported in the literature; furthermore, what significance this may have in the management of injured tissues is not completely understood.

Other physiological responses are associated with tissue heating, including increased metabolic activity, increased circulation, increased inflammation, increased tissue elasticity and decreased viscosity, and sweating. Although these responses occur in the dermis, deeper tissues are much less affected because of the insulating effects of adipose tissue. Except in superficial joint structures, superficial heating does not alter deeper tissues. Thus, superficial heating does little to the metabolism or blood flow of deeper damaged tissues.

With regard to neuromuscular effects, superficial heat applied to the knee joint did not improve activation of the quadriceps in patients with AMI (Warner et al. 2013), nor did the application of menthol (Huffman et al. 2010). Muscle strength and function are generally not affected by the application of superficial heat. A better method to "warm up" the muscles would be to do light, repetitive exercise. Pedaling a stationary bike or using an upper body ergometer or other device would be a more effective way to increase the temperature and prepare the body for specific exercise.

In general, superficial heat relieves pain and decreases muscle spasms. Clinicians should follow the same two rules (as suggested with cryotherapy) in any rehabilitation exercise program: (1) pain that alters normal movement patterns indicates that the person is not ready to perform the exercise, and (2) the person should be able to do tomorrow what was done today. Clinical experience will refine the clinician's ability to judge the appropriateness of integrating a superficial heat modality into the rehabilitation program.

Does Superficial Heat Improve Treatment Outcomes?

The literature on the outcomes of treatment with superficial heat, like that on cold therapy, is limited. What is available, however, suggests that superficial heat does have a clinically useful analgesic effect. French et al. (2006) concluded that "There is moderate evidence in a small number of trials that heat wrap therapy provides a small short-term reduction in pain and disability in a population with a mix of acute and sub-acute low-back pain, and that the addition of exercise further reduces pain and improves function." Nadler et al. (2002) reported that continuous heat wrap application was more effective in reducing pain than oral administration of acetaminophen or ibuprofen. Akin et al. (2001) found similar treatment as effective as ibuprofen in the treatment of dysmenorrhea. Nadler et al. (2003a, 2003b) reported on two trials of continuous heat wrap in the treatment of acute low back pain. In both trials the heat wrap was more effective than placebo medication or oral ibuprofen. Superficial heat applied for 20 min has also been reported to reduce the sensitivity of active myofascial trigger points. Robinson et al. (2002) concluded that superficial moist heat can be used as palliative therapy in the treatment of rheumatoid arthritis.

On the basis of the available literature we can conclude that long-duration (8 h), low-level heat can be recommended in the management of acute low back pain, and that shorter-duration moist heat can be used clinically to reduce myofascial pain as part of a more comprehensive treatment session. More investigation is needed to examine the effect of the use of superficial heat on recovery from other musculoskeletal conditions. When it is used safely, however, the clinician can expect that 20 or more minutes of superficial heat will reduce pain and thus likely stiffness in patients with musculoskeletal injuries and arthritic conditions.

CONTRAST THERAPY

Several physiological effects have been proposed to explain the benefits of contrast therapy. Many have suggested that contrast therapy results in cycles of vasodilation and vasoconstriction, thus creating a "pumping action" to reduce swelling or "wash out" local chemical mediators. However, tissue temperatures are not affected by contrast treatments (Myrer, Draper, and Durrant 1994; Myrer et al. 1997; Higgins and Kaminski 1998). The brief exposure to cold and the fact that superficial heating has minimal effect on deep blood flow suggest that there is little vascular response to contrast therapy.

Even though there is no good explanation for the effects of contrast therapy, this approach has been used to treat some physically active people. For example, contrast therapy may be effective in reducing edema in subacute foot and ankle injuries. When swelling limits range of motion several days after injury, contrast therapy along with active range of motion appears to reduce swelling. The sharp sensory contrast between heat and cold appears to reduce pain and therefore muscle spasm. Models of descending influence over dorsal horn processing of nociceptive input certainly offer a plausible explanation for the analgesic response to contrast. A decrease in pain and spasm, combined with active, pain-free range of motion, would in turn increase lymphatic drainage from the area and decrease swelling.

As with many therapies, there has been little investigation of the effectiveness of contrast treatments. Cote et al. (1988) reported that swelling increased in sprained ankles after contrast therapy administered over 3 days after acute lateral ankle sprain. Certainly, these results suggest that contrast therapy should not be administered early in the plan of care. Kuligowski et al. (1998), however, found that contrast or cold therapy had more effect on pain and loss of motion associated with delayed onset muscle soreness than superficial heat. Further investigation is needed on this treatment approach to identify if and when it should be applied.

A Word on Counterirritants

The subject of counterirritants (analgesic balm) designed for superficial application does not fit with any specific chapter on therapeutic modalities. Although the topical application of some of these agents results in a sensation of cooling or heating (often implied in the product name), topical counterirritants do not result in clinically meaningful changes in tissue temperature (decrease or increase).

The lack of a thermal response does not mean, however, that these agents are clinically useless. The chemical stimulation of cutaneous sensory receptors will alter sensory input into the dorsal horn of the spinal column. The pain modulation theories presented in chapter 6 offer some explanation for the soothing, analgesic benefits of counterirritants. The rubbing required for application and the stimulating effects of the counterirritant will increase large-diameter afferent input. Thus, the stimulation of large-diameter first-order afferent nerves offers a plausible explanation for a favorable response to topical counterirritants. Some topical products contain salicylates or nonsteroidal anti-inflammatory medications. Mason et al. (2004) concluded that products containing salicylates may reduce acute pain but have lesser effects on chronic pain. Topically applied NSAIDs, ketoprofen in particular, also appear to be safe and effective in reducing pain (Mason et al. 2004).

SUMMARY

This chapter is devoted to the use of cold and superficial heat in the treatment of musculoskeletal injuries. The physiological and therapeutic response to treatment with cold is discussed with emphasis on effectiveness of treatment. The common applications and safety concerns related to cold and superficial heat are presented in chapter 11. This chapter introduced and briefly discussed contrast (heat and cold) treatments and topical counterirritants.

1. *Describe the four energy transfer mechanisms used by therapeutic modalities.*

Thermal energy can be transferred to or from the body by four mechanisms: conduction, convection, radiation, and conversion. Conduction involves direct contact between a warm and a cool surface. Convection is heating or cooling through the movement of air or a liquid. Radiation involves exposure of a surface to radiant energy, such as lying in the sun or under a heat lamp. Conversion involves converting one form of energy, such as ultrasound, to thermal energy.

2. *Describe the thermal changes that occur with local cold and superficial heat application.*

Cold application cools the skin and deeper tissues. Cooling of the skin occurs more rapidly than cooling of deeper tissues, and the skin is cooled to lower temperatures than the deeper tissues. However, a 20 min cold pack application will decrease muscle temperature approximately 7°F (4°C) at a depth of over 2 cm. Superficial heat increases the temperature of the skin. Due to the insulating effects of adipose tissues, the superficial joint structures are the only deep tissues that are heated to a clinically significant degree.

3. *Discuss the effects of local cooling and superficial heat on blood flow, muscle, and the nervous system.*

Superficial heat increases cutaneous blood flow. However, because blood flow to deeper tissues such as muscle is regulated by metabolic demand rather than temperature, superficial heating has little effect on blood flow in deeper tissues. Therapeutic cold causes vasoconstriction in cutaneous and deep tissues. Both therapeutic cold and superficial heat can decrease muscle spasm. Therapeutic cold decreases the temperature of muscle spindles, relieving muscle spasm. Superficial heat has a similar effect; however, because superficial heating does not raise deep tissue temperature, the decrease in muscle spindle activity is thought to occur through reflex mechanisms. A 15 to 20 min application of cold will decrease nerve conduction velocity. Because the rate at which impulses are carried by small-diameter primary afferent nerves is slowed, fewer pain messages reach the central nervous system and less pain is perceived. Superficial heat stimulates thermal receptors, from which increased input may trigger descending analgesic mechanisms mediated by the release of beta endorphin.

4. *Discuss the evidence on the treatment outcomes of local cold and superficial heat application.*

Although the use of cold and/or superficial heat with musculoskeletal injury management is empirically accepted, the effectiveness of such practices remains to be demonstrated. At present there is limited evidence for beneficial effects on tissue healing and ultimate treatment outcomes, and it warrants further critique for quality and strength.

5. *Describe the application of cold in a program of cryokinetics.*

Cryokinetics is a treatment technique that combines cold application and active exercise. Cold is used to decrease pain and muscle spasm and allow for pain-free therapeutic exercise.

6. *Describe contrast therapy.*

Contrast therapy involves alternating therapeutic cold and superficial heating modalities. This technique is most commonly used to treat the foot, leg, and ankle by alternating immersion in a warm and a cold whirlpool or water bath.

Clinical Applications of Cold and Superficial Heat

OBJECTIVES

After reading this chapter, you will be able to

1 describe the common methods and parameters of applying therapeutic cold and superficial heat;

2 discuss the indications for cold application and the impact of cooling on arthrogenic muscle inhibition and acute inflammation;

3 describe the contraindications to cold application;

4 discuss the indications for superficial heat application and the impact of heating on arthrogenic muscle inhibition and tissue elasticity;

5 describe the contraindications to superficial heat; and

6 describe the application of cold in a program of cryokinetics.

A 43-year-old club hockey player is referred to your care for treatment of an acute recurrence of low back pain. The player states that he twisted his back when he collided with two opponents in a game early this morning. He experienced immediate pain and chose not to continue playing because there were only a few minutes left in the game. He was evaluated by his personal physician because he began experiencing increased pain and muscle spasm while at work. He was provided with analgesic medications and referred for treatment of "mechanical low back pain."

On presentation he is in obvious discomfort but states that the pain is well localized to the mid-lumbar spine. He denies radicular symptoms or significant medical problems except for one previous episode of back pain that he experienced while cutting wood last year. He received treatment on three occasions consisting of superficial heat, manual therapies, and therapeutic exercise, and his back pain resolved within 2 weeks.

You determine that relieving pain and muscle spasm is the first priority. Which modality is the best choice? Are any treatments contraindicated? Which treatments will facilitate completion of therapeutic exercises at home? This chapter addresses the application of cryotherapy and superficial heat as therapeutic modalities.

The decision to include cold and superficial heat modalities in the treatment plan should follow the same evaluative process as for all therapeutic modalities:

- Indications for use
- Application outcomes
- Contraindications
- Form of modality (mode of delivery)
- Application parameters (settings)

Chapter 10 describes general physiological responses to cold and superficial heat. In this chapter, we will discuss specific indications for when thermal modalities would be beneficial, along with expected application outcomes and contraindications. There are many devices available for delivering therapeutic cold and superficial heat. Their manuals contain instructions on how to use them. Here we wish to stimulate your thoughts about which modes of application will most benefit your patients and which application parameters are supported in the literature.

CRYOTHERAPY

The main reason cold is applied in clinical practice is pain relief. Although repeated applications of cold may affect secondary tissue injury (introduced in chapter 5), much more study is needed before we can fully understand this phenomenon and determine if the effects are beneficial or ultimately delay tissue repair. Cryotherapy is a simple, portable, and inexpensive means of relieving pain and muscle spasm after musculoskeletal injury. Cryotherapy can be used to manage pain during the acute inflammatory response, to allow for pain-free therapeutic exercise, and to manage some persistent pain patterns, particularly myofascial pain syndrome.

Applying Cold After a Musculoskeletal Injury

Multiple acronyms reflect evolving concepts about the initial care of acute musculoskeletal injuries. RICE refers to Rest, Ice, Compression, and Elevation; PRICE to Protection, Rest, Ice, Compression, and Elevation; and POLICE (Bleakley, Glasgow, and MacAuley 2012) to Protection, Optimal Loading, Ice, Compression, and Elevation. What do these recipes for care mean? The notion of protecting injured tissue from further damage and managing pain by limiting use of the injured tissue (rest) are intuitive. The innate response to injury causes us to guard, protect, and limit the use of injured tissues. The application of ice (or cold) in response to injury is not innate but has become engrained in care recommendations. There has been little study, however, of the effectiveness of cryotherapy. Despite a culture in which ice application is central to conventional care recommendations, the magnitude of pain relief achieved during and after treatment has not been quantified in acutely injured patients. There is also little evidence to suggest that a quicker recovery is facilitated by the use of cold. This should not be construed to suggest cryotherapy is ineffective, but it is rather a reminder that clinicians should evaluate the expected effects and the role cold application plays in the rehabilitation program. Considerably more investigation is needed to identify the optimal effects and purposes for cold application.

Limiting and Managing Swelling

Compression and *elevation* may limit the extent to which swelling may develop. Compression opposes arteriole hydrostatic pressure or the force pushing plasma out of the circulation (capillaries). However, effective levels of compression increase pressure around mechanical and polymodal free nerve endings and may increase pain. Elevation decreases arteriole and capillary hydrostatic pressure and opposes the development of swelling. Since no external pressure is involved, elevation may be the most comfortable position for the injured body region. Unfortunately, the benefits of elevation are reversed when the injured limb is lowered.

Rest Versus Loading for Injured Tissues

Optimal loading seems counter to the recommendations for protection and rest. In concept, optimal loading does not exceed the ability of tissue to resist force and therefore does not cause additional damage or increase pain. It is now better understood that mechanical signaling can promote repair by up-regulating anabolic cell pathways and promoting appropriate stem/progenitor cell differentiation (see chapter 16). In theory, optimal loading is necessary to facilitate tissue repair without increasing pain.

Pain Modulation

After considering what is known and not known about tissue repair processes and the effects of cryotherapy following acute injury, is cold application indicated? Although we cannot precisely quantify the amount required for pain relief, the analgesic effect of cold modalities is empirically accepted. The benefits of the analgesic response should be focused on the goal(s) set for the individual application—for example, while in my care, the patient will experience decreased pain and muscle spasm. Depending on the nature of the injury and the stage of tissue healing, pain relief may be the only (if not the most important) treatment goal for that session. Among the practitioner's many skills, the ability to relieve discomfort and pain is paramount, even if the relief is transient.

Clinical experience suggests that cold application can alleviate pain associated with musculoskeletal injury. It appears that the more severe the reported pain, the greater the extent of relief experienced. At first, relief may come from stimulation of the periaqueductal gray (PAG) mediated analgesic mechanisms. Over several minutes the conduction velocity of thinly myelinated and unmyelinated nerves (A-delta and C) slows, reducing nociceptive information being directed toward the sensory cortex. The clinician should also consider the origins of the nociceptive signals; pain originating from deeper tissues may require longer applications of cold as well as a modality that can maintain an effective temperature gradient.

Clinicians have often used commercial cold water circulating units after surgery (e.g., Cryo/Cuff, Aircast Inc., Summit, NJ; Game Ready, Concord, CA). Although the cuff is applied over the surgical dressing, these devices have been reported by some investigators to relieve pain (Ohkoshi et al. 1999) and to decrease the use of pain medication (Ohkoshi et al. 1999; Barber, McGuire, and Click 1998). Because there is less tissue cooling, the unit can be applied for an extended period of time. However, further study is needed to substantiate these reports and compare the costs to the benefits of these cooling units.

Treating AMI

Swelling as a result of musculoskeletal injury, surgery, or arthritis has been associated with marked weakness and muscle atrophy. Swelling results in inhibition of motor neuron pools and prevents the person from fully activating a muscle. Pain is a foundational component of the inflammatory response to soft tissue trauma; Knight (1995) described the association of pain with lack of function. The resulting muscle spasm (guarding) serves to protect the area from further loading and trauma, but it also contributes to dysfunction or a lack of function. In addition, swelling forms in the interstitial and intra-articular spaces following the actions of inflammatory mediators. Together, these events create an environment of dysfunction that hinders or delays the remaining processes of tissue repair.

This stagnant environment presents a dilemma to tissue movement (resolving swelling), motor control, and strength gains, as the patient cannot recruit from a complete motor neuron pool. In addition, arthrogenic muscle inhibition (AMI) has been linked to early onset of joint osteoarthritis (Freeman, Mascia, and McGill 2013). Restoring movement has been linked to increased structural strength and stiffness of ligaments, increased collagen synthesis in tendons, and increased proteoglycan content in articular cartilage. As the healing process progresses to resolving swelling or restoring range of motion and strength, the ability to create movement of local tissues is integral to engaging the lymphatic system and capillary exchange.

AMI has been observed extensively with injury to the knee and ankle joints (Hopkins et al. 2002; Kuenze, Hertel, and Hart 2013; Pietrosimone et al. 2010; Rice, McNair, and Dalbeth 2009; Palmieri et al. 2004; Sedory et al. 2007). Experts describe AMI as a presynaptic, ongoing reflex inhibition of muscula-

ture surrounding a joint after distension or damage to that joint (Hopkins et al. 2002; Stokes and Young 1984; Young, Stokes, and Iles 1987). It is worth mentioning that, in studies of AMI, researchers have used a joint effusion model that does not produce pain, thereby attributing inhibitory effects to distention of the joint capsule. It is postulated that an excitation of mechanoreceptors in the involved joint capsule results in stimulation of Ib inhibitory interneurons; this inhibition is reflected by a decrease of available motor neurons within the muscle pool. Conversely, Doeringer, Hoch, and Krause (2009) state that an overfacilitation in motor neuron excitability could result in a constraint of the muscles surrounding the joint, thereby decreasing the freedom typically experienced by the joint and diminishing functional capabilities.

Cryotherapy has been shown to negate or diminish the affects of AMI at the knee and ankle. Two mechanisms have been said to result in the *disinhibitory* effect: a decrease in nerve conduction velocity and stimulation of Ia interneurons. First, local cooling with ice packs has been shown to decrease intra-articular temperature; Oosterveld et al. (1992; Oosterveld and Rasker 1994) described a decrease of 9.4°C after a 30 min application of ice. The change in temperature is attributed to decreasing the nerve conduction velocity and slowing the discharge rate of the aberrant mechanoreceptor excitation. This results in less information delivered to the spinal cord and a decreased stimulation of Ib inhibitory interneurons, hence disinhibition. Second, it is suggested that cold stimulates cutaneous receptors (mechanoreceptors and thermoreceptors) that may play a role in facilitating the motor neuron pool. The stimulated quick-adapting mechanoreceptors excite Ia interneurons, resulting in excitation of the motor neuron pool, which counteracts inhibition mediated by the Ib interneurons. It is also suggested that supraspinal centers are involved with the diminished inhibition observed with cold application, as the effects have been monitored to continue for 30 to 45 min after removal of the cold modality (Hopkins et al. 2002).

While the exact mechanism of AMI may not be completely understood, the beneficial influence of cold modality is apparent. These findings suggest the inclusion of local cold application in those patients who demonstrate swelling and muscle weakness or dysfunction. These effects are transient, and the long-term benefits of cryotherapy on AMI have not been demonstrated. As with using cold to modulate pain, benefits of the disinhibitory response should be focused on the goal(s) set for the individual application—for example, the patient will be able to perform volitional contractions that will assist with swelling reduction or restoring range of motion. Depending on the nature of the injury and the stage of tissue healing, not all patients with swelling will develop AMI.

Performance Enhancement and Recovery

Cryotherapy is often used to facilitate recovery from exercise, and coaches often suggest that cold immersion can be used to prevent soreness and fatigue, particularly in the lower extremities. Cold tanks are being installed in many athletic facilities to permit the use of this popular recovery modality. The science of cold immersion for recovery is still lacking, however. Several researchers have measured various factors, including vertical jump height (power), sprint times, and performance on an exhaustive exercise test to determine the effect of cryotherapy on subsequent physical tests (Rupp et al. 2012; Versey, Halson, and Dawson 2013). Most research has not shown that a single cold immersion treatment affects repeated performance better than controls. However, when looking at physiological factors such as inflammatory blood markers and even heart rate, there may be beneficial factors in using cold. More research is needed to determine the parameters associated with cold immersion and whether repeated treatments would have a cumulative effect on performance.

Cautions and Contraindications

A deleterious effect of cold modalities on the tissue healing process may be of concern. In chapter 4, we learned the inflammatory response is synonymous with tissue healing; acute inflammatory responses (i.e., vasodilation, chemical mediators, leukocyte infiltration) create a physiological environment for the eventual repair of damaged tissue and structures. While these physiological responses do not occur as individualized stages, they do build upon each other and establish a continuum of events. In chapter 10, we discussed the physiological effects of cold modalities: decreased cellular metabolism and activity, vasoconstriction, increased fluid viscosity. One can assume that the use of cryotherapy during the acute inflammatory response would interrupt the continuum, thereby impeding or halting the healing process. For example, cold-induced vasoconstriction and decreased membrane permeability reduce chemotactic signaling of neutrophil chemotactic factor (NCF) as well as diapedesis of neutrophils; this results in diminished attraction of macrophages and subsequent fibroblasts and hence deficient production of collagen tissue. This adverse effect of cold is theoretical, however, and at present there is no data supporting this paradigm.

Concerns may be alleviated by reviewing the clinical applications of cold. Current data and literature indicate that the physiological effects of cold are transient; changes remain for a limited time between 15 and 45 min after application. In addition, cold modalities are applied for a limited amount of time (e.g., 20 min) as well as inconsistently throughout the course of the day. Perhaps this mechanism may act to moderate the inflammatory response rather than retard it. Nevertheless, this speculation warrants further investigation into both the beneficial and detrimental contributions of cryotherapy.

Cold should not be applied in the presence of conditions worsened by treatment (Brown and Hahn 2009; Mailler-Savage and Mutasim 2008). Some medical conditions result in significant adverse reactions and contraindicate the application of cold (table 11.1). The most common condition in this category is vasospastic disorders, of which Raynaud's phenomenon is the most common. Raynaud's phenomenon is characterized by cold-induced constriction of arteries and arterioles in an extremity, most commonly the fingers, toes, and nose. The restriction in blood flow results in a blue, gray, or purplish discoloration of the skin accompanied by burning or tingling sensations or numbness. Raynaud's phenomenon is most common in women and usually develops during the early teen years. The symptoms and signs are transient; however, many people with Raynaud's phenomenon experience such discomfort that cold cannot be applied long enough to have a beneficial effect. Thus, cryotherapy is contraindicated.

Cold application is also very likely to worsen pain in patients suffering CRPS, complex regional pain syndrome (discussed in chapter 6). A clinician should also question the advisability of cold application in patients who report more, rather than less pain with treatment. There is no evidence that withholding cold negatively affects repair or recovery from injury. Some patients might obtain greater relief from modalities such as transcutaneous

Table 11.1   Indications, Contraindications, and Precautions for Cold

Indications	Contraindications	Precautions
Relieve pain	Raynaud's phenomenon	Application over superficial nerves
Control swelling and protect injured tissues (when combined with rest, elevation, and compression)	Cold urticaria	Diminished sensation
Decrease muscle spasm	Cryoglobulinemia Paroxysmal cold hemoglobinuria	Poor local circulation Slow-healing wounds Medically unstable

electrical nerve stimulation (TENS) or prescription medications. The lack of compelling evidence for the effectiveness of cold suggests that the patient's preferences should weigh heavily in the plan of care. Certainly, those who do not find relief with cold are unlikely to self-administer treatment even when advised to do so.

Cold urticaria, an allergic reaction to cold exposure, also contraindicates cryotherapy. When cold is applied to someone susceptible to cold urticaria, an **anaphylactic reaction** occurs. Hives break out in the cooler area and are accompanied by intense itching. Failure to recognize the problem and discontinue the cryotherapy could result in a more systemic reaction and could affect respiration and consciousness.

Cold-induced hemoglobinuria (urticarial cold hemoglobinuria) and cryoglobulinemia are two rare conditions that also contraindicate cryotherapy. Hemoglobinuria occurs when the rate of red blood cell breakdown exceeds the rate at which hemoglobin combines with other proteins. The excess hemoglobin is excreted in the urine. The condition is characterized by darkened urine and back pain. Cryoglobulinemia is a condition in which an abnormal clumping of plasma proteins (cryoglobulin) is stimulated by cold application. The symptoms include skin discoloration and dyspnea. These conditions may occur in conjunction with Raynaud's phenomenon or cold urticaria. Although these conditions are rare, you must keep them in mind. Initially cryotherapy is uncomfortable, but most people accommodate and tolerate it well. Be certain that discomfort during cryotherapy is not associated with any of these conditions.

Some other situations warrant caution. Some large nerves emerge from deep tissue and pass just below the skin and adipose tissue layers; because there is less tissue to insulate the nerve, it can be injured by cold or pressure during ice pack application. These injuries, referred to as cold-induced nerve palsy, are preventable. For example, the ulnar nerve as it passes through the ulnar groove and the peroneal nerve as it passes through the posterior lateral aspect of the knee are most susceptible. The lateral femoral cutaneous nerve can also be injured by cold applied in the area of the femoral triangle. Prolonged cold application (as little as 20 min) can damage these structures, leading to a loss of sensory and motor function. Protect these nerves by applying a dry cloth over the nerve, and limit cold application in the area to 20 to 30 min.

Special caution is also warranted when using cryotherapy to treat people who are frail, are suffering from significant medical problems, have slow-healing wounds, or have diminished circulation or sensation. The first law of therapeutics is "Do no harm." Thus, if you are uncertain about the safety of any modality, do not administer the treatment.

Mode of Delivery

Common forms of cold modalities used in the clinical setting include ice packs, whirlpools, garments and pumps, ice massage, and vapocoolant sprays. Access to the various forms is often dictated by the financial capability and resources of the particular setting, but the principles of energy transfer apply to all application modes.

Following acute injury, cold is most commonly applied by placing crushed ice in a bag. Cold water immersion (e.g., whirlpool) can be used to cool an extremity, such as the foot and ankle, while allowing for simultaneous therapeutic exercise (cryokinetics). Immersion of more surface area becomes increasingly uncomfortable. Ice massage offers an alternative that cools tissue and permits rapid initiation of exercise when sufficient response (numbness) is reported. The use of vapocoolant spray is only indicated for rapid relief of relatively minor injuries such as contusions.

Ice Pack

Ice packs can be created in several ways. The simplest and most common ice pack consists of crushed or cubed ice in a plastic bag or waterproof reusable pouch (figure 11.1). Crushed ice is often preferred because it conforms to the body more readily than cubed ice. An individual ice pack effectively cools a focal or localized area; multiple packs must be used to affect larger body parts. This is an inexpensive treatment that can be combined with compression and elevation of the injured part. If the injury involves an extremity, the bag can be secured over the injured area with a velcro strap, elastic bandage, or plastic film (e.g., Flexiwrap, Cramer). If the patient is suffering from low back, thoracic, or neck pain, it may be easier to lay the bag of ice directly on the body surface. Cooling with an ice pack is improved with the use of crushed ice and an elastic bandage applied over the ice pack (Knight 1995).

A couple of variations on the standard ice pack are worth mentioning: "wet ice" and "towel packs." Various researchers have described the concept and effectiveness of wet ice, in which crushed ice is combined with water. This approach allows for better heat exchange by maximizing the properties of phase change (from solid to liquid) of the ice. At present, there is no recommendation for an exact wet ice protocol, but Dykstra et al. (2009) described

effective gains using 2,000 mL of crushed ice with 300 mL of room temperature water. Towel packs consist of ice placed directly onto a dry towel, which is then folded to form an envelope surrounding the ice. Again, no exact recipe is available, but testimony by clinicians and patients reveal a favorable response to the comfort and conformability of the pack.

Commercial cold packs are also commonly used, but they do present varying concerns. The construction of some commercial cold packs does not allow them to conform well to the body. In addition, commercial cold packs stored in a freezer may be considerably colder than crushed ice, which is about 32°F (0°C). Because of the greater temperature difference between a commercial cold pack and the skin, cooling is more rapid and may result in frostbite. An insulating layer of plastic or cloth is recommended between commercial cold packs and the skin in order to prevent frostbite. However, available data suggest the properties of the insulating layer should be considered because it affects heat exchange (Tsang et al. 1997; Tsang and Truglio 2012). Conversely, commercial cold packs that are used often throughout the day may not present with the same temperature properties later in the day.

Cold Water Immersion

Cold water immersion and cold whirlpools are used to administer cryotherapy to cool tissues by convection (figure 11.2). Whirlpool units generally consist of a stainless steel tub (available in varying sizes) and a motorized turbine that circulates water within the

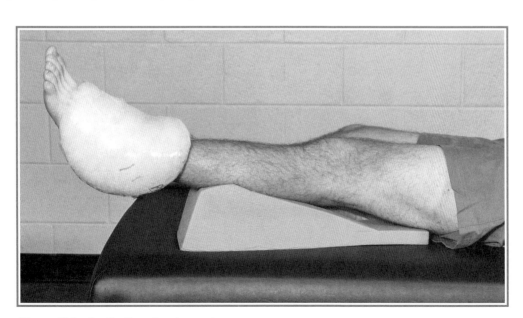

Figure 11.1 Application of an ice pack.

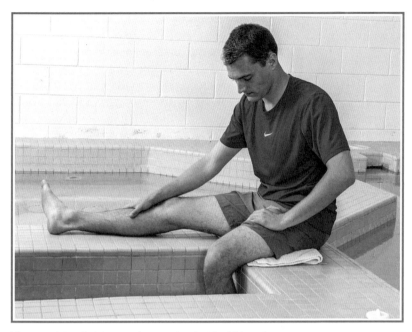

Figure 11.2   Cold water immersion/cold whirlpool.

tub. Water temperature is controlled by the amount of ice added to the tap water; this should be monitored throughout the day, as the temperature will rise as the whirlpool is used and as the ice melts. Immersion in 4 to 10°C (40-50°F) water or in a 10 to 15°C (50-60°F) whirlpool will cool tissue as well as an ice pack will (Pritchard and Saliba 2014), but cold immersion keeps the temperature lower for a longer period of time. Warmer water can be used in a whirlpool because the movement of the water continually breaks down the thermopane, the boundary layer of

water around the body part that is warmer than the cold bath (figure 11.3). Loss of the thermopane allows tissues to cool more rapidly. This application method offers a couple of advantages, including treatment of a larger body segment or multiple joints and the integration of cryokinetics with active exercise during the cooling process. Cold water immersion is also commonly used after intense exercise or competition in an attempt to minimize the effects of exercise-induced muscle damage and to facilitate recovery; these efforts have not been substantiated in the research literature but are common in clinical practice.

A common trend observed with modern facilities is the use of a walk-in pool for cryotherapy/cryokinetic treatment. These units are often Jacuzzi tubs or exercise pools that have been reconfigured with a refrigerant unit. This method offers a few additional advantages over standard whirlpools: large capacity for simultaneous treatment of multiple patients, active movements of multiple body segments, and minimal maintenance. In addition, the commercial refrigerant feature allows for ease in establishing and maintaining an optimal treatment temperature and gradient without the need to continually add ice.

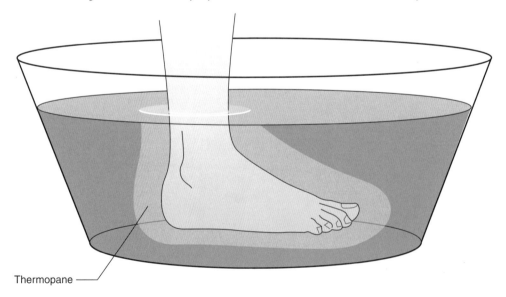

Thermopane

Figure 11.3   The foot immersed in cold water. The skin warms the surrounding water, forming a thermopane on the boundary layer, which is warmer than the cold bath.

Garments and Pumps

Cold water circulating units (figure 11.4), also called cryocuffs (a term derived from the trade name Cryo/Cuff), are similar to ice packs in that a cold surface is placed on or near the skin through preformed garments that are shaped to general anatomical segments, such as ankle, shank, and shoulder. Garments permit the treatment of a larger area than that achieved with an ice pack. Cold water is circulated through the garment, either gravity feed or with a mechanical pump. Standard units incorporate a chamber where ice is added to chill the water before circulation through the garment; advanced devices use a refrigerant unit to cool the water. Elevation of the extremity is more easily achieved with units that operate with a mechanical pump in comparison to gravity feed units. Some current models also offer the feature of added compression. Although less tissue cooling is achieved with this method when compared to direct application of an ice pack, tissue temperature does reach therapeutic levels (Tsang and Trulio 2012). A beneficial feature of these units is their application under the elastic wraps, dressings, and splints that are often applied postoperatively. The cold water circulating unit may lessen postoperative pain and the need for analgesic medications. These devices have also been reported to lessen blood loss following total knee arthroplasty (knee replacement surgery) (Levy and Marmar 1993; Leutz and Harris 1995). The cold water circulating unit provides hours of mild cooling without the need to remove braces and wraps and without the mess of ice packs.

Ice Massage

Ice massage is perhaps the most inexpensive form of cryotherapy (figure 11.5); water is frozen in a paper or foam cup, which is then used to cool and massage the skin. Reusable cup forms with handles are also available, making the application process even easier, although the melting ice does create a little bit of a mess. Ice massage is incompatible with elevation or compression and treats a very limited tissue area. However, ice massage has been reported to reduce pain before therapeutic exercise and may relieve postexercise discomfort.

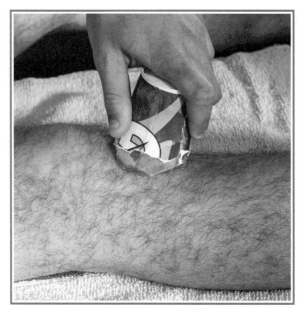

Figure 11.5   Ice massage.

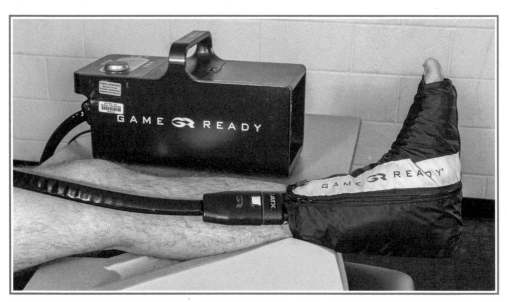

Figure 11.4   Cold water circulating unit.

This technique can also be used to desensitize trigger points in people who have myofascial pain syndrome, and it is easily incorporated with home-based treatment.

Vapocoolant Sprays

One more method of cold application warrants brief mention, vapocoolant or "cold sprays." These devices generally consist of a volatile liquid, such as ethyl chloride, fluorohydrocarbon, or alkane mixtures (butane, propane, and pentane) that evaporate upon being dispensed. When applied to the skin, the rapid evaporation produces a decrease in tissue temperature that is very superficial and localized (figure 11.6). There is virtually no temperature change below the epidermis; however, overspraying may cause frostbite of the superficial tissue. Vapocoolant sprays may temporarily interrupt ascending neural signaling (nociception and sensation) through the desensitization of receptors or the activation of ion channels. The anesthetic effect is brief but may be effective in the management of tender trigger points associated with myofascial pain syndrome (Travel and Simons 1983).

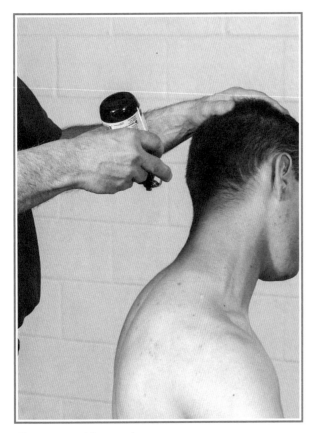

Figure 11.6 Vapocoolant spray.

Application Parameters

A summary of the literature on the physiological effects of cold reveals a target tissue temperature range of 13 to 15°C (55-60°F). Regardless of the mode of application (excluding vapocoolant sprays), all cold modalities will have to possess a similar temperature, such as a whirlpool circulating 13°C water. In addition, the ability of the modality to maintain the operational temperature will optimize heat transfer and tissue cooling. Certain application modes may be more desirable and efficient than others (for example, whirlpool versus multiple ice packs), especially in the treatment of multiple patients or in a large treatment area.

Treatment Time

Empirical evidence reveals most cold modalities are commonly applied for 15 to 20 min. This recommended time period appears to stem from earlier concerns about cold-induced vasodilation, more commonly known as the "hunting response" or "Lewis reaction" (Lewis, 1930). Lewis (1930) described the process of alternating vasoconstriction and vasodilation in extremities when exposed to cold. This was seen to occur within 10 to 20 min of exposure (dependent on the mode of exposure); therefore, to avoid the pro-inflammatory effect, clinicians adopted the limited treatment time. With advancements in technology, Knight et al. (1980) were able to reexamine this environment and found that the local vasodilation only lessened initial vasoconstriction; therefore net vasoconstriction remained.

Some have suggested that cold applied at intervals of 10 min is more effective than a sustained 20 min application (Bleakley et al. 2006). While there is no other literature that substantiates or contradicts the standard application time period, a recommendation may come from a practical viewpoint. As the cold modality is applied, the patient should be evaluated for the desired physiological response, such as pain relief. Regardless of how much time has elapsed, if the application goal has been attained, the application may be ended and the patient progressed to the next exercise or treatment. Further investigation into the effects of treatment applications of varying durations is needed to improve the efficiency of cold modalities.

Cryokinetics

Pain, swelling, and joint instability alter the ability to coordinate movement. The link between pain and muscle spasm (aka a pain–spasm cycle) is well recognized. Muscle spasm represents facilitation in motor activity. Patients experiencing low back pain, for example, often have palpable spasm of the paraspinal muscles. Cold may reduce muscle spasm by lessening the sensitivity of muscle spindles and thus allow for greater active motion. Increasingly the benefits of pain-free motion as well as the deleterious effects of rest following injury have been recognized. Not only is mechanical loading vital to tissue repair as previously discussed, limiting activity may promote AMI. Sound clinical judgment, however, must be used in initiating cryokinetics.

When treating an acute musculoskeletal injury, the clinician must be aware of the potential to further damage tissue and exacerbate symptoms with overly aggressive movement and tissue loading. With relatively minor injuries, such as a grade I lateral ankle sprain with injury isolated to the anterior talofibular ligament, cryokinetics can be initiated 1 to 2 days after injury. Activities such as walking and jogging do not stress the injured ligament. Thus, the injured person can return to daily activities when his or her function allows, provided that the ankle is protected from forced inversion. However, if the ankle injury is more severe and involves, for example, injury to the syndesmosis (articulation between the distal tibia and fibula), walking and jogging must be delayed until greater repair of the damaged ligaments permits pain-free, functional movement.

In general, cold decreases sensation and relieves pain but does not provide **anesthesia**. If exercise during cryotherapy is painful, it should be discontinued. Cold can be reapplied before resuming exercises after analgesia has returned. Clinical judgment is needed to know when it is best to end the exercise session. Pain managed by cryokinetics requires operational definition. In the context of cryokinetics, pain should be thought of as reported discomfort or discomfort that alters normal, functional movement patterns. Some patients may report little or no discomfort but may demonstrate a limp or other aberrant movement. Practiced aberrant movements likely foster, rather than reverse, AMI. Additionally, if the injured person becomes too aggressive with a therapeutic regimen, pain, spasm, and swelling may increase. An increase in symptoms on the day following therapeutic exercise slows the rate of recovery. It may take 1 to 3 days to manage the symptoms that are the source of the AMI the treatment was intended to reverse. Two good rules in any rehabilitation exercise program are as follows: (1) pain that alters normal movement patterns indicates that the person is not ready to perform the exercise, and (2) the person should be able to do tomorrow what was done today. Clinical experience will refine the clinician's ability to judge the appropriateness of an exercise for each person, but these rules are common-sense guidelines for the progression of therapeutic exercise, especially cryokinetics.

Video 11.1 demonstrates the use of cryokinetics for an ankle sprain.

SUPERFICIAL HEAT

Superficial heat is soothing; most people have found relief of sore muscles and joints in a hot shower, hot tub, or application of a heating pad. However, when is it appropriate to recommend the application of superficial heat in the treatment of musculoskeletal injury? Returning to the concepts that formed recommendations for treatment with cold, the use of superficial heat should be goal directed and do no harm. Superficial heat can be used during the latter stages of the inflammatory response to relieve pain and muscle spasm or tightness before therapeutic exercise. In addition, heating permits passive or active range of motion exercises that increase lymphatic drainage and reduce swelling. Superficial heat can also be used to treat restrictions in superficial joints.

Applying Superficial Heat After a Musculoskeletal Injury

As described in chapter 10, superficial heating increases blood flow in local tissues via vasodilation, increased membrane permeability of capillaries, and decreased fluid viscosity. During the acute response to injury, these physiological events are already in process due to the mechanisms of inflammation. Application of superficial heat during this stage would only serve to magnify the proinflammatory response and exacerbate pain and swelling. In addition, an increase in local cellular metabolism rate (nutrient demand and waste production) would further strain the injured tissue environment and contribute to secondary injury. Hence, the use of superficial heat is not advisable in patients who are experiencing physiological responses of acute inflammation.

Pain Modulation

Superficial heat alleviates pain, likely through the activation of pathways descending from the raphe nucleus to the dorsal horn of the spinal column. The magnitude of pain relief following superficial heat application has received limited attention. Denegar et al. (2010) reported slightly greater pain relief with circulating superficial heat (22% on average) or a heating pad in comparison to cold application (15%) in patients with knee osteoarthritis. Data from the same investigation revealed that superficial heat was preferred by twice as many patients as cold application; however, patients who preferred cold experienced more relief (33% reduction in pain). These data highlight the importance of patient preference in forming recommendations for care.

Muscle Spasms

Superficial heat has also been shown to reduce muscle tightness. Lewis et al. (2012) observed reduced paraspinal muscle activity in patients with low back pain following the application of a heat wrap. Interestingly, the application of superficial heat has little impact on the temperature of muscle, and thus the relaxation of muscle is likely due to the inhibition of pain, which in turn decreases activity in gamma motor pathways.

Again, the context of the complete injury environment must be considered in choosing to use superficial heat to decrease muscle spasms. Take, for example, muscle spasms that have developed as a result of dehydration. Applying superficial heat would transiently reduce muscle spasms and provide relief but at the same time would compound heat stress and the complications of electrolyte and fluid loss. Muscle spasms would undoubtedly return, probably in greater magnitude.

Tissue Elasticity

Limitations in range of motion may develop following musculoskeletal injury as a result of changes in the properties of ligaments, joint capsules, and tendons. Heat modalities increase the temperature of local tissues, but only for 3 to 5 min post application (Draper and Ricard 1995). Concomitant heating and loading (stretching) of these tissues have been demonstrated to restore functional range of motion. The joints of the hand, wrist, foot, and ankle respond best to superficial heat because there is little adipose tissue over these joints. However, ultrasound and diathermy result in a more vigorous heating and are the modalities of choice for heating tissue before mobilization and stretching. Knight et al. (2001) reported that the application of superficial heat did not enhance the effect of stretching of the plantar flexor muscles, while a 7 min ultrasound treatment was an effective adjunct.

Treating AMI

The effects of superficial heat application on AMI have not been extensively examined, and consequently the treatment is scarcely practiced in the clinical environment. Warner et al. (2013) reported a lack of effect on the quadriceps central activation ratio and knee extension torque. In this study, a moist heat pack was applied to the knee joint in patients with a history of knee injury or surgery and experiencing AMI. Most other studies on this topic use healthy participants who undergo an effusion protocol to induce an AMI response.

Regardless of methodology, the application of superficial heat to treat AMI appears counterintuitive. Inhibition demonstrated with AMI is caused by the excitation of mechanoreceptors in the involved joint capsule, resulting in stimulation of Ib inhibitory interneurons; this inhibition decreases the available motor neurons within the muscle pool. Superficial heat increases the conduction velocity and decreases the depolarization threshold of neural tissues; the increased temperature would only add to the volley of ascending neural signaling, thereby reinforcing inhibition. In addition, an overfacilitation in motor neuron excitability could result in a constraint of the muscles surrounding the joint, thereby diminishing functional capabilities (Doeringer, Hoch, and Krause 2009). This analysis, while theoretical, illustrates our limited understanding of AMI and reinforces the need for further investigations; given the strength of the available evidence, the application of cold or TENS is recommended in treating AMI. Further exploration of the management of AMI, especially in pathological patients, such as those with osteoarthritis, is warranted.

In summary, when the goal of treatment is the relief of pain and muscle tension, the application of superficial heat is a viable option. When properly administered (see "Cautions and Contraindications"), superficial heat is safe and often preferred by patients. Prolonged application through products such as Thermacare 8 Hours Heatwraps (Pfizer Consumer Healthcare, Kings Mountain, NC) has been reported to improve function (Tao and Bernacki 2005) and sleep quality (Nadler et al. 2003). These products are safe and warrant consideration when aching pain affects sleep or daily function.

Cautions and Contraindications

Clinical experiences, the limited research data available, and communication with the patient form the basis of decisions about the application of superficial heat. However, an acute inflammatory state is considered a contraindication to heating. The consequences of heating too soon after acute injury are largely unknown, but clinical observation suggests that in patients reporting higher levels of pain, heat will further exacerbate symptoms. During the initial response to injury, heating does not accelerate tissue healing; instead it exaggerates the inflammatory response, thereby hindering the healing processes. Superficial heating does result in increases of intra-articular temperature and skin temperature as well as small increases in muscle tissue temperature. Even small increases in blood flow will likely increase hydrostatic pressure and thus may increase swelling. Since the goal of heat application is primarily pain management, and other modalities and strategies for pain management are available, heat is not recommended as an alternative to cold in acute management.

Burns

Unlike the situation with cold, there are no rare complications associated with superficial heat (table 11.2). This does not imply, however, that superficial heat is completely safe. In fact, burns from superficial heating are far more common than cold-induced injuries. Burns, the primary risk of superficial heating, can be prevented by providing adequate insulation around moist heat packs, controlling whirlpool and fluidotherapy temperatures, and screening out individuals at risk for burns due to loss of sensation or circulatory problems. In addition, caution is needed when anyone lies on a moist heat pack because heat cannot escape, and it builds up more rapidly than it would otherwise. Extra insulation with toweling is needed if the injured person is to lie on the heat pack. Clear instructions are needed to prevent injury caused by superficial heating modalities during self-administered treatment.

Cardiovascular Stress

Heat also stresses the cardiovascular system. The heat stress from a superficial heat application combined with a warm, humid environment can be lethal for someone with coronary artery disease or multiple medical problems. These problems are not equally encountered in all health care settings. It is important for the clinician to be ever mindful that modalities routinely used with young, healthy people are not safe for everyone.

Mode of Delivery

Moist heat packs and warm whirlpools are the most commonly applied superficial heating modalities. Other forms—paraffin baths, heat lamps, and fluidotherapy—are also classified as superficial heating devices. The mode used to apply superficial heat varies by region of the body being treated, location of treatment, and intended purpose. As with cold modalities, the principles of energy transfer must be considered regardless of which application mode is selected.

Table 11.2   Indications, Contraindications, and Precautions for Superficial Heat

	Indications	Contraindications	Precautions
Superficial heating in general	Decreased pain Decreased muscle spasm	Diminished sensation Poor local circulation	Medically unstable Coronary heart disease
MODALITY SPECIFIC			
Whirlpool	Heat very superficial joint capsules	Open wounds	
Fluidotherapy	Heat very superficial joint capsules		
Paraffin	Heat very superficial joint capsules	Open wounds	

Moist Heat Pack

The most common form of superficial heating is a moist heat pack, usually a hydrocollator pack (figure 11.7); other forms include microwave safe heating packs and electric heating pads. Moist (hydrocollator) packs are convenient in clinical care, as the packs can be reheated often throughout the day; these heat packs are filled with a gel that retains heat. These packs are placed into a hydrocollator tank, a water tank equipped with a heating element that heats and maintains water at 76.6°C (170°F).

At the elevated temperature, direct contact could burn the skin; therefore a barrier should be used to wrap the pack (terry cloth covers or layered cotton towels). When using heat packs with patients who are at risk for skin injury (i.e., those with circulatory compromise) and in circumstances when a person lies on a hot pack, be certain to provide sufficient

Video 11.2 demonstrates proper clinical application of a hydrocollator pack.

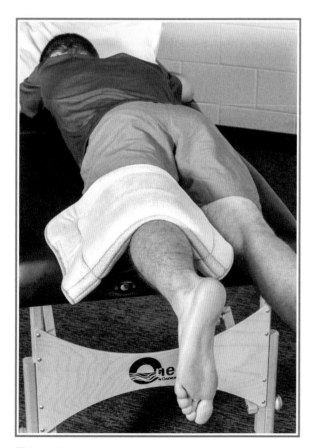

Figure 11.7   A hydrocollator pack application.

insulation. However, incorporating a barrier will decrease energy exchange, and therefore treatment time may need to be adjusted.

Superficial heating at home is more commonly done with packs that can be heated in a microwave oven or with an electric pad. Burns can occur with any form of superficial heating, but special caution is advised with electric heating pads. The devices do not cool over time when in use, posing greater risk with prolonged exposure such as when a patient falls asleep during treatment.

Video 11.3 demonstrates proper at-home application of a heating pad.

Warm Water Immersion

Warm water whirlpools are another common form of superficial heat (figure 11.8); they achieve heat exchange via convection. Whirlpools permit heating around an entire limb or joint. They also allow for active or passive motion during heating. The motion of the water subtly massages the tissue, which may add to the analgesic and antispasmotic effects of superficial heating. The same whirlpool units used for cold water immersion can be used for warm water immersion. Whirlpool units consist of a stainless steel tub (available in varying sizes) and a motorized turbine that circulates water within the tub. Water temperature is controlled by the amount of hot tap water used to fill the tub. These units are not equipped with a heating element; therefore water temperature will drop rapidly and must be adjusted throughout the day.

The temperature of the water must be maintained at a therapeutic level but also within a safe range. Water that is too hot can scald the skin; therefore whirlpool temperatures should never exceed 46°C (115°F). Treatment in a whirlpool also stresses the body's ability to dissipate heat and can result in hyperthermia and heat illness. The larger the portion of the body immersed in the whirlpool, the greater the heat stress. Table 11.3 provides reasonable guidelines for maximum whirlpool temperatures for various areas of the body. If the whirlpool is located in a poorly ventilated area, greater caution is advised. The whirlpool should be visible from all areas of the treatment facility, and no one should use a whirlpool unsupervised. Use extra caution when treating people who are prone to heat illness or who

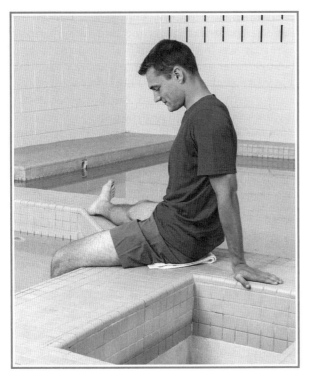

Figure 11.8 Whirlpool immersion.

have medical conditions that compromise the body's ability to withstand hot, humid environments.

However, thermal injury is not the only concern associated with whirlpool use; bacteria thrive in warm, moist environments. Whirlpools should be thoroughly cleaned and disinfected after each use. In facilities where many people are treated, the whirlpool may not be properly cleaned between uses. Under these circumstances, identify people with open wounds and take extra precautions to prevent the spread of infections.

Jacuzzi or hot tubs are commonly installed in modern facilities for superficial heat treatment. These units were originally designed to operate with heated water; therefore the only reconfigura-

tion is to the shape and size of the units. The same configuration has been applied to walk-in exercise pools. These units offer additional advantages over standard whirlpools, including their large capacity for simultaneous treatment of multiple patients and active movements of multiple body segments. In addition, the built-in heating element allows for ease in establishing and maintaining optimal treatment temperature and gradient without the need to continually add more hot tap water.

Paraffin

Paraffin baths are filled with seven parts paraffin wax and one part mineral oil heated to 51.6 to 52.7°C (125–127°F). Due to the lower specific heat of wax compared to water, higher temperatures are used than with whirlpool baths. Paraffin uses conduction to exchange heat energy and is most commonly applied in treating the hand and wrist, as it conforms around the fingers and hand to heat uniformly. Before application, the body area should be washed to minimize surface dirt and oils. Application protocol consists of dipping the body part into the paraffin (figure 11.9), then removing it until the wax hardens. This procedure is repeated four or five times until there is a thick layer of warm wax around the treated area. A plastic bag or oven mitt is placed over the treated area; the plastic bag allows you to remove the wax at the end of treatment without making a mess, but the oven mitt holds heat longer. Generally the paraffin is left on for 20 to 30 min. Paraffin has limited applications

Table 11.3   Maximum Whirlpool Temperature by Body Part*

Body part	Degrees F	Degrees C
Wrist and hand	112	44.4
Foot and ankle	110	43.3
Elbow	108	42.2
Knee	106	41.1
Thigh	104	40.0

*Assuming well-ventilated whirlpool area and absence of medical conditions that require precaution in warm, humid environments.

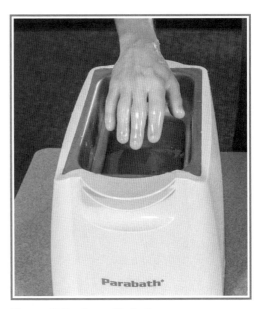

Figure 11.9 A paraffin bath.

and is not readily available in many settings, but it is valuable in treating hand pain and loss of hand function. Paraffin cannot be used if there is an open wound, and it should be used with caution if the person has sensory or vascular compromise in the area to be treated.

Heat Lamps

Heat lamps were once commonly used to provide superficial heat. Because of cost and convenience, heat lamps have been replaced by moist heat packs. A heat lamp positioned over a moist towel will increase the temperature of the skin. The amount of heating is dependent on the strength of the bulb and the distance between the lamp and the towel (inverse square law). The heat lamp provides the same benefits as a moist heat pack. However, each lamp can be used on only one person at a time, whereas many people can be treated simultaneously with inexpensive moist heat packs.

Fluidized Therapy

Fluidized therapy has been referred to as a dry warm whirlpool (figure 11.10). A fluidized therapy unit contains ground cellulose material that can be heated to 48.8 to 51.6°C (120-125°F) and then circulated within an enclosed chamber with forced air. The result is heating through convection and a subtle massage. Fluidized therapy is similar to paraffin in that the most common region treated with these devices is the wrist and hand. These units allow passive or active movement during treatment. Individuals with properly dressed open wounds can be treated with fluidized therapy without the risk of contamination. In contrast to what happens in treatment of an extremity in a whirlpool, with fluidized therapy the treated limb does not sit in a gravity-dependent position.

Application Parameters

A summary of the literature on the physiological effects of superficial heat reveals a target tissue temperature range of 40 to 45°C (104-113°F). Depending on the mode of application, caution is advised with heat modalities that possess a temperature higher than 46°C (115°F) due to the potential for scalding the skin. Mechanized units are often preferred because they can maintain the treatment temperature, optimizing heat transfer. In addition, certain application modes may be more desirable and efficient than others (e.g., whirlpool versus moist heat packs), especially in the treatment of multiple patients or in a large treatment area.

Treatment Time

The duration of heat application needed to alleviate pain and muscle tension has not been established. Clinical and personal experiences suggest that treatment goals can be attained with applications of 20 min or more. Empirically, very brief (a few minutes) application seems to have little effect. Heat wrap application provides a more sustained warming and favorable outcomes. Therefore it seems reasonable to recommend that superficial heat be applied at a comfortable temperature for 20 or more minutes as desired for the relief of pain and muscle tension. When applied to a joint before therapeutic exercise, joint mobilization or stretching, a similar duration is recommended.

CONTRAST THERAPY

As discussed in chapter 10, there is little research on the effectiveness of contrast therapy, and guidelines for application are based on clinical experiences and expert opinion. Contrast is most easily administered to the foot, ankle,

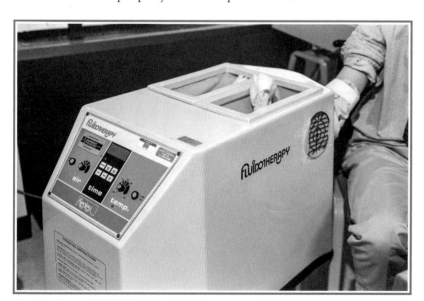

Figure 11.10 Fluidotherapy.

and leg, with alternating exposure to cold and heat. Most commonly, separate cold and warm whirlpools are used for this application (figure 11.11). The temperature of the cold bath and warm whirlpool should be within the ranges described in this chapter. The literature provides several recommendations about the length of time cold and heat should be applied, as well as the number of cycles of heat and cold that should be completed during a treatment (Walsh 1996; Bell and Prentice 1998). A cold-to-warm ratio of 1 to 3 min or 1 to 4 min appears reasonable based upon clinical observations and experience. There is no definitive literature to guide decisions about beginning or ending treatment with heat or cold. In general it is reasonable to recommend ending with heat if further activity is planned in comparison to ending with cold if the treatment is the last activity for the session. Due to the limited investigation of contrast treatments, it is not possible to provide guidelines about which patients might benefit. Contraindication for exposure to cold and heat should be observed, and as with all water-based treatment, any open wound must be protected from infection.

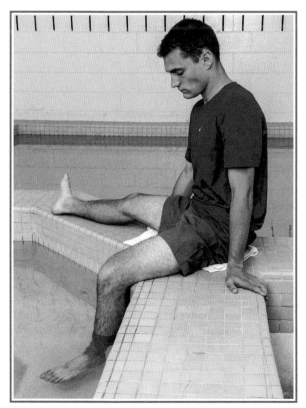

Figure 11.11   Contrast therapy.

SUMMARY

This chapter is devoted to the application of cold, superficial heat, and contrast therapy in the treatment of musculoskeletal injuries. The common applications and safety concerns related to cold and superficial heat are discussed.

Pain and muscle spasm indicate the use of cryotherapy, superficial heat, and contrast treatment. This raises the question, which is best? There is no simple answer. The clinician must consider several factors when selecting a modality, weighing the potential benefits against potential risks. Contraindications are the first consideration in selecting a therapeutic modality. If the injured person suffers from Raynaud's phenomenon (cryoglobulinemia, hemoglobinuria) or cold urticaria, then cold and contrast cannot be used. As noted, heat is not recommended during an acute inflammatory response to injury. Cold can be used to manage pain and muscle spasm associated with acute events. If cold is contraindicated, TENS and medication offer alternatives to manage pain, and there is no evidence that failing to treat with cold compromises recovery from injury. Combining cold with protection, elevation, and compression is generally recommended.

If neither heat nor cold is contraindicated and the condition is not acute, you must consider other factors in choosing between cryotherapy, superficial heat, and contrast therapy. The most important considerations are the severity of pain and muscle spasm, and patient preference. Cold is likely a better choice when pain and muscle spasm are severe. However, the patient's preference is also important. If a certain treatment has helped a person in the past, he or she is likely to believe that the treatment will work again and is likely to actively participate in a plan of care that includes that treatment.

Compliance by the injured person is especially important in a sports medicine clinic. The clinician often must develop home treatment programs for patients who are treated in the clinic only once or twice per week, or may be away from a school-based facility. Certainly someone who prefers not to be treated with cryotherapy is unlikely to use cold at home unless provided with a very convincing argument about why such treatments are essential to his or her recovery. Thus, the ease of application and the probability of compliance with home use are also considerations when you are choosing between cryotherapy and superficial heat.

1. *Describe the common methods and parameters of applying therapeutic cold and superficial heat.*

   Therapeutic cold can be applied with an ice pack, ice massage, a cold whirlpool, cold water immersion, or a vapocoolant spray. Superficial heat can be applied with a hot pack, a heating lamp, a warm whirlpool, paraffin, or fluidized therapy.

2. *Discuss the indications for cold application and the impact of cooling on arthrogenic muscle inhibition and acute inflammation.*

   Cold is primarily used to relieve pain and muscle spasm. Cold may also limit swelling after musculoskeletal injury. Following an acute injury, cold application will be maximally effective when combined with compression, elevation, and protection of injured tissues. Cold has also been shown to disinhibit neuromuscular pathways in patients exhibiting arthrogenic muscle inhibition. The application of cold to the affected joint, such as a knee, prior to exercise involving the quadriceps can result in better motor unit recruitment than can be achieved without cold application.

3. *Describe the contraindications to cold application.*

   Some medical conditions result in significant adverse reactions and contraindicate the application of cold (table 11.1). The most common condition in this category is vasospastic disorders, among which Raynaud's phenomenon occurs the most frequently. Cold urticaria, an allergic reaction to cold exposure, also contraindicates cold application. Cold-induced hemoglobinuria (paroxysmal cold hemoglobinuria) and cryoglobulinemia are two rare conditions that also contraindicate cryotherapy. Hemoglobinuria occurs when the rate of red blood cell breakdown exceeds the rate at which hemoglobin combines with other proteins. Cryoglobulinemia is a condition in which an abnormal clumping of plasma proteins (cryoglobulins) is stimulated by cold application. In addition, cold can injure superficial nerves such as the ulnar and common peroneal. Thus, extreme caution is required when cold is applied near or over these structures.

4. *Discuss the indications for superficial heat application and the impact of heating on arthrogenic muscle inhibition and tissue elasticity.*

   Superficial heat is used to relieve pain and muscle spasm. The choice between using heat and cold depends on a number of factors, including contraindications, degree of pain and muscle spasm, and preference.

5. *Describe the contraindications to superficial heat.*

   The primary concern with the use of superficial heat is burns. The clinician must be sure that the patient can sense heating and tolerate warming of the skin. In patients for whom the application of heat is deemed safe, heat should not be applied during an acute inflammatory response. If patients self-apply heat at home, it is important to review safe application procedures. Burns can be prevented through the use of insulating materials and instructing patients in the appropriate positioning for and duration of treatment.

6. *Describe the application of cold in a program of cryokinetics.*

   Cryokinetics literally means cold and movement. When neuromuscular control is lost and AMI is exhibited after an injury, cold can be used to alleviate pain and reduce muscle spasm. In some cases (e.g., weeks after anterior cruciate ligament reconstruction) AMI persists after pain and muscle spasm resolve. In these cases cold can be applied until numbness is achieved (typically 15–20 min) in preparation for therapeutic exercises appropriate for the condition being treated. For example, following a lateral ankle sprain, cold application may precede weight bearing and walking to facilitate restoration of a normal, pain-free gait.

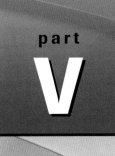

Ultrasound, Electromagnetic Fields, and Laser Therapies

Part V provides an understanding of the physical principles and applications of three somewhat related therapeutic modalities, in that they all have a role in biostimulation. Therapeutic ultrasound has been applied in the treatment of musculoskeletal conditions for decades. Ultrasound can increase the temperature of subcutaneous tissues and affect cell function. The parameters of the acoustic signal can alter the tissues' responses, and they vary with the goal of the treatment. The clinical benefits of treatment with ultrasound have been questioned. These issues are discussed in the context of contemporary considerations of effectiveness and costs. Diathermy is similar to ultrasound in its ability to heat deeper tissues without elevating skin temperature. Diathermy exposes the target tissue to an electromagnetic rather than acoustic energy field. Similar to the discussion of ultrasound, the physical principles, potential benefits, contraindications, and safety considerations of diathermy are presented. A brief discussion of pulsed electromagnetic fields in fracture care is also provided.

Laser is a somewhat newer therapeutic modality. In clinical care, nonheating, low-power lasers are used for therapeutic benefit. Chapter 14 explains the physical principles of lasers. Clinical application, considerations for safety, and a review of the clinical research related to the outcomes of treatment with laser are provided in chapter 15.

Principles of Ultrasound and Diathermy

OBJECTIVES

After reading this chapter, you will be able to

1. describe how therapeutic ultrasound is generated by the treatment unit;

2. define beam nonuniformity ratio (BNR) and effective radiating area (ERA);

3. identify and describe the use of effective conducting media for ultrasound treatments;

4. define dose, duty cycle, treatment duration, and frequency as parameters of therapeutic ultrasound;

5. describe the thermal effects of therapeutic ultrasound;

6. describe the treatment parameters and physiological effects of pulsed ultrasound;

7. discuss the technique and effectiveness of phonophoresis;

8. describe the differences between therapeutic ultrasound and diathermy;

9. identify the two mechanisms through which diathermy can be used to heat deep tissues; and

10. describe the potential uses of diathermy and pulsed electromagnetic field therapy in the treatment of musculoskeletal injuries.

Two people are awaiting treatment at a university sports medicine clinic. The first is a 22-year-old track athlete who sustained a strain of the biceps femoris 3 weeks ago. The second is a 36-year-old tennis player suffering from limited left wrist range of motion after suffering a distal radius and ulna fracture in a motor vehicle accident 10 months ago. Is treatment with ultrasound or diathermy indicated in the treatment of either athlete? What parameters should be selected with the use of the modalities? How is the energy transmitted into the tissues? This chapter examines current uses and the evidence of efficacy of ultrasound and diathermy and pulsed electromagnetic fields.

This chapter focuses on therapeutic ultrasound and, to a lesser extent, the therapeutic use of diathermy and pulsed electromagnetic fields. Ultrasound and diathermy can be administered by clinicians to heat deeper tissues including muscles, tendons, ligaments, joint capsules, and scar tissue. Unlike the superficial heating modalities discussed in chapter 10, acoustic energy generated by ultrasound devices and electromagnetic fields generated by diathermy units penetrate the skin and subcutaneous fat. Thus, ultrasound is considered a deep-heating modality.

Not all of the purported benefits of ultrasound are attributable to thermal effects. When ultrasound is pulsed, less heating occurs than when treatment time remains the same. Responses to pulsed ultrasound are believed to be due to the effect of the sound energy at the cellular level as opposed to tissue heating.

Sound energy also has been used to drive medication through the skin. This process, known as **phonophoresis**, has been used commonly in athletic training and physical therapy despite very little evidence of efficacy. These issues are explored in greater detail later in this chapter.

At one time diathermy was a popular deep-heating modality. Because diathermy is more cumbersome to apply and has more contraindications than ultrasound, diathermy is now less commonly used in clinical practice. However, new diathermy devices have come on the market, and diathermy is available in more facilities than it was a few years ago. Diathermy allows for heating of larger areas of tissue.

ULTRASOUND

Ultrasound differs from the modalities discussed in the previous three chapters in that it transmits energy that falls within the acoustic, rather than electromagnetic, spectrum. Ultrasound is used in medicine for imaging as well as in the treatment of musculoskeletal conditions. Different frequencies of ultrasound are used for each application. The ultrasound units used in the practice of athletic training and physical therapy emit sound energy at frequencies between 800 kHz (800,000 Hz) and 3 MHz (3,000,000 Hz). Modern high-quality ultrasound units allow the clinician to select the treatment frequency. Typically a clinician can choose frequencies near 1 MHz and 3.3 MHz. Some units are also adjustable to 2 MHz (figure 12.1). The importance of frequency and the applications of ultrasound at various frequencies will be discussed in detail. Initially, it is important to understand that therapeutic ultrasound uses acoustic energy, delivered at very specific high frequencies.

Ultrasound machines use electrical current to create a mechanical vibration in a crystalline material housed in the "head" of the unit. Vibration of the crystalline material produces a wave of acoustic energy (ultrasound) (figure 12.2). The crystalline material in modern ultrasound devices is synthetic, although natural crystals were once used. The sound energy emitted from the ultrasound head travels through tissues and is absorbed.

Ultrasound technology is now used extensively for diagnostic imaging. Ultrasound in the range of 3.5 MHz to 15 MHz is used to image organs of the abdo-

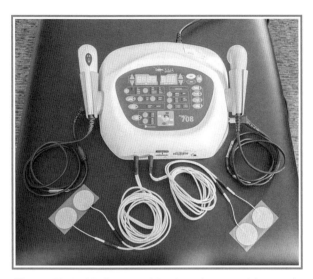

Figure 12.1 Modern combination ultrasound, laser, and electrotherapy device.

men and thorax as well as musculoskeletal tissues (Whittaker et al. 2007). Ultrasound is also routinely used for prenatal examination. Through ultrasound, some correctable birth defects can be identified, and the sex of the fetus can also be determined.

In musculoskeletal care, ultrasound can be used to detect muscle strains, ligament sprains, and degenerative changes in tendon. The sound energy used for imaging differs in frequency and pulse characteristics from that used for therapeutic purposes.

Beam Nonuniformity Ratio and Effective Radiating

Two terms describe the size and quality of an ultrasound crystal found in *therapeutic* ultrasound devices.

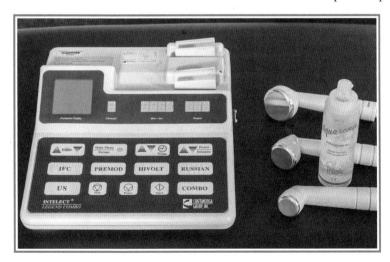

Figure 12.2 Components of an ultrasound unit.

Effective radiating area (ERA) is the area that receives at least 5% of the peak sound energy. This is essentially the size of the area to which sound energy is conducted when the head of the ultrasound unit contacts the skin. The ERA is somewhat smaller than the surface area of the sound head.

The beam of sound energy emitted from a crystal is not uniform but rather is characterized by areas of high intensity and lower intensity (figure 12.3). **Beam nonuniformity ratio (BNR)** is the ratio of the average intensity of the ultrasound beam across the ERA divided by the peak intensity of the ultrasound beam; the lower the BNR, the more uniform the intensity of the sound wave.

$$BNR = \frac{\text{spacial peak intensity}}{\text{spacial average intensity}}$$

A low BNR minimizes the risk of developing "hot spots" and allows the clinician to deliver higher doses of ultrasound without causing pain and discomfort. The BNR must be listed by the manufacturer on all units. Ideally, the BNR would be 1; however, this is impossible, and the acceptable range is between 2 and 6.

Unfortunately, BNR and ERA may not adequately define how an ultrasound unit will function. Holcomb and Joyce (2003) reported significant differences in the change in tissue temperature between two ultrasound units with a BNR of 3.7 and 2.3 and an ERA of 4.9 and 4.6 cm, respectively. These authors speculated that the area of peak intensity or peak area of the maximum beam nonuniformity ratio (PAMBNR) as described by Draper (1999) might explain why two ultrasound units differ in performance. Certainly a small spike of peak amplitude as illustrated in figure 12.4 will deliver less energy and therefore have less thermal effect than that provided by a larger area of peak amplitude. Johns, Straub, and Howard (2007) and Straub, Johns, and Howard (2008) reported considerable variability in ERA and special average intensity in 3 and 1 MHz ultrasound units, respectively, from different manufacturers. Differences between reported and actual ERA values were identified for all but one manufacturer when 3 MHz sound heads were evaluated (Johns, Straub, and Howard 2007). Demchak, Straub, and Johns (2007) noted differences in the rate but not peak heating of the calf muscles using three different 1 MHz ultrasound

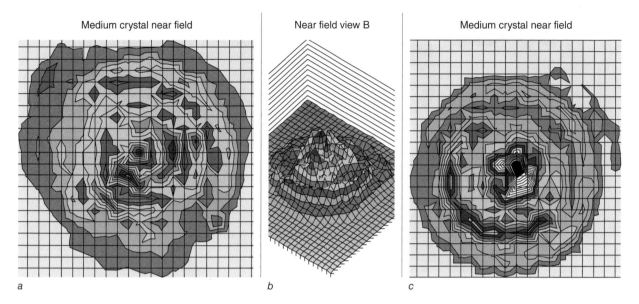

Medium crystal near field   Near field view B   Medium crystal near field

a   *b*   *c*

Figure 12.3   Beam scan of a crystal with a beam nonuniformity ratio (BNR) of 2.32, *(a)* top view and *(b)* side view. When tested on 40 subjects, the ultrasound transducer housing this crystal produced a very comfortable treatment at 1.5 to 2.0 watts per cm² (W/cm²). Beam scan of a crystal with a BNR of 7.75, *(c)* top view. When this was tested on 40 subjects, the ultrasound transducer housing the crystal produced an uncomfortable treatment at 1.5 W/cm² and was not tolerated at 2.0 W/cm².

Courtesy of Brigham Young University Sports Injury Research Center.

transducers. Johns et al. (2007), however, have reported greater heating with 1 MHz sound heads with more concentrated energy fields. The issue of equipment performance across parameters requires further study. Variability in the characteristics of the acoustic energy field may yield differing treatment effects and perhaps pose a risk of adverse events. Frye et al. (2007) reported blistering of the anterior shin after ultrasound to the calf muscles in laboratory experiments employing common clinical treatment parameters.

a   *b*

Figure 12.4   The area of peak intensity, *(a)* small and *(b)* larger, may affect the performance of ultrasound devices.

Conducting Media

Air is a poor conductor of ultrasound energy. To maximize delivery of sound energy to the tissues, a conducting medium must be used. Several substances have been used to conduct ultrasound, including ultrasound gel, gel pads, mineral oil, lotions, and water. The amount of sound energy conducted varies substantially between conducting media. Commercial ultrasound gel (Draper 1996; Draper et al. 1993; Klucinec et al. 2000) and gel pads (Klucinec et al. 2000; Klucinec 1996) (figure 12.5) are superior conducting media. Water is not as good a conducting medium (Draper 1996; Draper et al. 1993; Klucinec et al. 2000; Klucinec 1996; Forrest and Rosen 1989, 1992), attenuating as much as 65% of the sound energy (Klucinec et al. 2000).

Rubley et al. (2008) reported smaller differences (approximately 15%) in Achilles tendon tissue heating when comparing gel and degassed water as conducting media. Differences in research methods and ultrasound equipment may explain the estimated magnitude of differences between conducting media. Collectively, however, the research suggests that ultrasound

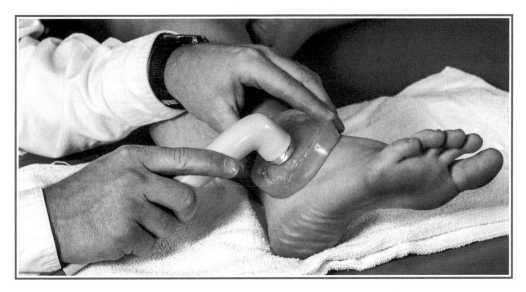

Figure 12.5 Ultrasound gel and gel pads.

gel is the conducting medium of choice for clinical administration of therapeutic ultrasound. The conducting capacities of most gels and creams have not been established. However, some have been shown to be very poor conductors of sound energy (Cameron and Monroe 1992; Draper 1996; Draper et al. 1993; Forrest and Rosen 1989, 1992; Klucinec 1996; Klucinec et al. 2000). When applying ultrasound, use gels and gel pads known to be effective conductors.

Parameters of Treatment with Ultrasound

As with electrotherapy, you can alter the treatment parameters of ultrasound depending on the desired effect. Fortunately, the number of adjustable parameters is smaller. You can control the amplitude of the sound waves and therefore the amount of sound energy being emitted from the sound head. The sound energy emitted by the crystal is measured in watts (W). The dose of sound energy delivered is based on the amount of energy being emitted divided by the radiating area of the crystal measured in square centimeters (cm^2). Thus, ultrasound dose is measured in W/cm^2. You can also adjust the duty cycle, duration of treatment, and frequency.

Duty cycle refers to the process of interrupting delivery of the sound wave so that periods of sound wave emission are interspersed with periods of interruption. Figure 12.6 depicts pulsed and continuous ultrasound.

Often you can select between several duty cycles. Duty cycle is calculated by dividing the time during which sound is delivered by the total time the sound head is applied. For example, if ultrasound is

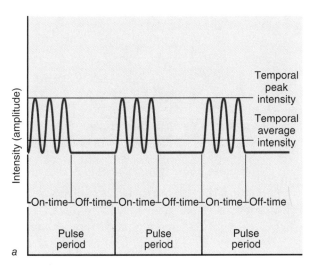
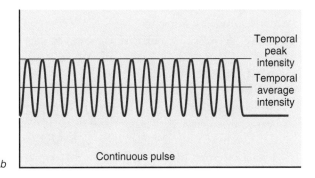

Figure 12.6 *(a)* In pulsed ultrasound, energy is generated only during the "on" time. Duty cycle is determined by the ratio of "on" time to pulse, in this case 50%. *(b)* Continuous ultrasound is shown.

transmitted for 150 ms out of every second of treatment, then the duty cycle is 150/1,000, or 15%. When the emission of sound energy is not interrupted, the duty cycle equals 100%, and the ultrasound is referred to as continuous ultrasound.

Much has been learned about the treatment duration needed to elevate tissue temperatures. An interaction among the frequency, dose, and treatment duration has also been found. Some recipes for duration and intensities of ultrasound treatments used in the past do not increase tissue temperature sufficiently.

The frequency of the sound waves affects the depth at which the greatest amount of ultrasound energy is absorbed, as well as the time required to increase tissue temperature. Ultrasound units typically allow for treatment with more than one frequency, but older units had a single fixed frequency of 1 MHz. Treatments with higher frequencies are usually more appropriate for musculoskeletal injuries.

Sound Energy Absorption in Tissues

The amount of acoustic energy absorbed by tissues is influenced by many factors. The tissue characteristics, as well as the frequency, dose (W/cm²), duty cycle, and duration of treatment with ultrasound affect the amount of acoustic energy absorbed. When continuous ultrasound is delivered, the greater the energy absorption, the greater the tissue heating. Tissues with greater protein density have a higher rate of absorption, whereas tissues with a higher water content have lower absorption rates. Thus, tendon, ligament, and muscle tissue absorb more sound energy than skin and adipose tissue. Superficial bones and nerves absorb the most energy.

Ultrasound at a higher frequency (3 MHz) is absorbed more rapidly than that at a lower frequency (1 MHz) (figure 12.7). Therefore, ultrasound at higher frequencies affects tissues that are more superficial, whereas at a lower frequency less energy is absorbed superficially and more is available to penetrate into tissues. Thus, if the goal of treatment is to heat the capsular tissue at a joint such as the elbow with ultrasound, a 3 MHz frequency is appropriate. Temperature increases of up to 8°C have been reported with 3 MHz ultrasound at 1 W/cm² in 4 min in superficial tissues such as the

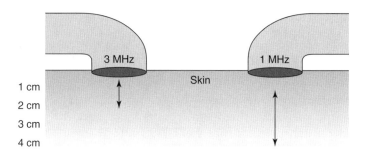

Figure 12.7 A great depth of heating is achieved with 1 MHz. The specific depth of heating is device dependent, and the values provided represent a range rather than specific limits of thermal responses.

patellar tendon (Chan et al. 1998). If the target tissue is deep tissue, a lower frequency (1 MHz) is necessary; 10 min of continuous 1 MHz ultrasound at 2.0 W/cm² will elevate temperature about 4°C at a depth of 2.5 cm (Draper, Castel, and Castel 1995). There is likely considerable overlap in tissue heating between 1 and 3 MHz ultrasound, as heating of tissues at 2.5 cm depths with 3 MHz ultrasound has been reported (Hayes et al. 2004). The interactions between ultrasound parameters and thermal response are discussed further shortly.

Thermal Effects of Ultrasound

Many of the benefits of ultrasound have been attributed to tissue heating. This section examines the effects of parameter adjustments on the thermal response to ultrasound. Draper (1996) suggested that an increase of 1°C (mild heating) increases metabolic activity; a 2° to 3°C increase reduces muscle spasm, increases blood flow, and reduces chronic inflammation; and a 4°C increase alters the viscoelastic properties of collagen.

An increase in temperature increases metabolic activity in deeper tissues. When these tissues are more active, the demand for oxygen is increased, which, in turn, increases local blood flow. Thus, one of the effects of ultrasound is to increase local blood flow. The issues of tissue repair and treatment efficacy with ultrasound are discussed later in this chapter.

The analgesic and antispasmotic responses to ultrasound are not as great as those following cryotherapy, superficial heating, and transcutaneous electrical nerve stimulation. The primary effects of continuous ultrasound are increases in collagen elasticity in response to increased tissue temperature. By properly selecting treatment parameters you can increase temperature more than 4°C in the target tissue.

Duty Cycle and Tissue Heating

Continuous ultrasound results in therapeutically beneficial amounts of tissue heating. Pulsed ultrasound may have therapeutic benefits in certain circumstances (see "Efficacy of Ultrasound Therapy for Musculoskeletal Conditions" later in the chapter), but these effects are nonthermal. Certainly the sound energy delivered with a pulsed ultrasound treatment is absorbed into the tissues at depths determined by the frequency of the sound wave. However, the total energy delivered during pulsed ultrasound is less than with continuous ultrasound at the same intensity and duration. Thus, less local tissue heating occurs.

Dose and Tissue Heating

The greater the dose of sound energy, the greater the amount of energy delivered to the tissues. Thus, with continuous ultrasound, a higher dose results in greater tissue heating in less time. Many clinicians administer ultrasound at a low dose, often 1.5 W/cm², because they were instructed in school to do so. This practice may have come about because older units caused discomfort at higher doses due to the characteristics of the crystal. Although higher doses of ultrasound, greater than 2.5 to 3.0 W/cm², can damage tissue, you should not limit the dose to 1.5 W/cm².

Treatment Time and Tissue Heating

There is an interaction among frequency, dose, and the time required to increase tissue temperature. At a frequency of 3 MHz, 4 to 5 min is sufficient to achieve a 4°C increase in local tissue temperature at a dose of 1.5 W/cm². However, when a 1 MHz frequency is applied, a 10 min treatment at a dose of 2.0 W/cm² is required to achieve the same increase in tissue temperature (Draper 1996; Draper, Castel, and Castel 1995). Although no minimum dose has been established for obtaining specific levels of heating, longer applications are needed when lower intensities of ultrasound are used. For example, a 1 MHz frequency continuous ultrasound treatment at 1.5 W/cm² requires 12 min to increase tissue temperature 4°C as opposed to the 10 min needed at 2 W/cm² (Draper 1996).

Treatment Area, Sound Head Movement, and Tissue Heating

The parameters outlined in the previous sections to heat deeper tissues are predicated on treatment over an area no greater than three times the ERA of the crystal and a slow, controlled movement of the ultrasound head. When larger areas are treated, the amount of acoustic energy reaching any single area is decreased. In addition, heat buildup is allowed to dissipate from the target tissue. Thus, there is less temperature increase during treatment and therefore less change in tissue elasticity and local blood flow during and after treatment.

Treating larger areas such as the lower back has little or no effect on the tissues, although there may be a placebo effect. Thus, ultrasound should not be applied over large areas. Currently, the best recommendation for treatment technique suggests covering a treatment area two to three times the ERA with the sound head covering less than two times the ERA per second (ERA/s).

Moving the sound head slowly prevents hot spots from developing in areas of peak amplitude and helps you maintain good contact with the skin or gel pad surface. With higher-quality, lower BNR rating crystals, the sound head can be moved more slowly, resulting in more uniform heating and greater patient comfort. Rapid, sloppy movement of the sound head with frequent breaks in contact between the skin or gel pad decreases the thermal response to treatment.

Tissue Cooling

Tissue temperatures fall fairly rapidly following ultrasound therapy. Draper and Ricard (1995) reported that when 3 MHz ultrasound was used to heat muscle tissue at the depth of 1.2 cm to an average of 5.3°C, the tissue cooled 2°C within the first 3.5 min. Rose et al. (1996) reported that tissues at 2.5 and 5 cm depth, heated 4°C by 1 MHz continuous ultrasound, cooled 2°C in less than 7 min. From these studies it is apparent that the thermal response to ultrasound is short-lived and that superficial tissues cool more rapidly than deeper ones. Thus, any stretching or manual therapies should be performed immediately following treatment or even initiated in the last few minutes of treatment when possible if the benefits of heating from ultrasound are to be realized.

Nonthermal Ultrasound and Repair

Therapeutic ultrasound, as described so far, relates to clinical applications commonly provided by athletic trainers, physical therapists, and other health care providers. When ultrasound is pulsed or administered at low amplitude, little or no heating occurs. However, pulsed ultrasound has been shown to affect tissue healing in some circumstances and to alter cellular activity in vitro. Research has demonstrated that low doses of ultrasound, electrical energy, and light energy can speed healing in some patients. Reports on the use of pulsed ultrasound in treating human patients with chronic ulcers suggest that pulsed ultrasound has a physiological impact (Callam, Harper, and Dale 1987; Dyson and Suckling 1978; Erikson, Lundeberg, and Malm 1991). However, the subjects of these studies differ from healthy athletes in many respects, and we must use caution in generalizing these results to the treatment of musculoskeletal injuries. More recently, Loyola-Sánchez (2012) reported that active ultrasound therapy administered using a 1 MHz ultrasound device with a therapeutic dose of approximately 0.2 W/cm^2 (112.5 joules per cm^2 (J/cm^2) avg amplitude = 1.0 W/cm^2, ultrasound pulsed to 20% for 9.5 min, treatment 3 times per week for approximately 8 weeks [24 treatments]) increased medial tibial cartilage thickness in patients with mild to moderate osteoarthritis. The clinical implications of this work as well as the precision of the estimate of magnitude of thickening and optimal parameters require further investigation. These findings, however, offer evidence of a treatment effect when ultrasound is applied in the management of degenerative musculoskeletal conditions. The responses to ultrasound cannot be solely attributed to a thermal response.

Low intensity, pulsed ultrasound (LIPUS) has been shown to speed fracture healing in human patients and animal models (Bashardoust Tajali et al. 2012; Walker, Denegar, and Preische 2007; Urita et al. 2013; Kristiansen et al. 1997). The parameters of LIPUS differ from conventional ultrasound. For example, Urita et al. applied a commercially available LIPUS device (Sonic Accelerated Healing System 2000, Smith & Nephew, Memphis TN) that provided ultrasound delivered at a frequency of 1.5 MHz, modulated to 30 mW/cm^2 daily for 20 minutes to patients recovering from forearm osteotomy procedures for up to 12 weeks postoperatively. They reported a 27% reduction in time to cortical union and an 18% reduction in time to endosteal union. Others have reported similar effects in acute and nonunion fractures. It is important to note the very low energy levels and longer duration of treatment that define LIPUS. Similar responses to higher doses of energy delivered by conventional clinical ultrasound devices to facilitate fracture repair have not been reported.

Research on the impact of ultrasound in tissue repair has primarily focused on cases of poor or delayed repair, such as skin ulcers and nonunion and acute fractures. Considerable work has also been done on animal models, including studies of acute inflammation and the treatment of tendon and ligament injuries. The application of pulsed ultrasound has been studied following silver nitrate–induced inflammation in animal models. Pulsed ultrasound treatments of 2 to 4 min at low doses may transiently decrease capillary leakage (Fyfe and Chahl 1980). However, greater leakage of plasma over 24 h followed by a more rapid resolution of effusion has also been reported by the same investigators (Fyfe and Chahl 1985). The mechanism by which pulsed ultrasound affects swelling has not been fully explained, and further study of mechanism and dose response is needed before pulsed ultrasound is routinely used following acute soft tissue injury.

In animal studies, investigators have found that after treatments with pulsed ultrasound, tissue repair is expedited (Dyson and Pond 1970) and tensile strength of healing tissues increased (Dyson and Pond 1970; Enwemeka, Rodriquez, and Mendosa 1989; Friedar 1988; da Cunha, Parizotto, and Vidal Bde 2001). Takakura et al. (2002) reported that pulsed ultrasound enhanced early repair of medial collateral ligament injuries in rats but did not result in improved load to failure, stiffness, or energy absorption at 3 weeks into the healing process. Saini et al. (2002), however, reported that 10 min of 0.5 W/cm^2 of continuous ultrasound on the third postoperative day and continuing for 10 days resulted in differences in the repair of severed Achilles tendons in a small sample of dogs until 120 days postoperatively. Treated animals also subjectively recovered from lameness more rapidly.

Ying, Lin, and Yan (2012) provided a summary of research that demonstrated accelerated healing at bone-tendon junctions. All of the reviewed work involved animal models, but it is consistent with research that reports accelerated fracture repair. The mechanical stimulus of the acoustic wave as a mechanism for enhanced cell responses is emphasized by these authors. Warden et al. (2008), however, found no additional benefit of ultrasound in patients with patella tendinopathy who participated in a rehabilitative exercise program that emphasized eccentric loading of the affected tendon. Little is known about the potential for ultrasound in general and LIPUS more specifically to promote ligament repair. No human trials were identified in our literature review, although El-Bialy, Alhadlaq, and Lam (2012) reported that LIPUS has an anabolic effect on human periodontal ligament cells in vitro. These results and the similarities in repair across musculoskeletal connective tissue identify the need for additional research and ultimately human clinical trials.

Mechanisms of Effect: Acoustical Streaming and Stable Cavitation

The mechanisms that may explain the nonthermal effects of ultrasound are not fully understood. Historically, the literature on the nonthermal benefits of ultrasound attributed most of the effects to acoustical streaming and **stable** cavitation (figure 12.8). Acoustical streaming is the movement of fluids along cell membranes due to the mechanical pressure exerted by the sound waves. The movement occurs only in the direction of the sound wave. Acoustical streaming facilitates fluid movement and may increase cell membrane permeability. More recent research, done in the context of **mechanobiology**, suggests that the fluid shear created by ultrasound serves as a mechanical stimulus to the cell. The transduction of mechanical signals is discussed in earlier chapters. The most plausible current explanation for the facilitation of repair through pulsed ultrasound and LIPUS is up-regulation of anabolic cell signaling pathways and facilitation of stem/progenitor cell differentiation favoring repair (Kumagai et al. 2012). Angle et al. (2011, pp. 286-287) summarized the effects of LIPUS: "LIPUS, in essence a wave of alternating pressure, is translated into an extracellular mechanical force at the cell membrane, where it is transduced into intracellular electrical and/or biochemical signals."

Cavitation is the formation of gas-filled bubbles. Ultrasound produces pressure changes in tissue fluids that create the bubbles and cause them to expand and contract. Stable cavitation refers to a rhythmic cycle of expansion and contraction during repeated pressure changes over many acoustic cycles. Unstable cavitation refers to a collapse of the gas bubbles. Unstable cavitation, which is most associated with low-frequency, high-intensity sound waves, is believed to damage tissues. Stable cavitation, which occurs with therapeutic ultrasound, is thought to facilitate fluid movement and membrane transport. Stable cavitation may also represent a mechanical stimulus at the cell membrane.

An increased movement of fluid and dissolved nutrients to and across cell membranes may also play a role in tissue repair. Certainly acoustical streaming and stable cavitation also occur during continuous ultrasound. Continuous ultrasound, as noted previously, is usually applied in higher doses of energy to heat tissues prior to stretching or manual therapy.

Contraindications to Ultrasound

Ultrasound is a relatively safe, easy-to-use therapeutic modality with few contraindications. Of greatest concern are the use of ultrasound in people with cancer and the impact of therapeutic ultrasound on fetal development. Ultrasound has been reported to promote growth (Sicard-Rosenbaum et al. 1995), and perhaps metastasis, of malignant cells in laboratory animals and should not be used near tumors. The impact of therapeutic ultrasound on fetal development in humans is not fully known. Thus, therapeutic ultrasound should not be applied near the abdomen during pregnancy or to women of childbearing age who could be pregnant. The energy delivered to the tissues by therapeutic ultrasound is much greater than that of diagnostic ultrasound, which is commonly used during pregnancy. Ultrasound also should not be applied over an infection.

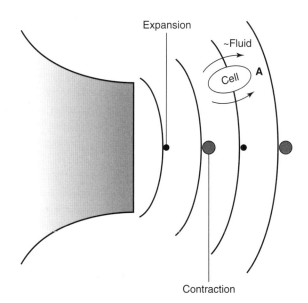

Figure 12.8 Acoustical streaming and cavitation. Acoustical streaming is the movement of fluids around cells by sound waves. Cavitation is the expansion and contraction of air bubbles because of pressure changes in surrounding fluid due to acoustic energy.

Despite considerable confusion in the literature over the years, ultrasound can be applied safely over metal implants such as plates and screws. Gersten (1958) and Lehmann, Delateur, and Silverman (1966) concluded that it is safe to apply ultrasound over joint replacements that contain metal and synthetics such as polyethylene and are held in place by methyl methacrylate cement. However, because low-frequency ultrasound is used to loosen prostheses for removal and revision, and because the long-term impact of ultrasound on joint replacements is not fully known, it should not be used over joint replacements.

Ultrasound should not be applied over the heart or in the area of a cardiac pacemaker. Ultrasound should also not be applied over the eyes or genitalia. The use of ultrasound directly over open epiphyses should be minimized because the impact of such exposure is not fully known and may involve accelerated closure of epiphyses. However, adolescents and children rarely experience problems for which ultrasound is indicated. Ultrasound is often used to treat back conditions. The use of ultrasound should be restricted to an area no more than three to four times the ERA to increase tissue temperature to therapeutic levels. Exposure of the spinal cord to ultrasound should be minimized. In patients who have had a laminectomy, do not apply ultrasound directly over the area of the cord that is no longer protected by bone. Although these precautions and contraindications should be observed, they rarely affect the selection of ultrasound as a therapeutic modality.

Phonophoresis

Phonophoresis is similar to iontophoresis, discussed in previous chapters, in that a modality is applied to drive medications into the tissues. Phonophoresis uses sound energy, as opposed to electromagnetic energy, to drive the medication; thus, the medications driven into the tissues do not have an electrical charge in solution.

Hydrocortisone and dexamethasone are administered with phonophoresis. These medications are mixed with ultrasound conducting gel or other media. Many of the creams, gels, and ointments that have been used to study and administer hydrocortisone with phonophoresis in the treatment of musculoskeletal conditions are poor conductors of ultrasound energy (Cameron and Monroe 1992). Phonophoresis cannot effectively deliver hydrocor-

tisone or other active ingredients unless the gel used is a good conductor of acoustic energy. Cagnie et al. (2003), for example, found that phonophoresis enhanced the delivery of ketoprofen (a nonsteroidal anti-inflammatory medication) into synovial tissues when mixed in Fastum gel (Industrie Farmaceutiche Riunite srl, Florence, Italy). These investigators found higher levels of ketoprofen following ultrasound at a frequency of 1 MHz at 1.5 W/cm^2 at a 20% duty cycle for 5 min than with continuous ultrasound. Ketoprofen levels were higher in synovial than in adipose tissues, and little change in plasma concentrations was observed within 120 min of application.

Similarly, Saliba et al. (2007) reported that pulsed ultrasound (1.0 W/cm^2, or 50% pulsed, at an output frequency of 3 MHz for 5 min) enhanced the absorption of dexamethasone applied for 30 min before ultrasound delivery under an occlusive dressing. Serum concentrations of greater than 10 ng/dl were reported 10 h after treatment. Recent research suggests that phonophoresis with dexamethasone is more effective in reducing pain and restoring nerve conduction velocity and pinch strength than iontophoresis in the treatment of carpal tunnel syndrome (Bakhtiary et al. 2013). These investigators, however, did not compare either treatment to no-treatment control.

Despite a few papers suggesting possible benefit, perhaps the greatest similarity between phonophoresis and iontophoresis is the lack of evidence about its efficacy. Very little research evidence supports the practice of phonophoresis. The work of Griffin et al. (1967; Griffin and Touchstone 1972) first suggested the potential for phonophoresis in treating musculoskeletal conditions. Interpretation of the clinical research is complicated by the unknown bioavailability of phoresed medications. Investigations into the efficacy of phonophoresis (Cicone, Leggin, and Callamaro 1991; Darrow et al. 1999; Oziomek et al. 1991) have not demonstrated benefit. Penderghest, Kimura, and Gulick (1998) also reported that phonophoresis (pulsed) did not affect responses to therapy consisting of cryotherapy and exercise in the treatment of tendinopathy. As noted by Cagnie et al. (2003), "Changes in tissue levels of drugs used in phonophoresis do not necessarily indicate that a particular drug will have a therapeutic effect."

As with iontophoresis, the exact amount of medication reaching target tissues following phonophoresis is often unknown. Thus, the clinician does not know whether a pharmacologically effective dose of medication has been administered. The concerns about the pathophysiology of the tissue raised in the discussion of iontophoresis should also be considered in connection with phonophoresis. It now appears that corticosteroids (e.g., hydrocortisone and dexamethasone) interfere with tissue repair processes despite potentially reducing the symptoms (such as pain) associated with inflammation and tendinopathy.

Although iontophoresis and phonophoresis have potential as medication delivery mechanisms, much more work must be done to identify conditions that may respond to treatments. The optimal parameters for delivery must also be established. Finally, the efficacy of treatments must be investigated through clinical trials before their continued use in the management of musculoskeletal injuries and conditions is warranted.

EFFICACY OF ULTRASOUND THERAPY FOR MUSCULOSKELETAL CONDITIONS

The use of ultrasound in the treatment of musculoskeletal conditions has been studied through clinical trials, allowing for the preparation of several systematic reviews. A search of the Physiotherapy Evidence Database using the search term "ultrasound" revealed dozens of systematic reviews, practice guidelines, and review papers related to ultrasound in the treatment of arthritic and soft tissue conditions. Many clinical trials are also referenced.

We cannot review all of these reports in this chapter. In summary, however, there is little evidence to support the use of ultrasound in the treatment of some musculoskeletal conditions. Systematic reviews have concluded that there is a lack of evidence to support the use of ultrasound in the treatment of patellofemoral pain syndrome (Brosseau et al. 2001), osteoarthritis of the knee (Welch et al. 2001), acute ankle sprain (Van der Windt et al. 2002), or plantar heel pain (plantar fasciitis) (Crawford, Atkins, and Edwards 2000). Randomized controlled clinical trials have shown a lack of benefit from ultrasound therapy for lateral epicondylalgia (tennis elbow) (Hacker and Lundeberg 1991), generalized shoulder pain (pulsed ultrasound) (Nykanen 1995), acute lateral ligament sprains of the ankle (Nyanzi et al. 1999), subacromial bursitis (Downing and Weinstein 1986), and patellar tendinopathy (Warden et al. 2008).

From a broader perspective, reports by Gam and Johannsen (1995), Van der Windt et al. (1999), and Robertson and Baker (2001) concluded that there is a lack of evidence to substantiate the use of ultrasound in treating musculoskeletal disorders. Robertson and Baker summarized the issue well when they wrote, "There is little evidence that active therapeutic ultrasound is more effective than placebo ultrasound for treating people with pain or a range of musculoskeletal disorders or for promoting soft tissue healing."

Does this lack of evidence mean that the reader should disregard all of the information in the earlier sections of this chapter? Draper (2002), in a letter to the editor in response to the paper by Robertson and Baker (2001), pointed out that the investigators in several studies that have been mentioned used inappropriate treatment parameters. In fact, two well-controlled clinical trials have shown that pulsed ultrasound improves treatment outcomes for patients with calcific tendinitis of the shoulder and carpal tunnel syndrome. Ebenbichler et al. (1998) used ultrasound at 0.89 MHz, 20% duty cycle, at 2.5 W/cm^2 for 15 min, five times per week for 3 weeks and then three times per week for 3 weeks in patients with calcific tendinitis. At 9-month follow-up, resolution of the calcific lesion was found in 42% of patients treated with active ultrasound and in only 8% treated with placebo. Reduction in the calcific mass was found in an additional 23% of the treated patients as compared to 12% of the placebo-treated group. Ebenbichler et al. (1999) applied 1 MHz ultrasound at 1 W/cm^2, 20% duty cycle, for 15 min five times per week for 2 weeks and then twice per week for 5 weeks in patients with carpal tunnel syndrome. Those receiving ultrasound had less pain and more normal electrodiagnostic studies at 6-month follow-up. Huang et al. (2005) reported that treatment with both pulsed and continuous ultrasound enhanced the benefits of isokinetic exercise in patients with osteoarthritis of the knee. Specifically, when ultrasound preceded exercise, there were greater improvements in range of motion, self-reported pain and function, gait velocity, and knee extensor force production. The use of ultrasound before activity differs from ultrasound as an isolated treatment, which has been found to be ineffective for the treatment of knee and hip osteoarthritis (Robinson et al. 2001).

Furthermore, there is little evidence on which to base decisions about the use of ultrasound prior to tissue mobilization or stretching when range of motion is restricted. Draper et al. (1998) reported greater gains in dorsiflexion range of motion immediately after treatment in subjects who received continuous ultrasound before stretching. However, after 10 treatments distributed over 5 days, there were no differences between subjects treated with ultrasound and those who just performed stretching. Draper (2010, 2011, 2014) has reported success in improving long-standing motion restrictions at the wrist and elbow when ultrasound or diathermy (discussed later in this chapter) is applied prior to joint mobilization. These results are important because (1) previous interventions had failed to reverse substantial limitations in functional range of motion, and (2) once restored, the motion gains were maintained. These results strongly suggest that ultrasound may be a beneficial adjunct to stretching and manual therapy in patients with motion restriction. Thus, the issue with the application of ultrasound and diathermy, as well as other modalities, is appropriate patient selection. Future clinical trials and case series reports will better guide decisions about ultrasound administration.

The preceding discussion focuses on the traditional use of therapeutic ultrasound. The evidence for the effectiveness of LIPUS in the treatment of acute and delayed-union fractures is more compelling.

Ultrasound should not be abandoned completely as a therapeutic modality. However, the liberal use of ultrasound in the management of a multitude of conditions without replicating parameters shown to produce results cannot continue either. Further research is clearly warranted to identify how this modality can be used to effectively treat athletes and others with musculoskeletal injuries.

DIATHERMY AND PULSED ELECTROMAGNETIC FIELDS

Electromagnetic fields are found in two applications in the treatment of musculoskeletal injuries: diathermy and pulsed electromagnetic fields (PEMFs). The same principles apply to each application. The difference is that diathermy involves heating of tissues and PEMFs result in no tissue heating. The next two sections describe how heat is generated by diathermy and explain why PEMFs do not cause heating.

Diathermy

Diathermy is the therapeutic generation of local heating by high-frequency electromagnetic waves. Most diathermy units are classified as shortwave diathermy and generate an alternating current at 27.12 MHz. When the body is placed in an electrical field, known as the capacitance technique, heating occurs due to the rapid rotation of **dipoles** (structures with positive and negative poles) (figure 12.9). As the current alternates between positive and negative, the dipoles rotate to align with the electrical field. The mechanical friction and the movement of electrons result in local heating. Tissues with large numbers of dipoles, such as skin and muscle, have a greater capacitance to store an electrical charge. Thus, more current must be generated to cause dipole motion in these tissues. The greatest heating occurs in tissues with fewer dipoles, particularly fatty tissues. Thus, capacitance technique diathermy heats the subcutaneous fat more than the underlying muscle.

Heating of tissue in a magnetic field, also known as the inductance technique, differs in that the body is not placed in an electrical field. Instead, magnetic waves are generated as an electrical current is driven through a coiled wire (figure 12.10). The magnetic field creates small currents in the tissues. The greatest heating occurs in tissue with low impedance, especially muscle. Thus, the inductance technique is preferable for heating deeper tissues.

Like ultrasound, diathermy is effective for heating deeper tissues, but it can heat larger areas. Unlike ultrasound, pulsed diathermy can heat the deep tissues by 3 °C to 4 °C (Draper et al. 1999, Hawkes et al. 2013), although intra-articular temperatures rise to

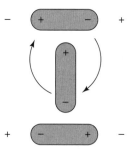

Figure 12.9 Dipole rotation in an alternating electromagnetic field.

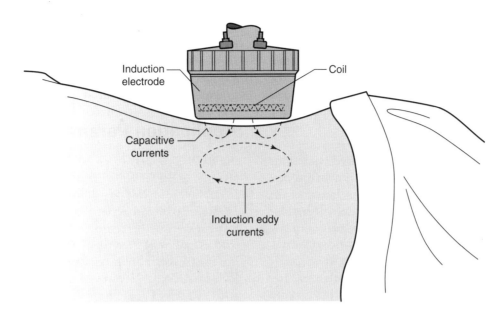

Figure 12.10 With magnetic field diathermy applicators, eddy currents are induced in the tissues having the highest conductivity.

a lesser extent (Oosterveld et al. 1992). However, diathermy units are expensive and can be used on only one person at a time. In addition, diathermy carries a number of precautions and contraindications. All metal should be removed from the patient. In the past, metal implants and cardiac pacemakers were considered absolute contraindications for treatment with diathermy. Several investigators have studied the use of diathermy in the treatment of patients with knee osteoarthritis (OA). Atamaz et al. (2012) reported reduced medication use, while Fukuda et al. (2011) and Trock et al. (1993) reported improved function and quality of life in patients with knee OA. Akyol et al. (2010) and Rattanachaiyanont and Kuptniratsaikul (2008), however, found that diathermy did not enhance the benefits of an exercise program in similar patient groups. Work by Ozgüçlü et al. (2010); Clarke et al. (1974); Svarcova, Trnavsky, and Zvarova (1987); and Moffett et al. (1996) also does not support treating patients with knee OA with diathermy. Additional research is needed to identify patients who might benefit from treatment with diathermy and to identify the optimal combination of palliative treatments and therapeutic exercise.

Diathermy has also been applied in combination with manual therapy in efforts to restore joint motion following injury. Seiger and Draper (2006) and Draper (2011) found that pulsed diathermy in conjunction with joint mobilization was effective in restoring range of motion at the ankle and elbow

in patients with long-standing impairment. It is important to note that Seiger and Draper (2006) reported no adverse effects following the use of pulse diathermy (27.12 MHz, 800 pps, 400 μs [48 W]) over metallic fixation of fractures around the ankle. Thus, the presence of metal should not be considered an absolute contraindication to the use of diathermy, but caution is advised until the range of safe parameters is better established. Diathermy must not be used near the uterus of a pregnant woman or near the abdomen or back of a woman of childbearing age who could be pregnant. Finally, diathermy should not be used on people with infections; acute inflammation; moist, open wounds; malignant tumors; or large joint effusions.

In addition to the studies already cited about the application of diathermy for patients with knee osteoarthritis and motion loss following injury, other clinical trials and systematic reviews of diathermy are available. Belanger's text (2002) identified reports from controlled trials of diathermy on the treatment of neck pain and ankle sprains. None of the trials showed benefit in treating sprained ankles with diathermy (Pasila, Visuri, and Sundholm 1978; Barker et al. 1985; McGill 1998). McCray and Patton (1984) reported decreased trigger point sensitivity following diathermy treatment. While the longevity of this improvement was not addressed, a decrease in trigger point sensitivity may allow patients with myofascial pain to complete therapeutic exercise regimens central to their plan of care that would otherwise be painful. Foley-Nolan et al. (1990, 1992) reported less pain and greater cervical range of motion in patients with chronic (>8 weeks) neck pain and whiplash treated with PEMF therapy (1990) and less pain after 2 and 4 weeks in patients suffering from acute whiplash who were provided a collar emitting a PEMF (1992). These patients were treated, however, with nonthermal levels of PEMF therapy. Thus, there is little evidence that diathermy alone enhances treatment outcomes in patients with musculoskeletal conditions. As noted in the discussion of ultrasound, this is not a reason to abandon all consideration of diathermy but rather indicates the need for clinical trials to identify situations in which treatment with diathermy will enhance care. Draper et al. (2004) also reported substantially greater gains in hamstring flexibility after 15 min treatments with 27.12 MHz diathermy pulsed at 800 bursts per second with 400 μs burst duration. Subjects received treatments for 5 days and retained substantially more flexibility at 3 days after the final treatment than subjects who completed the same stretching protocol without diathermy treatment. These results suggest that diathermy enhances treatments directed at soft tissue stretching.

Pulsed Electromagnetic Fields

Although diathermy is used on a limited basis in clinical care, the underlying technology has been used to promote tissue healing. Like ultrasound, diathermy can be pulsed to decrease the total energy transmitted to the tissues. Pulsed shortwave diathermy can be adjusted to provide a thermal response or to produce no tissue heating. When shortwave diathermy is adjusted to a low frequency (less than 600 pps) with a short phase duration (65 μs into the nonthermal range), it is often classified as pulsed electromagnetic field (PEMF) or pulsed radio frequency energy (PRFE). This reclassification is important because diathermy implies heating, whereas the labels PEMF and PRFE imply a nonthermal therapy.

PEMF has been used mainly to treat nonunion fractures. Although more research is needed, there is evidence that these modalities can promote heal-ing in these difficult-to-manage cases (Bassett 1984; Holmes 1994; Sharrard 1990; Walker, Denegar, and Preische 2007; Assiotis et al. 2012; Shi et al. 2013). PEMF has also been studied in patients with osteoarthritis. Ryang We et al. (2013) completed a systematic review that included 14 studies and 482 patients with knee OA. These investigators reported that when high methodological trials were analyzed, there was a modest improvement in pain function after 4 and 8 weeks of treatment when compared to a control group not receiving PEMF.

Pulsed electromagnetic field therapy has been investigated with regard to tissue healing; some studies have suggested that PEMF may speed wound healing (Brown and Baker 1987; Goldon et al. 1981; Itoh et al. 1991). However, not all reports agree, and the use of PEMF in treating soft tissue injuries warrants further investigation. Warden et al. (2008) reported no benefit in the treatment of chronic patella tendinopathy with PEMF. At present there is not enough information to recommend PEMF in the treatment of soft tissue injuries sustained by athletes.

SUMMARY

Therapeutic ultrasound is commonly applied in the management of musculoskeletal conditions. This chapter describes how therapeutic ultrasound is generated and addresses concerns about beam non-uniformity ratio (BNR) and the area of tissue that can be affected during treatment. The parameters of ultrasound, including dose, duty cycle, treatment duration, frequency, and conducting media, are defined and discussed. Depending on the parameters selected, ultrasound may or may not increase tissue temperature. The thermal and nonthermal effects of ultrasound are discussed. Ultrasound to induce phonophoresis and therapeutic diathermy are described with reference to evidence of treatment effectiveness. Contraindications and precautions for treatment with therapeutic ultrasound and diathermy are emphasized. The chapter concludes with a brief discussion of the application of pulsed electromagnetic fields and pulsed ultrasound to stimulate the healing of fractures.

KEY CONCEPTS AND REVIEW

1. *Describe how therapeutic ultrasound is generated by the treatment unit.*

Ultrasound is generated through vibration of a crystal in an electrical circuit with alternating current. The rapid vibration of the crystal generates the emission of sound waves that are directed into tissues to achieve therapeutic effects.

2. *Define beam nonuniformity ratio (BNR) and effective radiating area (ERA).*

BNR and ERA stand for beam nonuniformity ratio and effective radiating area, respectively. Because the crystals used in ultrasound equipment are not perfectly uniform, some parts of a crystal emit more sound energy than others. BNR is a ratio of the peak sound energy emitted from an ultrasound head divided by the average intensity emitted over the entire radiating area. ERA is simply the area of the crystal that emits at least 5% of the peak sound energy produced by the crystal.

3. *Identify and describe the use of effective conducting media for ultrasound treatments.*

Because air is a poor conductor of ultrasound energy, a conducting medium must be used between the ultrasound head and the skin. Commercial ultrasound gels are designed to transmit ultrasound energy. Ultrasound gel is inexpensive and clearly the best transmitter of sound energy. Other conducting media, such as mineral oil, have been used but are substantially less efficient. A water bath has been recommended for ultrasound treatment over uneven surfaces such as the knuckles of the hand. Water, however, is also not an ideal conductor of high-frequency sound energy. Uneven surfaces are best treated with a gel pad, with ultrasound gel placed between the sound head and the pad and between the pad and the skin.

4. *Define dose, duty cycle, treatment duration, and frequency as parameters of therapeutic ultrasound.*

Ultrasound dose is measured in watts of energy over the ERA, or W/cm^2. The frequency of therapeutic ultrasound ranges from 0.8 to 3 MHz, with higher frequency (3 MHz) used to treat more superficial tissues. When pulsed ultrasound is used, the duty cycle refers to the amount of time ultrasound is transmitted in relation to total treatment time. For example, a 20 ms burst of ultrasound followed by an 80 ms interruption would create a 20% duty cycle. Treatment duration is simply the length of time an ultrasound treatment is applied. To achieve optimal increases in tissue temperature, a longer treatment of continuous (no duty cycle) ultrasound is required at 1 MHz than at 3 MHz (8–10 min versus 4–5 min).

5. *Describe the thermal effects of therapeutic ultrasound.*

When 8 to 10 min of continuous 1 MHz ultrasound is delivered, temperature increases 4°C in deeper (2.5–5 cm) tissues. A similar increase in temperature can be achieved at 1 to 2.5 cm with 4 to 5 min of continuous 3 MHz ultrasound.

6. *Describe the treatment parameters and physiological effects of pulsed ultrasound.*

The primary parameter of pulsed ultrasound is duty cycle, which may vary from 10% to 90%. Pulsed ultrasound has been shown to increase the metabolic activity of fibroblasts in vitro and to speed healing of slow-to-heal skin lesions such as decubitus ulcers.

7. *Discuss the technique and effectiveness of phonophoresis.*

Phonophoresis is the use of ultrasound energy to drive medications through the skin. Although some studies have reported that medication can be driven through the skin, it is unknown whether pharmacologically effective doses can be delivered. There is little evidence that phonophoresis is clinically effective in treating musculoskeletal conditions.

8. *Describe the differences between therapeutic ultrasound and diathermy.*

Diathermy heats deep tissues with electromagnetic energy as opposed to acoustic energy. Modern diathermy units are considerably more expensive than ultrasound but have similar heating effects and can heat larger areas of tissue.

9. *Identify the two mechanisms through which diathermy can be used to heat deep tissues.*

Diathermy can heat tissues by means of capacitance, in which the patient becomes part of an alternating-current electrical field. The continuous reversal of the position of dipoles (structures with positive and negative poles) creates friction and therefore heat. Diathermy can also heat tissue by means of inductance. When an electrical current is passed through a wire, magnetic or eddy currents are generated. This technique brings about the greatest heating in tissues with low impedance, such as muscle.

10. *Describe the potential uses of diathermy and pulsed electromagnetic field therapy in the treatment of musculoskeletal injuries.*

Pulsed electromagnetic fields (PEMFs) are used to treat nonunion and acute fractures; PEMF may also speed healing following injury or surgery to tendons and ligaments and may relieve persistent pain. More study is needed to determine the best use of PEMF in treating musculoskeletal injuries.

chapter 13

Clinical Application of Ultrasound and Diathermy

OBJECTIVES

After reading this chapter, you will be able to

❶ identify patients who might benefit from the application of therapeutic ultrasound and diathermy;

❷ identify contraindications for treatment with therapeutic ultrasound and diathermy;

❸ describe the administration of therapeutic ultrasound and diathermy in the treatment of musculoskeletal injuries; and

❹ discuss the potential benefits and applications of LIPUS and PEMF in the management of fractures.

A 24-year-old graduate student presents to a university student health clinic for treatment of her left elbow on the recommendation of a physician. She reports that she played collegiate volleyball and suffered a fracture or dislocation of her elbow in a rock climbing accident 10 months ago. Although she has little pain, she lacks 25° of elbow extension, which limits her ability to play club volleyball. The physician suggested a course of therapy to try to regain extension range of motion. In reviewing her history, you learn that she did receive some therapy about 6 weeks after her injury and does do some stretching exercises to improve elbow extension. How could you combine treatment with ultrasound or diathermy and joint mobilization to address this patient's impairment? How would these treatments be administered?

Chapter 12 describes how ultrasound and diathermy devices transmit acoustic and electromagnetic energy. Much of the chapter is devoted to a critical review of the effectiveness of ultrasound and diathermy devices found in athletic training and physical therapy clinical settings. Chapter 12 also describes the use of pulsed ultrasound and pulsed electromagnetic field devices in the treatment of fractures and, to a lesser extent, other musculoskeletal conditions. This chapter discusses the clinical application of therapeutic ultrasound and diathermy in clinical practice.

TREATMENT WITH THERAPEUTIC ULTRASOUND

As noted in chapter 12, the indications for and the evidence of effectiveness of therapeutic ultrasound are limited. There are, however, some circumstances when the application of therapeutic ultrasound can facilitate the achievement of treatment goals. Heating connective tissue before performing joint mobilization or stretching may be more effective in restoring range of motion than joint mobilization or stretching alone (Draper 2010). Furthermore, there is conflicting evidence related to the use of ultrasound in the treatment of carpal tunnel syndrome (Page et al. 2013) and limited evidence to support the application of ultrasound in the treatment of calcific tendinopathy (Ebenbichler et al. 1999). In patients with these conditions, the risks, costs, and benefits of treatment options need to be considered

in conjunction with the patient's desire and health status. When the broad scope of patients seeking care for musculoskeletal injuries is considered, the portion for whom ultrasound may be of benefit is small. Clinicians should critically appraise the potential for benefit before recommending therapeutic ultrasound as a part of the patient's plan of care.

Contraindications to Treatment With Ultrasound

As with all therapeutic interventions it is important to review a patient's medical history and presenting signs and symptoms to identify conditions that contraindicate a certain plan of care. Ultrasound is a relatively safe, easy-to-use therapeutic modality, but it might harm some patients (table 13.1), and it should not be applied to some areas of the body.

Ultrasound should not be used on patients with cancer unless approved by the treating physician. Ultrasound has been reported to promote growth (Sicard-Rosenbaum et al. 1995), and perhaps metastasis, of malignant cells in laboratory animals. Clearly the risk of complicating cancer treatment outweighs any potential benefit of the application of ultrasound.

The impact of therapeutic ultrasound on fetal development in humans is not fully known. Thus, therapeutic ultrasound should not be applied near the abdomen during pregnancy or to women of childbearing age who could be pregnant. The energy delivered to the tissues by therapeutic ultrasound is much greater than that of diagnostic ultrasound, which is commonly used during pregnancy.

Table 13.1   Indications and Contraindications for Ultrasound and Diathermy

	Indications	Contraindications
ULTRASOUND		
Continuous	Heat protein-rich, deeper tissue prior to manual therapies to restore range of motion Questionable benefit in treatment of carpal tunnel syndrome	Application over cardiac pacemaker, eyes, genitalia, joint replacements Pregnancy Cancer Infection Deep vein thrombosis Acute inflammation Minimize exposure over open epiphyses and spinal cord Diminished or absent sensation
Pulsed	Limited evidence of benefit in the treatment of calcific tendinopathy Questionable benefit in treatment of carpal tunnel syndrome	Application over cardiac pacemaker, eyes, genitalia, joint replacements Pregnancy Cancer Infection Deep vein thrombosis Minimize exposure over open epiphyses and spinal cord
DIATHERMY		
Continuous and pulsed	Heat large area of deeper tissue Increase blood flow in deep tissues Decrease pain and muscle spasm	Application over cardiac pacemaker, eyes, genitalia, joint replacements, and metal implants* Pregnancy Open wounds Cancer Infection Deep vein thrombosis Acute inflammation and joint effusion Diminished or absent sensation

*Evidence of safety over metal implants with pulsed diathermy (see Seiger and Draper 2006)

Ultrasound also should not be applied over an infection. There is potential to compromise the body's ability to contain and destroy bacteria. Ultrasound should also not be applied near the eyes or genitalia. Ultrasound should also not be applied over the heart or in the area of a cardiac pacemaker. Ultrasound should also not be applied if there is concern about deep vein thrombosis (DVT). It is theoretically possible that ultrasound could dislodge a thrombus, which can lead to a pulmonary embolism, heart attack, or cerebral vascular accident (stroke). More importantly, a DVT is a potentially dangerous, easily evaluated medical condition associated with limb pain (most often in the calf) and swelling.

The use of ultrasound directly over open epiphyses should be minimized because the impact of such exposure is not fully known and may involve accelerated closure of epiphyses. However, adolescents and children rarely experience problems for which ultrasound is indicated. Ultrasound has been used to treat back conditions, but evidence of effectiveness is lacking, and the treatment of low back pain with ultrasound is not recommended. Should ultrasound be applied over the spine, exposure of the spinal cord to ultrasound should be minimized. In patients who have had a laminectomy, do not apply ultrasound directly over the area of the cord that is no longer protected by bone. Although these precautions and contraindications should be observed, they rarely affect the selection of ultrasound as a therapeutic modality.

Despite considerable confusion in the literature over the years, ultrasound can be applied safely over metal implants such as plates and screws. Gersten (1958) and Lehmann, Delateur, and Silverman (1966) concluded that it is safe to apply ultrasound over joint replacements that contain metal and synthetics such as polyethylene. However, because low-frequency ultrasound is used to loosen prostheses for removal and revision, and because the long-term impact of ultrasound on joint replacements is not fully known, it should not be used over joint replacements. Lastly, since ultrasound heats tissues, it should not be used over areas where sensation is limited.

Patient Screening

Although there are limited indications for treatment with ultrasound, the process of identifying contraindications is central to a comprehensive evaluation of each patient. Cancer can cause symptoms that mimic musculoskeletal conditions such as mechanical low back pain, muscle strain, and stress fracture. The clinician must integrate information from the patient's medical, family, and social history, the history of the current condition, and the findings from the patient interview and physical examination when deciding if referral to a physician is warranted. Cancer is more common in older patients, but it also occurs in children, adolescents, and younger adults. A family history increases the risk of developing some cancers, as does environmental exposure to some chemicals and toxins (e.g., cigarette smoke, asbestos). A personal history of cancer also poses a risk of recurrence. Concerning findings from an interview include:

Changes in bowel or bladder habits

A skin lesion that has failed to heal normally (e.g., persists >6 weeks)

Unusual bleeding or discharge (blood in stool, urine, or unusual vaginal secretion)

Thickening or lump in tissue (breast or testicle, but may be found in musculoskeletal structures, including bone and muscle)

Indigestion or difficulty swallowing

Obvious change in mole or wart

Nagging cough or hoarseness

These warning signs can be recalled by connecting the first letter of each sign to spell CAUTION. Use caution in proceeding with treatment if any of these warnings are identified.

Physical examination findings that suggest that the origin of symptoms may not be musculoskeletal include

proximal or bilateral muscle weakness,

bilateral change in deep tendon reflexes (brisk or hypoactive), and

enlarged lymph nodes.

The patient's description of pain may also yield clues to the presence of nonmusculoskeletal conditions. Night pain—that is, pain that is described as worse at night or that causes wakening—may result from cancer. If night pain is accompanied by sweating, a nonmusculoskeletal source becomes more probable. Pain that is constant, intense (>7 on pain scale), and not relieved by changes in position is concerning, especially when the onset of pain cannot be traced to a recent event. When there is no clear history of an acute onset, the clinician should not assume symptoms have musculoskeletal origins. If there is doubt, you should refer the patient to another health care provider.

An infection is likely to develop fairly rapidly. Infections result in fever as well as localized warmth and pain. When infection is suspected, timely referral for definitive medical care is essential.

A DVT can develop after surgery and in patients with blood clotting disorders. Unexplained tenderness, muscle tightness, and swelling, especially in the calf, are common findings in patients with DVT. The concern, as noted previously, is that a thrombus or clot in a vein can dislodge and travel to the vessels of the heart, lungs, and brain. A DVT can be identified through diagnostic ultrasound and treated effectively with medication.

Contraindication related to implanted pacemakers and other medical devices and the possibility of pregnancy are identified through a review of the medical history and direct questioning of the patient. Diminished or absent sensation can be identified through interview and physical examination, and these generally preclude the application of any heating or cooling modality. Although uncommon in patients who might benefit from treatment with ultrasound, some contraindications are serious medical conditions that need to be identified. Timely referral for a definitive diagnosis and appropriate care can reduce the morbidity and mortality associated with cancer and DVT.

Preparation for Treatment With Ultrasound

When you elect to apply therapeutic ultrasound, there are several steps to complete. As with any intervention, the patient should know why the treatment is recommended and what to expect during treatment. Since ultrasound and diathermy heat deeper tissue through energy conversion, a sense of mild warmth is common when continuous ultrasound is applied for a sufficient duration. If pain is experienced, the amplitude of the ultrasound may be set too high or, more likely, the beam characteristics of the crystal in the device have created areas of high peak energy. To some degree this can be overcome with continued movement of the ultrasound head.

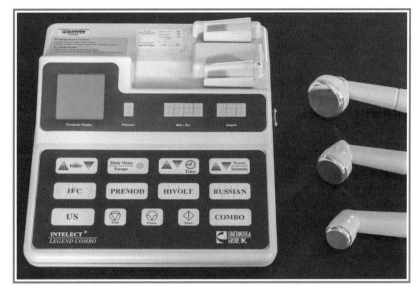

Figure 13.1 Some ultrasound devices have multiple sound heads, each with a different ERA.

It is important to recognize that the ultrasound head and the gel used during treatment can be a source of contamination. When these are applied over intact skin, the risk of transmitting infection is probably very low given the absence of literature on the issue. However, if the patient's skin is abraded or an open wound is present, the risks associated must be considered. Prior to treatment, the skin should be washed and the ultrasound head should be cleaned with a disinfectant. To minimize contamination of ultrasound gel, it should be applied to the area to be treated without making contact between the bottle and the skin.

Once the area to be treated is prepared and the ultrasound device turned on, the next step is the selection of treatment parameters. Ultrasound devices allow for the selection of treatment frequency and amplitude. Some permit selection of the size of the ultrasound head, and thus the effective radiating area (ERA) used (figure 13.1). If the target tissue is fairly superficial, such as the anterior capsule of the elbow, a higher frequency is recommended. The selection of the treatment time depends on the amplitude of the ultrasound delivered. At frequencies of 3 or 3.3 MHz, 3°C of tissue heating can be achieved with 5 min of treatment at 1.5 W/cm² and 3 to 4 min at 2 W/cm². If the target tissue is deeper (e.g., posterior capsule of the hip), a lower (1 MHz) frequency of ultrasound will result in heating of the target tissues. In this case the desired temperature increase can be achieved with a treatment time of about 10 min at an amplitude of 2 W/cm² and about 12 min at 1.5 W/cm².

In some cases the clinical literature might be used to guide parameter selection. For example Ebenbichler et al. (1999) reported that 24 fifteen-minute sessions of pulsed ultrasound (20% duty cycle, frequency 0.89 MHz, intensity 2.5 W/cm²) had a greater probability of resolving calcific lesions in tendons around the shoulder and reducing pain and disability after the last treatment than sham ultrasound. Similarly, Piravej and Boonhong (2004) applied ultrasound at 0.5 W/cm² to the palmar carpal tunnel for 10 min. Clinical parameters (e.g., pain) and EMG findings improved after a course of 20 treatments. While there are too few data to substantiate the results reported by Ebenbichler et al. (1999) or Piravej and Boonhong (2004), the potential benefit and low risk associated with ultrasound treatment should be taken into consideration, especially in patients who do not respond to or are not candidates for other treatment options.

Treatment Technique

Once the parameters have been selected, treatment involves positioning the patient for treatment (figure 13.2) and slowly moving the ultrasound head in an area no more than two to three times the ERA (figure 13.3). The clinician must maintain good

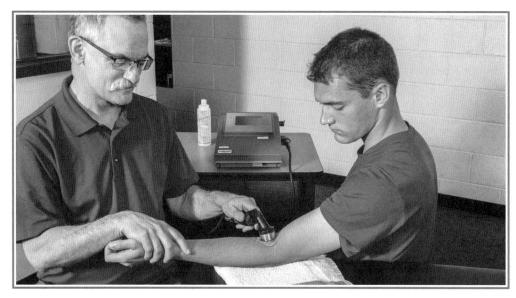

Figure 13.2   Proper technique for therapeutic ultrasound application to the volar aspect of the elbow in clinical practice.

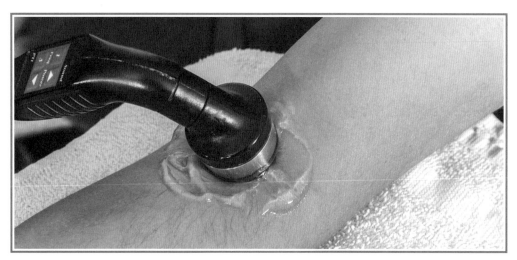

Figure 13.3   Treating an area two to three times the effective radiating area.

contact between the sound head and the skin and move the sound head steadily to prevent an area of high energy output from overheating a small area of the tissue and causing pain. Upon completion of the treatment, the sound head and the skin should be wiped off with toweling and the sound head disinfected. If joint mobilization or stretching is to be performed, it must be done immediately, as the tissue will cool rapidly (5–10 min, depending on the treatment parameters and depth of the target tissue).

Video 13.1 demonstrates the use of ultrasound on an anterior elbow.

Video 13.2 demonstrates the use of ultrasound on an ankle.

TREATMENT WITH DIATHERMY

Although diathermy is applied less often than ultrasound, it may be a better choice when the goal is to heat deeper tissue. The advantages to diathermy are that the extent of heating is not dependent on the technique of the clinician and larger areas of tissue can be heated. Like ultrasound, diathermy increases temperature in deeper tissues. Draper et al. (1999) reported temperature increases of greater than 3.5°C at a depth of 3 cm in the medial gastrocnemius at 15 and 20 min of treatment. At 27.12 MHz, pulsed diathermy was applied at a rate of eight hundred 400 μs bursts per second, generating an average of 48 W. Similar levels of heating were reported at a depth of 1 cm into the medial gastrocnemius (Draper et al. 2013) with a 30 min application of a ReBound continuous diathermy device (ReGear Life Sciences, Inc., Pittsburgh, PA) generating 35 W. These investigators reported an increase in temperature of more than 2.5°C after a 20 min application of a hydrocollator pad.

Patient Selection

The indications for and evidence of effectiveness of diathermy are similar to those described for therapeutic ultrasound. Draper (2014) reported on a case series of patients treated with diathermy and joint range of motion who suffered from persistent and substantial losses of elbow range of motion following fractures and dislocations. In five of the six cases, excellent restoration of motion was achieved, facilitating functional gains and return to participation in work and sport.

Very limited data are available about the use of diathermy in the treatment of carpal tunnel syndrome (Incebiyik, Boyaci, and Tutoglu 2014), tendinopathy (Szlosek et al. 2014), and calcific tendinopathy (Di Cesare et al. 2008). At this time there are too few data to suggest that diathermy is of greater benefit than other treatment options in the treatment of these conditions. Thus the application of diathermy cannot be recommended in clinical care at this time.

Patient Screening

Once the decision has been made to apply diathermy based on the desire to heat tissues, the first step is to identify contraindications. In general, the contraindications for treatment with therapeutic ultrasound also apply to diathermy due to the risk of an adverse event or a delay in the appropriate care of a nonmusculoskeletal condition. Unlike ultrasound, diathermy can heat moisture on the surface. While this is not a concern with appropriate preparation of a patient with intact skin moisture, it poses a risk for patients with open wounds. Thus, diathermy should not be directed on areas of damaged skin. The safety of diathermy over metal implants at an output above 48 W has not been established, so additional caution is warranted for patients on whom internal fixation or arthroplasty has been performed.

Preparation and Treatment

Patients to be treated with diathermy should be positioned comfortably on nonmetal chairs or tables. Although diathermy at an output of 48 W has been shown not to heat metal implants, jewelry and body piercings should be removed. The skin over the area to be heated should be exposed and inspected for sensation and general condition. The skin should be dry and an absorbent towel placed between the skin and the diathermy drum. The duration of treatment is best based on the parameters of the device and existing literature. For example, if a device emits an average of 48 W, then sufficient heating can be achieved in 15 to 20 min. The patient should be told that a comfortable, warm sensation can be expected. If the heating becomes uncomfortable, the treatment should be stopped. The patient must be able to communicate directly with the clinician throughout the treatment. As with ultrasound, heated tissue begins to cool rapidly. Post-diathermy joint mobilization or stretching should be initiated immediately.

LIPUS AND PEMF

Low-intensity pulsed ultrasound (LIPUS) (figure 13.4) and pulsed electromagnetic field (PEMF) (figure 13.5) devices were described in chapter 12. The best-established indication for these devices is in the management of fractures. Although treatment with LIPUS or PEMF does not assure faster healing or resolution of nonunion fractures in every case, there is mounting evidence of effectiveness. Hannemann et al. (2014) completed a systematic review with meta-analysis of studies involving PEMF and LIPUS on fracture management and concluded "PEMF or LIPUS can be beneficial in the treatment of acute fractures regarding time to radiological and clinical union. PEMF and LIPUS significantly shorten time to radiological union for acute fractures undergoing non-operative treatment and acute fractures of the upper limb. Furthermore, PEMF or LIPUS bone growth stimulation accelerates the time to clinical union for acute diaphyseal fractures." These same authors did not find evidence that these treatments decrease the risk of delayed healing or

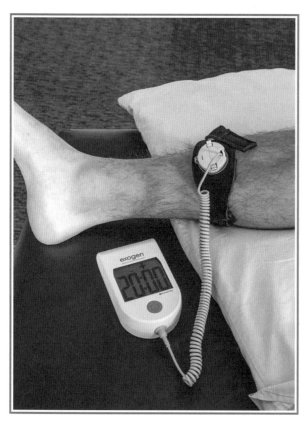

Figure 13.4 Low-intensity pulsed ultrasound for the treatment of a tibial fracture.

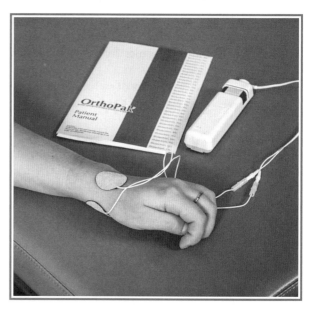

Figure 13.5 Pulsed electromagnetic field generator for the treatment of fractures.

nonunion; however, at present there are no known adverse responses to treatment or contraindications other than the use of these devices in the proximity of an implanted medical device such as a cardiac pacemaker. There is more limited evidence that PEMF and LIPUS can promote healing in nonunion fractures (Bashardoust Tajali et al. 2012; Walker, Denegar, and Preische 2007), but again no data suggest that such treatments pose any health risks.

The decision to prescribe LIPUS or PEMF therapy to accelerate fracture repair rests with the physician managing the case. Other health care professionals who treat musculoskeletal injuries may be called upon to instruct patients in the proper use of their devices. LIPUS devices have a fixed frequency, duty cycle, and amplitude. The duration of treatment is generally based on the recommendations of the manufacturer. A once-daily, 20 min application of LIPUS is typical. Since new devices may come on the market and devices may differ between manufacturers, patient instruction is best done by providing and following the manufacturer's recommendation. Exogen (Bioventus LLC, Durham, NC), for example, provides a thorough yet easy-to-follow set

of patient and physician materials (appropriate for allied health care providers) related to the use and potential benefits of LIPUS.

PEMF devices also have fixed parameters. Punt, den Hoech, and Fontijne (2008) described the treatment of nonunion fracture with PEMF pulse characteristics as follows:

Pulse amplitude 50 mV

Pulse width 5 ms

Burst width 5 ms

Burst refractory period 62 ms

Signal on time 24 h

Repeat repetition rate 15 Hz

In this study, nonunion was established at 8 months post-fracture. Patients who had little pain, no fracture site movement, bridging of two cortices by dense bone, and resolution of the fracture line were considered to have had treatment success. More than 75% of patients achieved success with varying lengths of continuous PEMF application.

LIPUS and PEMF devices are designed for patient self-administration. However, as with instruction in any home or self-care intervention, appropriate instruction in the use of LIPUS and PEMF devices should be routinely performed and documented.

As noted in chapter 12, the study of the effects of LIPUS and PEMF on the healing of soft tissues and the treatment of osteoarthritis is ongoing. At this time there is insufficient evidence from human patient trials to recommend treatment. However, new indications may emerge as the science of healing progresses and the results from clinical trials are reported.

SUMMARY

This chapter is devoted to the application of therapeutic ultrasound and diathermy. Although therapeutic ultrasound is available in most rehabilitation clinics, the best available evidence suggests that this modality should only be applied to manage specific diagnoses in selected patients. Clinicians must recognize and screen for contraindications for ultrasound if treatment with ultrasound is indicated. Appropriate preparation of the area to be treated, selection of parameters most likely to facilitate the achievement of treatment goals, and an appropriate treatment technique are essential. Diathermy provides an alternative approach to heating deeper tissues. Diathermy is used far less often than ultrasound but can heat larger areas of tissue. The setup and treatment are not dependent on clinician technique. As with ultrasound, it is important to carefully screen prospective diathermy patients for conditions that contraindicate treatment. LIPUS and PEMF devices may be prescribed to accelerate fracture repair or promote healing of nonunion fractures. Other applications to facilitate the repair of connective tissues may emerge. At present the use of these devices is primarily guided by physicians. Patients can self-treat with these devices, but all clinicians involved in the care of musculoskeletal injuries should understand the use of these devices and be able to instruct patients in their use.

1. *Identify patients who might benefit from the application of therapeutic ultrasound and diathermy.*

Patients who suffer from loss of joint range of motion, and thus loss of function, due to scar and tissue adhesions may benefit from the heating of the tissue before joint mobilization or tissue stretching procedures. There is conflicting evidence and opinion about the effects of ultrasound in the management of carpal tunnel syndrome and calcific tendinopathy. The addition of therapeutic ultrasound might be considered in cases where the patient is not improving at the expected rate.

2. *Identify contraindications for treatment with therapeutic ultrasound and diathermy.*

Ultrasound or diathermy should not be applied near a pacemaker or over the eyes or genitalia. The clinician must screen patients for signs of cancer and deep vein thrombosis (DVT). Patients with any signs of cancer, infection, or DVT should not be treated with any therapeutic modality, including therapeutic ultrasound or diathermy, until they are evaluated by a physician. Patients who are pregnant or might be pregnant should not be treated with ultrasound or diathermy.

3. *Describe the administration of therapeutic ultrasound and diathermy in the treatment of musculoskeletal injuries.*

When applying therapeutic ultrasound, the clinician must select the frequency of the acoustic energy emitted (usually either 1 or 3 MHz), the duty cycle (pulsed versus continuous ultrasound or diathermy—diathermy units may deliver only pulsed energy), the amplitude or dose, and the duration of treatment. The appropriate selection of parameters allows for an appropriate level of tissue heating. The parameters for diathermy are less complicated. The characteristics of the electromagnetic field generated by a device are not adjustable. It is important to know how much energy is produced in order to estimate the appropriate length of treatment. For example, a device generating 48 W of energy will warm tissues sufficiently in 20 min for joint mobilization or stretching.

4. *Discuss the potential benefits and applications of LIPUS and PEMF in the management of fractures.*

Low-intensity pulsed ultrasound (LIPUS) and pulsed electromagnetic field (PEMF) devices were developed for the management of fractures. These devices have a fixed frequency, duty cycle, and amplitude, and they can be self-administered by patients. There is evidence that LIPUS can speed the repair of acute fractures and that these devices can promote repair in delayed and nonunion fractures. While treatment with these devices is physician directed, clinicians who treat musculoskeletal disorders should be familiar with them and should be able to properly instruct patients in self-administration. Research may find additional applications for these devices in the treatment of other musculoskeletal conditions.

Principles of Low-Level Laser Therapy

OBJECTIVES

After reading this chapter, you will be able to

1 understand the evolution of light therapy;

2 describe the unique characteristics of laser energy;

3 discuss the types of lasers available for soft tissue treatment and compare their energy outputs with respect to power, dosage modifications, wavelength, and pulse frequency; and

4 understand the physiological effects of low-level laser therapy.

A 60-year-old golfer is referred to the sports medicine clinic by an orthopedic surgeon for treatment of carpal tunnel syndrome. The surgeon has prescribed laser therapy in addition to therapeutic exercise. What is low-level laser, and how does it enhance healing? This chapter explains laser energy and how it is proposed to affect healing.

The recognition and application of light energy for healing are not new. Light has been associated with worship, superstitions, and healing powers throughout the ages. The Phoenicians, early Hebrews, and Greeks had their sun god worship, and their reliance on the sun for health and healing (actinotherapy and heliotherapy) is well documented. When we think of the effects of light energy on biological tissues we can quickly appreciate the impact the sun has on photosynthesis and vision. These are two examples of biological processes that depend on the application and absorption of electromagnetic energy. Light energy has had many applications in health care throughout history, but as technological advancements occurred in medicine, its application diminished. Lasers are the most refined form of light energy and are now used extensively for medical and scientific purposes.

The use of lasers for soft tissue healing was discovered by accident. A Hungarian physician, Endre Mester, was researching the ability of ruby laser energy to destroy tumors in rats in the early 1960s (Mester, Szende, and Tota 1967). His laser was not nearly as powerful as he had originally thought, and as he applied this light energy, he noticed that the superficial surgical wounds he had imposed were healing more quickly than in the nontreated animals. Additionally, the hair grew back faster on the animals that received the laser therapy. Thus began the extensive investigation of using low-power lasers to heal soft tissue injury.

LASER is an acronym for light amplification of stimulated emission of radiation. Einstein conceived of the laser in 1917, but the first working laser was not built until 1960 (Van Pelt 1970). Lasers are commonplace now and are used in a variety of applications in fields such as communication, industry, and medicine. Therapeutic lasers used for wound healing and pain management have been called many things,

including soft lasers, cold lasers, low-power lasers, low-intensity lasers, and biostimulators, to list a few. At present, the most commonly used term is low-level laser therapy (LLLT). The principal criterion for this type of laser energy is that it does not raise the treated tissues above 36.5°C.

Low-level lasers have been used extensively in physical medicine throughout Europe and Canada for many years. Lasers were excluded in the first edition of this text because the U.S. Food and Drug Administration (FDA) had not approved the use of these devices for the treatment of musculoskeletal disorders in the United States. In 1999, however, the FDA started to evaluate Premarket Notifications 510(k) for these medical devices. The 510(k) approval is required for anyone who wants to market Class I, II, and some Class III devices and Class IV devices intended for human use in the United States. The 510(k) must be submitted to the FDA at least 90 days before marketing unless the device is exempt from 510(k) requirements. A 510(k) is a premarketing submission made to the FDA to demonstrate that the device to be marketed is as safe and effective as, that is, substantially equivalent (SE) to, a legally marketed device that is not subject to premarket approval (PMA). The 510(k) allows a specific laser device to be used for specific conditions. Approval means that the approved laser can be sold, but that the only claim the manufacturer can make is for the indication described in the 510(k).

As of January 2002, the FDA had granted the premarket notification for the application of LLLT for two clinical applications.

1. The "adjunctive use in providing temporary relief of minor chronic neck and shoulder pain of musculoskeletal origin." The laser is a 630-nanometer (nm) diode laser with a 10-milliwatt (mW) output.

2. The "adjunctive use in the temporary relief of hand and wrist pain associated with carpal tunnel syndrome." The approved device was a low-energy infrared laser containing a cluster of three 30 mW, 830 nm laser diodes.

In addition to those specific treatment parameters, several other laser companies have received premarket notification approvals for their devices for the same applications. One should be sure when purchasing a device that the company has obtained FDA approval for the product. Claims beyond those listed on the approval should not be marketed. Clinical data will most likely be generated and submitted to the FDA for approval that will further expand the application of LLLT. This assumption is based on the extensive research and clinical application of LLLT devices in other countries.

The FDA approvals offer certified athletic trainers and other health care providers another modality for the treatment of patients they serve. This was, to our knowledge, the first time that a therapeutic modality was approved only for the treatment of specific conditions. Although extensive applications of this modality for other maladies are described in the international literature, any use of a therapeutic laser for the management of other conditions is considered "off-label" application. We will review some of this literature later in the chapter. American clinicians should not bill for any application of LLLT other than those specifically approved, and the clinician bears full responsibility for any adverse effects.

Lasers come in many types and forms with differing applications. To understand the unique attributes of laser energy, some understanding of the electromagnetic spectrum and atomic theory

is necessary. The acronym LASER provides considerable insight into its production: Light energy, or **photons**, are amplified and then stimulated and emitted as radiant energy. Thus, as ultrasound involves acoustic energy, laser delivers light energy that is absorbed in the tissues.

ELECTROMAGNETIC ENERGY

Energy is the ability to do work. The electromagnetic spectrum is the total range of energy expressed in relation to the wavelength and frequency of this energy. Electromagnetic energy consists of photons that travel at the speed of light: 300,000,000 m/s. This spectrum ranges from long wavelengths such as radio waves that are measured in meters to the opposite end of the spectrum with gamma rays that are measured in femtometers (10^{-15} meters). Photons of different wavelengths have different energy levels (figure 14.1). Photon energy is proportional to its frequency—the higher the frequency, the higher the photon energy. The high-energy photons are in the gamma, X-ray, and ultraviolet end of the spectrum and are capable of ionizing atoms and molecules.

The electromagnetic energy emitted from the sun is transmitted to earth. The earth's atmosphere absorbs the high-energy photons (UVB and UVC) except for a portion of the ultraviolet range (UVA).

Photons are produced either naturally or artificially, but the two types have the same energy level and consequences. At wavelengths of 320 nm or shorter, the energy becomes ionizing, therefore dangerous for human exposure. Sunlight and light used for conventional illumination have a wide spectrum of electromagnetic energies. Neon lights are narrow-band lights that result in a predominant

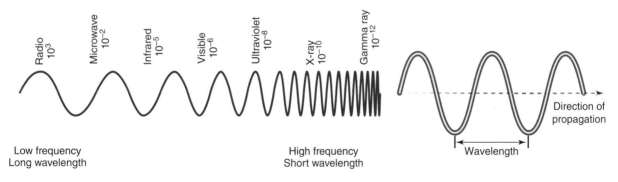

Figure 14.1   The electromagnetic spectrum is a continuum of energies categorized by their wavelengths and frequencies, which are inversely proportional. As the frequency increases, the wavelength shortens, and when there is a low frequency, the wavelength is long. The visible spectrum is within the electromagnetic spectrum and has wavelengths between 400 and 760 nm.

color. Light-emitting diodes (LEDs) use a relatively narrow band of electromagnetic energy that can result in a distinct color (red, yellow, green, or blue) or emit infrared frequencies that are invisible to the human eye. In contrast to the LEDs, which have a narrow band of electromagnetic wavelengths, laser light is very wavelength specific and therefore energy specific. Light-emitting diodes should not be confused with laser light, although the two terms are often used interchangeably.

LASER PRODUCTION

An atom has a nucleus consisting of protons and neutrons with electrons orbiting about in designated shells or valence levels. When energy is applied to an atom, the energy may be absorbed, causing one of the electrons to move and orbit in a higher shell. An atom in this state is labeled as "excited" and is unstable. The electron will return to a normal level of orbit (called **ground state**) as soon as possible.

When this occurs, the energy that caused the excited state is released as a photon (packet of light). In a normal state, electrons are absorbing energy and releasing photons continuously as the atoms try to remain in their most stable form (**spontaneous emissions**; see figure 14.2).

How is the light amplified? When a quantity of atoms is retained in a chamber **(lasing chamber)** and excited by the application of energy, photons are released in this confined area. As a photon strikes another excited atom, it stimulates the release of an additional photon as the electron returns to its resting orbit. As this occurs, the original photon is unaffected and continues to influence other atoms. Thus, as more and more photons are generated, increasing amounts of light energy are produced **(amplification)**. A lasing chamber is constructed with a semipermeable (also referred to as semi-reflective) mirror at one end. When the ability of the mirror to reflect light is exceeded, some laser light escapes from the chamber through the mirror (figure 14.3).

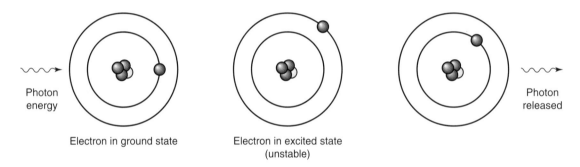

Figure 14.2 Energy (in photons) causes an atom to become excited, and an electron moves to a higher valence level. All matter seeks its most stable form, and thus it requires energy to be in an excited state. The matter releases an equal amount of energy as the atom goes back to its ground state. This process occurs naturally and is called spontaneous emission.

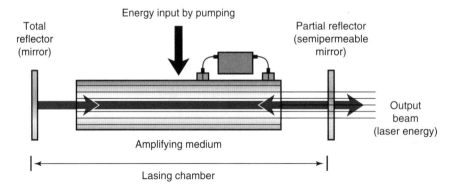

Figure 14.3 Basic production of a laser. Energy is applied to a closed chamber to allow amplification of photons. The energy is released at one end in the form of a laser.

PROPERTIES OF LASER LIGHT

What is unique about laser light? Laser light has three related properties: **monochromaticity**, **coherence**, and **collimation**. *Monochromic* means that the light is of one color or one wavelength that is specific to the energy level of the photon. The wavelengths of light energy range from 100 to 10,000 nm (billionths of meters). If the wavelength is less than 400 nm, the light falls into the ultraviolet spectrum. Visible light has wavelengths of 400 to 700 nm. The infrared spectrum lies between 700 and 10,000 nm. Two points can be drawn from this information. First, not all lasers emit light in the visible spectrum; second, when the light of a laser is visible, the light is of a single color since it is monochromic.

Coherent means that all of the waves of light energy are of the same length and are traveling in a similar phase relationship. This characteristic increases the wave amplitude characteristic (constructive interference). Furthermore, all of the energy is traveling in the same direction. This leads to the third characteristic of lasers, which is collimation.

Collimation refers to the degree to which the beam remains parallel with distance. A perfectly collimated beam would have parallel sides and would never expand at all. A laser beam does diverge somewhat and even obeys the inverse square law as the distance from the laser source is increased. The divergence of laser is minimal and varies with the type of laser (gas vs. diode), and can be modified with the use of lenses. The collimation of the laser is a safety concern for both the patient and the practitioner as the energy is concentrated to a thin beam. When the energy is focused on a small part of the retina, damage can result whether the laser is visible or not. Properties of laser and white light are compared in figure 14.4.

LASER CLASSIFICATION

Scientists have established safe exposure limits for different types of laser energy and developed a system of laser hazard classifications (American National Standards Institute [ANSI Z136.1-2000]) and a more recent revision was made available in 2007. The later version includes safety factors that are more consistent with international classifications. These classifications are separated by the *accessible emissions level* (AEL), which is the maximum power emitted during a specified duration of time.

There are five levels in the classification system: 1, 2, 3a, 3b, and 4. Categories 1, 2, and 3a are considered safe; 3b has certain risks; and 4 has the chance for serious risk. Standardized safety measures must be used to reduce the chance of adverse responses to laser exposure. Laser manufacturers are required to certify and label their devices in the appropriate category.

- Class 1 lasers: A Class 1 laser is considered to be incapable of producing damaging radiation levels and is therefore determined to be eye safe. These lasers are exempt from most control measures. Many lasers in this class are lasers that are embedded in an enclosure that prohibits or limits access to the laser radiation. Laser printers and CD players are Class 1 lasers.

- Class 2 lasers: Low-power visible lasers. Class 2 lasers are low-power lasers that also emit visible radiation (400 to 700 nm wavelength). These lasers do not exceed an AEL of 1 mW. The potential for an eye hazard exists if the exposure time is greater than 0.25 s. Bar code scanners are Class 2 lasers.

- Class 3 lasers: Medium-power lasers. Class 3 lasers are medium-power lasers or laser systems

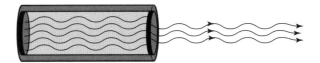

Coherent laser

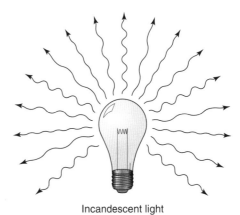

Incandescent light

Figure 14.4 Contrast the light emitted from a laser to that emitted from a light bulb. White light contains many different colors and therefore many wavelengths of light. Since the waves are of different lengths, they cannot remain in phase and they diverge. Thus, the light from a single bulb can illuminate a large area. The light emitted from a laser does not readily diverge, allowing travel over long distances and greater penetration.

Laser Components

There are thousands of types of lasers that are categorized by the way they are made. The four categories of lasers include gas (helium-neon), solid (ruby), liquid (dye), and semiconductor (diode).

The typical anatomy of a laser includes the following:

- Lasing medium: gas, semiconductor, liquid
- Power supply: energy source
- Resonating cavity: mirrored chamber

The lasing medium contains specific elements that will discharge photons of a specific wavelength and, therefore, energy. The power source applies energy to the lasing medium. The lasing medium stores the energy by raising the atom's outer electrons into a higher-valance orbit. This creates an environment where the majority of atoms are in their excited state, a condition that is called **population inversion.** When a photon of a specific energy identical to that being stored collides with an excited atom, an identical photon is produced. This photon, along with the incident photon, is released; the release is termed **stimulated emission** (figure 14.5). These photons further stimulate adjacent excited atoms, resulting in more photons being released. Depending on the elements of the lasing medium, the stimulated emission produces photons of a specific wavelength (monochromic) that are in a fixed phase relationship (coherent). The resonating chamber is composed of a chamber (gas), channel (diode), or rod (solid state) that further concentrates the production of the photons by the use of mirrors. The mirrors are placed at each end of the chamber. One mirror is totally reflective and the other mirror is partially reflective. As the photon concentration increases, the photons are emitted through the partially reflective end.

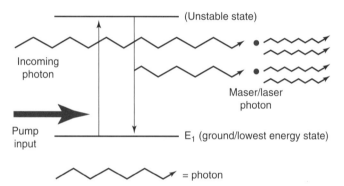

Figure 14.5   When energy is applied (pumping source), the atoms are in their excited state. When a photon strikes this atom, another photon is released in addition to the original photon. The additional photon causes more photons to be released when they strike additional excited atoms. This is termed stimulated emissions.

that require control measures to prevent viewing of the direct beam. Control measures emphasize preventing exposure of the eye to the primary or reflected beam.

- Class 3a lasers: Class 3a lasers have an AEL output power up to 5 mW. Viewing of the direct beam is normally not hazardous if it occurs for only momentary periods with the unaided eye. These lasers may present a hazard if viewed using collecting optics, which is any type of lens including glasses. Laser pointers and laser sights for firearms are examples of Class 3a lasers.

- Class 3b lasers: Class 3b lasers are medium-power lasers that have an AEL output power of 5 mW to 500 mW. Viewing these lasers under direct beam and specular reflection conditions is hazardous. The diffuse reflection is usually not a hazard except for higher-power Class 3b lasers. The Class 3b laser is not normally a fire hazard. Many of the LLLT devices are classified as 3b lasers.

- Class 4 lasers: High-power lasers. Class 4 lasers are high-power lasers that exceed an AEL of 500 mW. Direct beam, specular reflections, and diffuse reflections from these lasers present a hazard to both the eye and skin. A Class 4 laser can also present a fire hazard (radiant power > 2 W/cm^2 is an ignition hazard). In addition, these lasers can create hazardous airborne contaminants and have a potentially lethal high-voltage power supply. The entire beam path must be enclosed to reduce the potential hazards.

Lasers must be labeled appropriately to alert the user to potential hazards. Figure 14.6 demonstrates some standard labels for Class 2, 3, and 4 lasers.

Class 2 and Class 3a laser signs

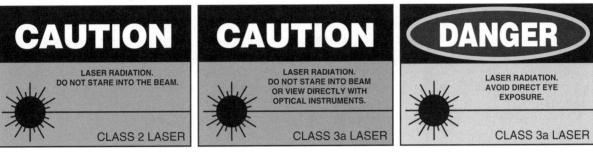

Class 3b laser signs

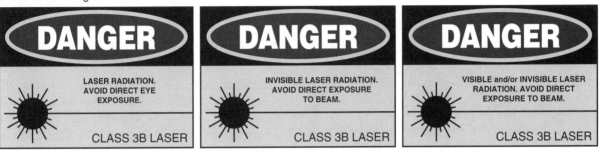

Class 4 laser signs

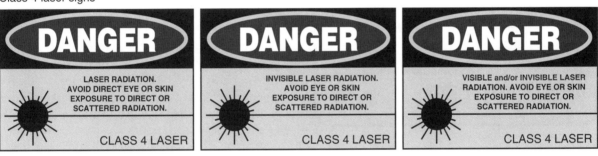

Figure 14.6 Lasers must be identified and marked according to their classification. The required labels need to be placed near the aperture to alert the user to potential hazards.

LASER PARAMETER SELECTION

Parameter selection is perhaps the most difficult aspect of LLLT since there are so many variables that must be considered. When one is determining the best-fit laser for therapeutic treatment, the following patient and laser parameters should be evaluated. Patient considerations include the type and condition of the tissue and acute or chronic condition, and even pigmentation may have an impact on the laser treatment outcome. Laser parameters that must be considered include wavelength, output power, average power, power density (intensity), and energy density (dosage). These factors are summarized in "Considerations for the Proper Selection of LLLT Treatment Parameters and Devices." It is import-

ant to understand these parameters to effectively operate different systems or to obtain comparable clinical outcomes. Many of the LLLT therapy devices marketed are menu driven, so selecting the tissue type and chronicity of the injury provides a specific treatment dosage.

One of the major problems with determining the efficacy of LLLT is that laser treatment is often poorly documented in the literature. Different laser types were used and dosages were varied or not reported. Therefore outcomes cannot be evaluated in a methodical manner. The equipment being marketed today is not well described, so the clinician may not know exactly what treatment parameters were delivered in a given study. It is important for the clinician to be aware of equipment features so that consistent energy levels can be delivered for a given condition.

Considerations for the Proper Selection of LLLT Treatment Parameters and Devices

The clinician should take into consideration both patient factors and the types of clinical lasers available. These factors are used to determine the best outcomes.

Patient Parameters

- Medical history and proper diagnosis: Diabetes or other medical conditions may alter clinical efficacy.
- Stage of the injury: Acute and chronic conditions require different dosages.
- Medications: Some medications, such as antibiotics, may make the patient photosensitive.
- Pigmentation of the tissues: Dark skin absorbs light energy more than light skin.

Laser Parameters

- Wavelength
- Output power
- Average power
- Intensity
- Dosage

photon energy and depth of penetration. The various elements used in the laser production result in the different photon energy levels emitted. The elements themselves are not introduced into the body. The types of lasers with LLLT have evolved to make the treatment application easier—the entire laser production can be housed in a handheld unit. When you are choosing a laser, factors to consider are the wavelength (which affects the depth of penetration), the ease of application, and the intensity or power density. Devices with multiple lasers in their surfaces make treating larger areas much more time efficient, but this feature adds to the expense.

Helium-Neon (HeNe)

The helium-neon laser was one of the first therapeutic lasers developed in the 1970s. It was initially a gas laser that emitted a red visible light with a wavelength of 632 nm. It is now available also as a semiconductor laser that eliminates the need for the gas chamber and fiber optics. Initially the typical power output was from 1 to 2 mW and was delivered by a fiber optic probe. Currently HeNe lasers are being produced with higher outputs, up to 25 mW. The depth of penetration with this wavelength is from 6 to 10 mm. The HeNe is commonly used for superficial wound care and dermatological problems (Shu et al. 2013; Dixit et al. 2012; da Silva et al. 2010).

A basic premise of electromagnetic energy is that the longer the wavelength (lower frequency), the greater the penetration. When determining the best-fit wavelength for laser application, the depth of the target tissue is an important consideration. Therefore, the helium-neon (HeNe) laser with a wavelength to 632 nm is more appropriate for dermatological (more superficial) conditions, and the gallium-arsenide (GaAs) with a wavelength of 904 nm is better for deeper structures. The ideal wavelength for specific problems has not been fully determined. Penetration is also affected by the power delivered (figure 14.7). Since energy can be absorbed while being transmitted, enough energy must be present at the target tissue to evoke a response.

Different types of lasers are available that allow the application of varied

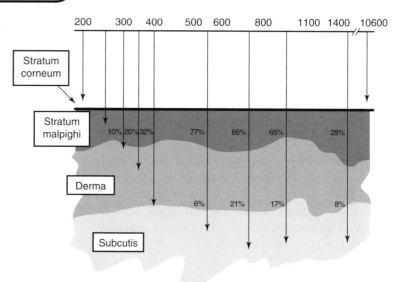

Figure 14.7 Depth of penetration. The wavelength of the laser is associated with the color (e.g., infrared, red) and the depth of penetration. Some laser energy is absorbed in the superficial, subcutaneous area, which decreases its ability to penetrate to deeper tissues.

Image from Lawrence Berkeley National Laboratory. Available: http://www.lbl.gov/ehs/pub3000/Skin_Effects.jpg

Indium-Gallium-Aluminum-Phosphide (InGaAlP or GaAllnP)

This type of laser is a semiconductor that emits a wavelength between 630 and 700 nm. It is gradually replacing the HeNe lasers in some applications because it does not require fiber optics. Semiconductor lasers have less coherence than gas lasers, so the treatment times need to be longer given the same output power. These lasers are commonly used for superficial wound care and dermatological problems (da Silva et al. 2010; Rodrigo et al. 2009).

Gallium-Arsenide (GaAs)

This is a semiconductor laser that uses an infrared wavelength of 904 nm, which is invisible to humans. It was first developed in the early 1980s and had an output power that ranged from 1 mW to 5 mW maximum output. The early GaAs lasers were pulsed and with the low output power provided minimal energy dosages. Currently, the output is up to 100 mW and can be superpulsed. Therefore, there is a short **pulsetrain** (burst) duration (100–200 ns) that is repeated up to 1,000 bursts per second. The depth of penetration has been reported to be 30 to 50 mm. This type of laser is being applied on deeper tissues such as tendons and ligaments as well as for the treatment of pathological conditions such as tendinopathies and osteoarthritis. (Alfredo et al. 2011; Tumilty et al. 2010).

Gallium-Aluminum-Arsenide (GaAlAs)

This is also a semiconductor laser in the infrared region with wavelengths that range from 780 to 890 nm but are most commonly between 800 and 830 nm. They are delivered in a continuous wave mode. This type of laser became more popular in the 1990s. The output power of these laser devices ranges from 30 to 100 mW, but the device has been manufactured with an output of up to 1,000 mW. Typically the gallium-aluminum-arsenide (GaAlAs) lasers are used for deeper ligament and tendon injuries. Higher output of the laser allows for shorter treatment times.

Combination Probes

Probes are produced that contain a grouping of several single-wavelength laser diodes in one probe. Cluster probes may combine LEDs with a single laser or may contain multiple laser diodes with a single LED. A single LED is often intended to be a visible signal when infrared (invisible) laser energy is being applied. The LED is often reported to be therapeutic, but this light is not a laser and cannot be compared to any LLLT reported in the literature.

COMPARING LOW-LEVEL LASER THERAPY TREATMENTS

Ultimately the tissues are going to respond to energy. There are several operational definitions that must be understood to appreciate how energy is varied with laser application. Although the photon energy that is intrinsic to a specific type of laser will not vary, the output power of the laser unit may affect the outcome. Descriptions of the power and how it is delivered to the patient must be consistent if one is to compare treatments. The dosage of the laser is determined by the intensity of the laser and the time of application. However, the number of application points and how close each irradiated site is to the next must also be consistent. The beam diameter varies with the type of laser (semiconductor vs. gas) as well as the equipment quality (fiber optics). Most LLLT equipment has narrow beam diameters, but the treatment is delivered per square centimeter. The rationale is that once the laser energy penetrates the skin, there will be absorption, reflection, refraction, and transmission of the energy. The narrow beam might be irradiating a larger diameter within the tissues. Furthermore, this generalization to a 1 cm treatment area makes the application easily reproducible.

The dosage of laser therapy is determined by the total amount of energy applied to the tissues. Microchip technology has simplified the calculations that the clinician must make so that the only variable is the time per irradiated area. The computations in the next section seem complex, but you will see that determining the dosage involves minimal math skill. Generally the higher the power of the laser, the shorter the time required to deliver the same dosage. The following definitions provide the basis for making laser treatments more consistent so that treatment outcomes can be compared when different types of lasers are used.

Output Power

The power of laser energy is measured in watts (W) or milliwatts (mW = 10^{-3} W). The output power is important in categorizing the laser for safety and should be clearly described with each device. The output power is not adjustable by the clinician.

The laser equipment you own will change with age; the stated output of the laser does not stay consistent over time. You should use a power meter to determine the output power of your device to make dosage applications correct. This factor is determined by the calibration of the therapeutic device.

Power Density

The power density of the laser is much like the power output or average power, but this parameter takes into consideration the actual beam diameter. Power density is also termed "irradiance" or "intensity," which is the average power per unit area in square centimeters (watts or milliwatts per cm^2 [mW/cm^2]).

$$\text{power density} = \text{intensity} = \text{power (W)} / \text{beam diameter in cm}^2 = \text{W/cm}^2$$

If the light is spread over a larger area, this will result in a lower power density (intensity) than if it were concentrated on a smaller area. The beam diameter determines the power density; therefore, it is affected by the degree of collimation the beam contains. Gas lasers have less divergence than semiconductor lasers. However, the use of fiber optics will increase the degree of divergence. The power density is usually programmed in the laser unit and reported simply as W/cm^2 or mW/cm^2 (beam diameter).

Average Power

Laser energy can be applied in a continuous or pulse-train (burst) frequency mode (figure 14.8). Knowing the average power is important in determining dosage when you are using a pulsed laser. If the laser is delivered in a continuous (cw) mode, then the average power is equal to the peak output power of the device. If the laser is pulsed (burst), then the average power is equal to the peak output power multiplied by the duty cycle. Therefore, if the peak power output of a laser is 5 mW (0.005 W) with a 25% duty cycle, then the average output is 1.25 mW (0.00125 W).

Different methods are used to create the pulsing of a laser, but with low-level lasers the most common method is by creating a duty cycle. However, low-level lasers may have a single pulse.

If a laser delivered output power of 50 mW in a continuous mode, it would take 20 s to deliver

1 joule (J) [(50 mW = 0.050 W) × 20 s = 1 J]. If the laser were pulsed to a 25% duty cycle, then it would take 80 s to deliver 1 J (0.050 W × 0.25 = 0.0125 mW × 80 s = 1 J). A longer time is needed to obtain the same dosage when the laser is pulsed. Pulse-train frequencies should not be confused with the **carrier frequency** of the laser, which is wavelength dependent.

If the desired treatment dosage were 2 J, then the treatment time would be peak output power × duty cycle.

$$0.005 \text{ W} \times 0.25 = 0.00125 \text{ W average power}$$

$$\text{dosage} = \text{joules (W/s)/cm}^2$$

$$\text{joules/average power} = \text{treatment time per cm}^2 \text{ of treatment area}$$

For example, 2 J / 0.00125 W = 1,600 s (26.67 min/cm^2). If the laser device was not pulsed, for example, 2 J / 0.005 W = 400 s (6.67 min/cm^2).

Treatment Duration

The treatment duration is really dependent on total energy, which is the product of power and time. Therefore, from a mathematical perspective, it would seem reasonable to justify a claim that a clinician can double the power and halve the time. This method assumes that the same amount of total energy would

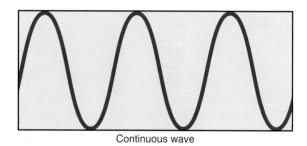

Continuous wave

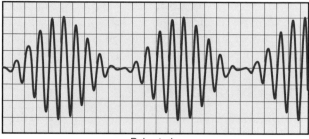

Pulse train

Figure 14.8 Continuous wave versus pulse train.

be applied, which is correct. However, there may be some biological responses that are affected by the rate of energy delivery. For example, if a high-power laser is applied for a shorter duration, it may burn or cause other damage to the tissues, but when the same total energy is pulsed or delivered over a longer duration, the treatment may produce a positive response.

Energy Density or Dosage

Energy density is the most important treatment parameter, describing the amount of energy applied per unit area. Dosage is measured in joules (a joule is equal to 1 watt per second). Therefore if the wattage or power is known, then the number of joules is affected by the treatment time per irradiated area. Treatment outcomes are dosage dependent, so this parameter must be consistently determined.

The difference between power density and energy density (dosage) is the time component.

$$\text{Power density or intensity} = \text{watts / beam area in cm}^2$$

$$\text{dosage} = \text{intensity} \times \text{irradiation time (seconds)} = \text{joules / cm}^2 \text{ treatment area}$$

The grid technique of irradiating each square centimeter of affected tissue is typically used. Therefore the total treatment time is affected by the intensity of the laser and the size of the treatment area. For example, if the laser is applied over a small area such as the transverse carpal ligament, then the treatment time will be significantly less than in treating the paraspinal musculature.

Recommended Dosage Range

The Arndt-Shultz principle is highly applicable with this type of modality. This principle suggests that some energy may elicit a small response in biological tissues. While more energy could have improved the result, too much energy negates the beneficial effect of the treatment.

The range of laser dosage that has elicited a reported therapeutic response is between 0.001 J/cm^2 and 10 J/cm^2. There is believed to be a minimal "window threshold" of energy needed to elicit a response. This explains why supermarket cashiers can get carpal tunnel syndrome despite the scanners! An excessive dose may result in a suppressive effect. It has been recommended that dosage between 0.5 and 1.0 J/cm^2 be used for open wounds and between 2.0 and 4.0 J/cm^2 with intact skin (table 14.1) (Law et al. 2015).

Pulsing Frequencies

Although there are different methods of pulsing lasers that will vary the power output, there is some interest in the impact that pulsing frequencies have on the outcome of laser treatments. Research is under way to determine if this parameter may affect therapeutic outcomes. Questions exist about whether the pulsing frequencies interfere with the resonating frequencies inherent in the tissue or whether the depth of penetration of the energy may be altered. Further research is needed to determine the relevance of this parameter.

Table 14.1   Treatment Dosages Recommended in the Literature Using a 780–860 nm GaAlAs Laser and a 904 nm GaAs Laser

Clinical condition	Dosage (joules)
Wound healing	4–35
Revascularization	2–3
Pain relief	1–7
Muscle spasms	2
Circulation	1–3
Nerve stimulation	0.1–0.5
Nerve cell regeneration	2
Inflammatory condition	1–3
Chronic conditions	3–6

Treatment Frequency

There is considerable variation in responses to laser therapy, so treatments should be individualized to the patient. The general recommendation is to use the least amount of energy that elicits the most benefit. Generally, laser treatments delivered three to four times a week with moderate doses are more effective than higher doses fewer times per week. Acute conditions should be treated more frequently than chronic conditions, but not more than once daily. Laser energy has a cumulative effect, so small doses spaced farther apart have elicited more effective outcomes.

PHYSIOLOGICAL EFFECT OF LOW-LEVEL LASER THERAPY

The potential use of LLLT in sports medicine would be to enhance wound healing and pain management after injury. It would be helpful to find a modality that could be applied acutely and one that would expedite the return of an athlete to competition by providing these outcomes. Low-level laser therapy has been reported to expedite the inflammatory process, decrease pain, and promote tissue healing. Studies have suggested that lasers promote fibroblast proliferation (Hawkins and Abrahamse 2006), promote the synthesis of types I and III procollagen mRNA (Abergel et al. 1984), hasten bone healing (Ozawa et al. 1995), and help in the revascularization of wounds (Kovacs, Mester, and Görög 1974). To understand how these proposed outcomes occur, we need to examine what is happening physiologically to the tissue once a laser treatment has been administered.

ATP Production

The proposed mechanism of action of laser therapy is associated with the ability of the cell to absorb the photon and transform the energy into adenosine triphosphate (ATP). The ATP is a form of energy that the cell uses to function. The cell must absorb the light energy for this process to occur. We know that certain cells have the capacity to absorb light energy, as in the skin reacting to sunlight. These light-absorbing components of the cells are termed chromophores or photoacceptors and are contained within the mitochondria and cell membrane (Huang et al. 2009). Examples of chromophores are cytochrome c oxidase, hemoglobin, myoglobin, porphyrins, and flavins (Karu 1987, Karu 1999).

The production of ATP is essential to cell function. Normally ATP is produced by the mitochondria, using oxygen as the primary fuel via oxidative phosphorylation. When laser is applied, the cells in the mitochondria react to the monochromatic light, resulting in altered biological processes (Karu 1998). The main biological process occurs in the electron transport chain, where a chromophore, cytochrome c oxidase, absorbs the photons, resulting in an increase in the oxidative metabolism within the mitochondria (Xu et al. 2008; Silveira, Streck, and Pinho 2007). This excitation leads to an increase in ATP production, which results in the synthesis of DNA, RNA, enzymes, and cells responsible for repairing damaged tissue (Xu et al. 2008; Brown 1999; Karu et al. 2001).

Nitric Oxide Release

The mitochondrion produces nitric oxide normally with increased production following exercise and stress (Giulivi, Poderoso, and Boveris 1998). The nitric oxide produced competes with oxygen to bind to many different receptors in the cell; the most common receptors are the c oxidase receptors and specialized hemoglobin and myoglobin receptors (Shiva and Gladwin 2009). With the increased availability of nitric oxide binding to these receptors, the oxygen cannot bind, which produces an inhibition of ATP synthesis (Lane 2006; Sarti et al. 2003). Laser has been suggested to release the nitric oxide from these receptors due to a process called **photodissociation**, allowing the oxygen to resume binding to the receptors, which returns the mitochondria's ability to synthesize ATP (Huang et al. 2009; Lingard et al. 2007; Lane 2006).

Reactive Oxygen Species

Reactive oxygen species (ROS) are molecules such as oxygen ions, free radicals, and hydrogen peroxide that are metabolic by-products of oxygen use in the mitochondria (Huang et al. 2009). While low levels of ROS are beneficial, elevated levels of ROS can result in cell damage. Low dosages of laser have been shown to lower the levels of ROS, increasing ATP production and producing increase in gene transcription at the cellular level (Huang et al. 2013).

Laser stimulation has been shown to enhance the production of ATP by forming singlet oxygen, reactive oxygen species (ROS), or nitric oxide, all of which influence the normal formation of ATP (Derr and Fine 1965; Lubart et al. 1990). The proposal that laser energy merely promotes normal cellular function rather than changing cell function explains why injured tissues respond to laser therapy while there is little effect on noninjured cells. This is in contrast to the application of high levels of laser energy or excessive doses that cause damage to cells. Again, the effect of the laser is dependent on the intensity of the energy, the exposure time, and the irradiated area. The wavelength of the laser affects the depth of penetration of the energy.

SUMMARY

Low-power laser, although used in physical medicine for many years, has been approved for use in the United States for less than a decade. This chapter reviews the evolution of laser and laser therapy and describes the unique characteristics of laser energy. Many types of laser exist; this chapter focuses on the types of lasers available for treatment of musculoskeletal conditions. The use of commercially available devices in clinical practice is described with attention to safety and contraindications of low-level laser therapy. The proposed mechanisms for response to treatment with laser are reviewed.

KEY CONCEPTS AND REVIEW

1. *Understand the evolution of light therapy.*

   Clinicians through the ages have used actinotherapy or light therapy to heal wounds and sicknesses without understanding the physiological impact of the application of light. Modern-day uses of light therapy include ultraviolet light and laser therapy. Laser applies the most refined photon or light energy.

2. *Describe the unique characteristics of laser energy.*

   Laser energy is composed of photons with the same energy, and it is only one color (monochromatic). These photons all have the same wavelength and frequency and travel parallel with each other, making them collimated. The photons are also in phase with one another, or coherent. These factors—monochromaticity, coherence, and collimation—are unique characteristics of laser light.

3. *Discuss the types of lasers available for soft tissue treatment and compare their energy outputs with respect to power, dosage modifications, wavelength, and pulse frequency.*

   There are different types of lasers made from a variety of elements, each producing a laser with a certain wavelength. Some types of lasers are more powerful than others, and some must be pulsed to be categorized for LLLT. Considering the variables in production, it is important for the clinician to understand how to compare clinical outcomes using the available parameters. The power is used to categorize the laser and is not adjustable by the clinician. The dosage takes into consideration the total amount of energy delivered and is calculated as the power (intensity) times treatment time. Dosage is measured in joules per square centimeter since most LLLT applications apply the energy over a 1 cm^2 area. Wavelength and pulse frequency are also parameters that are not controlled by the clinician but affect the depth of penetration and the amount of energy delivered.

4. *Understand the physiological effects of low-level laser therapy.*

   The physiological effects of LLLT are the result of the ability of the body to absorb energy from the photon application. Specifically, the application of low levels of light energy causes an increase in the production of ATP. Cell proliferation is enhanced when a stimulus exists, as in an inflammatory state. Low-level laser therapy can be used in sports medicine to promote tissue healing and to relieve pain.

chapter 15

Clinical Application of Low-Level Laser Therapy

OBJECTIVES

After reading this chapter, you will be able to

1. describe the indications, contraindications, and safety considerations of LLLT;

2. describe the application techniques during various phases of healing and the unique characteristics of laser energy; and

3. perform a laser treatment using a commercially available device.

A soccer player reported to the clinic with tenderness in his anterior thigh. He had been kicked during a match the day before and he now complains of tenderness, restriction in motion, and pain when he tries to run. There is an area approximately 6 cm in diameter where there is point tenderness. Clearly this is a contusion, and added protection is indicated. However, perhaps low-level laser therapy could facilitate healing and promote pain reduction. What factors should be considered when applying low-level laser therapy, and how is it administered? This chapter addresses the application of low-level laser therapy (LLLT) for musculoskeletal conditions.

Chapter 14 addressed the biophysical properties of laser energy and how that energy is absorbed by the body to produce its effects. This chapter presents the various uses of laser from an evidence-based perspective. Common impairments such as pain, swelling, and loss of motion, for example, are presented, and mechanisms to treat those impairments are discussed. Using clinical research is important to determine when and how a tool can be used to maximize its effectiveness. At times, there may be little support to use particular treatments, and being able to discern why a modality or treatment did not add benefit is also important.

LLLT is most commonly used as a bioenergy to promote healing and to reduce pain. A thorough musculoskeletal evaluation is used to help determine the cause of the problem and to focus therapy on the correct cause. Although pain and loss of function are the result of other inflammatory factors, the clinician should focus on the impairments. The use of LLLT to treat various conditions is described. Finally, the procedure for applying laser is addressed to improve outcomes and to make sure the treatment is consistently delivered and documented.

BIOLOGICAL EFFECTS OF LASER

Low-level laser therapy has been studied for over 40 years, with mixed outcomes reported. The applications have been extensive, involving dermatology, respiratory conditions, arthritic conditions, soft tissue and bone healing, pain, and nerve lesions, to name a few. Conclusions on efficacy are difficult to ascertain because many of the reported outcomes are in non-peer-reviewed literature, anecdotal reports, uncontrolled studies, or published abstracts, or controlled studies have poorly described methodology or show contradictory outcomes. The FDA must rely on clinical data as it considers whether to allow an expansion in the applications of LLLT. Ideal studies are from multiclinical sites and are randomized, blinded, placebo-controlled studies that verify safety and efficacy. As far as the FDA is concerned, the safety considerations have been largely satisfied, but further research is needed to determine efficacy with medical conditions other than carpal tunnel syndrome and neck pain.

APPLICATION TECHNIQUES

There are different methods of applying laser energy during the treatment. The various techniques are described next, and combinations of the techniques may be used when indicated clinically.

Point Application

Point application is used in treating acupuncture or trigger points; the laser is applied directly over a point, and the dosage is delivered. Power density considerations make the cosine law and the inverse square law (especially with highly diverging laser

Tips for Effective Application of Treatment

The following suggestions should be considered when one is administering laser treatment to ensure the most effective and consistent outcomes.

- The laser should be positioned perpendicular to the treatment surface.
- Firm contact should be maintained with the treatment site unless an open wound is present. If contact is not appropriate, then the laser should be held as close to the surface as possible.
- Determine the appropriate treatment dosage for the individual points as well as the total treatment dose, for example, 1 J/cm^2 for a total of 20 J.
- Treatment should be minimal at first, and the dosage and treatment frequency should gradually increase as tolerated to obtain the optimal outcomes.
- Treatment application can use one of several techniques:
  - "Surround the dragon": This technique uses point application around the perimeter of the pain site or lesion.
  - Grid technique: Fill in the pain area or lesion using point application in an imaginary 1 cm^2 grid (figure 15.1).
  - Acupuncture point: Use an acupuncture chart to locate appropriate points at which to treat involved structures or pain syndromes.

- Ask the patient to report any sensations or changes in his or her condition during treatment.
- Establish pre- and posttreatment changes in pain, edema, or functional capacity.
- Ask the patient before the next treatment about reaction to the previous treatment.
- Adjust the dosage according to the response elicited from the previous treatment:
  - Decrease the dosage if undesirable outcomes occurred.
  - Increase the dosage if there were no results.

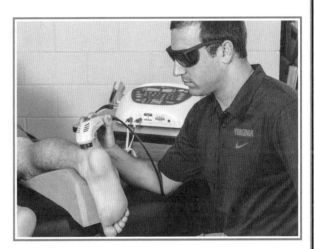

Figure 15.1   Grid laser application technique.

---

beams) very relevant with laser application. The laser application should be positioned in firm contact with the skin when appropriate or as close to the skin surface as possible. The applicator should also be positioned so it is perpendicular to the treatment surface. This will reduce energy loss due to diffusion or reflection.

There can be a considerable variation in the beam characteristics between lasers, but in the application of point stimulation the point is generally considered to be in a 1 cm^2 area. Although the beam may have a spot contact 2 mm in diameter, there will be a spread effect of up to 1 cm within the tissues. To treat trigger points or acupuncture points, the treatment is applied to individual points and then moved to the next point. When a surface area is being covered, two methods can be used to apply the laser energy—scanning and grid technique.

Scanning

In the scanning technique, the laser head is held close to the tissue surface and moved in a slow and steady manner over the treatment area. The scanning lines are approximately 1 cm apart, and the treatment is continued until the dosage is completed. There are expensive commercially produced laser devices that apply a scanning technique. The patient lies under the lasing head, which mechanically moves over the treatment area.

Grid

With the grid technique, the treatment area is determined and a grid matrix in 1 cm squares is imaged over this area. Point application is used for a specified dosage per square centimeter, which will ultimately distribute the total dosage over the area in the treatment grid. This technique is considered to be more accurate than the scanning technique. Firm contact should be made with the skin unless there is an open wound; in this case a 1 to 2 mm distance is maintained.

Of the methodological flaws noted, dosage has been and remains a significant pitfall in research. Frequently, studies used very low doses of laser. Following are the treatment parameters that should be documented to allow consistency in further research:

- Laser model
- Laser type and wavelength
- Probe description (single or cluster)
- Output power
- Pulsing and pulsing duration
- Pulse frequency
- Dosage
- Power density (intensity)
- Treatment technique (distance)
- Treatment time
- Treatment frequency

Video 15.1 shows application of a laser treatment to the Achilles tendon.

Video 15.2 shows application of laser for treatment of carpal tunnel symptoms.

INDICATIONS FOR LOW-LEVEL LASER THERAPY

Laser is indicated for a variety of impairments. Many studies have been conducted, primarily in Europe since LLLT is more commonly available in those countries. Much of the research on clinical populations, however, becomes confusing, especially since the parameters and power of the laser can vary. It is important that researchers describe the parameters consistently. For example, manufacturers and researchers must describe the power of the laser, specifically the total output and how that laser is modulated. The wavelength and time of exposure, which control the total energy delivered, are also important and should be reported.

Pathologies present with specific impairments that should be addressed as part of a comprehensive treatment plan. The evaluation should identify those impairments, and the clinician should choose the best course of treatment to address each one. For example, if the chief complaint is tenderness or pain, the clinician may decide to use electrotherapy, ice, or another agent to minimize pain so that rehabilitation can begin. LLLT is often used for a variety of impairments based on the stage of inflammation. Researchers propose mechanisms that are involved in treating these impairments so that clinicians may decide whether LLLT could be useful in each case. This method of evaluating the literature as a guide to practice is evidence-based medicine. Using evidence or research helps clinicians to determine when a therapy is predicted to have a benefit. The clinician uses his or her judgment to apply the therapy.

Inflammation

LLLT was once reported to be proinflammatory rather than anti-inflammatory due to the degranulation of mast cells that results in histamine production (Kana and Hutschenreiter 1981). However, recent research has found reduced inflammation following laser treatment (Bjordal 2006; de Morais et al. 2010; Alves et al. 2013). Laser has been shown to reduce prostaglandin E2 and inhibit cyclooxygenase 2 within cells, both of which are responsible for inflammation (Sakurai, Yamaguchi, and Abiko 2000). Prostaglandin E2, a hormone formed due to cell damage, attracts leukocytes and is responsible for increasing vascular permeability, while cyclooxygenase 2, an enzyme, is responsible for the formation of prostaglandins (Gomez et al. 2013). The effect of laser on inflammation suggests that LLLT may begin early in the injury process and may be combined with RICE (rest, ice, compression, elevation) as an initial intervention.

Pain

The FDA is allowing the marketing of approved LLLT devices for the treatment of symptoms associated with carpal tunnel syndrome and for adjunctive use in providing temporary relief of minor chronic neck and shoulder pain of musculoskeletal origin. The effect of LLLT on other painful conditions has been reported, but the effectiveness is equivocal. Numerous studies have shown that LLLT is effective in reducing pain, but the exact mechanisms are still to be determined. The production of endogenous opioids, nitric oxide, serotonin, and acetylcholine has been reported to be a source of analgesic effects elicited from laser radiation (Laakso et al. 1994; Choi, Srikantha, and Wu 1986). These mechanisms need further study. Another proposed mechanism for pain reduction is a direct effect on nerve conduction velocity and somatosensory evoked potentials. These changes have been measured after the application of LLLT, but their ability to influence pain is not well understood.

Wound Healing

Wound healing has been enhanced with the application of laser energy (Woodruff et al. 2004; Enwemeka et al. 2004). The most promising investigations have involved using laser to promote the healing of ulcers and other injuries to the skin. Research outcomes have varied for different reasons, including the use of different wavelengths and dosages and the use of healthy animal models.

Laser radiation results in **biomodulation**, meaning that it can stimulate or inhibit. This is compared to sunlight and tanning. Some energy is effective in stimulating melatonin production, producing a suntan, but excessive sunlight results in damage, causing sunburn. Low-dosage laser would be ineffective, while excessive energy might inhibit rather than stimulate healing. Acute injuries can be treated more often (daily) than chronic wounds, which should be treated only two or three times per week. Chronic wounds do not respond to aggressive interventions.

Laser energy is more effective in treating pathological states; therefore, when healthy subjects are used, the outcomes may be subdued. Although tissue healing is accelerated, no hyperplastic effects have been reported (Bosatra et al. 1984). During the course of healing, lased wounds had more collagen and had a higher tensile strength than the controls, but by day 14 the wounds were similar (Abergel et al. 1987; Kana and Hutschenreiter 1981; Surinchak et al. 1983). This shows that laser energy catalyzes normalization rather than creating a supernormal effect.

Systemic effects from laser therapy have been reported (Mester et al. 1971; Kana and Hutschenreiter 1981). This is why research using laser treatments on one body part and using another site on the same subject or animal as the control may give misleading results. These systemic effects are not always observed in the research but should be considered.

Blood Circulation

LLLT has been found to have an increase in both localized and limb blood flow in soft tissue structures. The improved circulation is theorized to help improve healing following injury by controlling ischemia, edema, and hypoxia (Leadbetter 2001; Maegawa et al. 2000). Increases in arteriolar dilation and microcirculation have been found within hours of a laser treatment, and these increases are maintained for up to three days following treatment (Ihsan 2005). Larkin et al. (2012) found a dose-response effect on increasing soft tissue blood flow with a Class 4 laser and a 3 W output power, 50% duty cycle, 1.5 average power or treatment, and a dose of 360 J compared to a sham and two other dose protocols. While the parameters used vary between studies and further research is needed, LLLT appears to have potential for positive effects on post-injury blood circulation.

Muscle Function

Laser has been investigated for its effects on many different components of muscular function, such as performance, fatigue, and recovery (Ferraresi, Hamblin, and Parizotto 2012). As you learned in chapter 14, the monochromatic properties of LLLT target the chromophores located in the mitochondria. This interaction has been theorized to increase ATP production on many different pathways. Researchers have focused on this reaction because it may show that LLLT has a positive effect on muscle function.

Muscle performance following LLLT is directly related to the increase in ATP synthesis. Two systematic reviews have recently examined the effect of laser on exercise performance when an LLLT treatment was administered before exercise. Both studies found that a treatment with power outputs between 50 and 200 mW and doses between 5 and 6 J per point had positive effects on increasing the number of repetitions before fatigue and decreasing the strength deficits during the exercise protocols

(Leal-Junior at al. 2013; Borsa, Larkin, and True 2013). These two authors also found benefits on muscle damage following exercise when measured through biomarkers. They reported improvement in the removal of blood lactate and decreases in metabolic by-products following exercise, specifically creatine kinase and C-reactive protein. Other functions of muscle performance have been measured: muscle power (Leal-Junior 2009), maximum voluntary contraction (Baroni et al. 2010), and electromyography activity (Kelencz et al. 2010), to name a few. However there are few studies on these variables, and more research is needed.

Adjunctive Therapy

Other modalities in addition to LLLT can be beneficial, although thermal devices should be used after the laser treatment. Blood, specifically the hemoglobin, absorbs laser energy, so any modality that increases blood flow could make LLLT less effective. Generally it is recommended that tissues be cooled before laser treatment and heated afterward if these therapies are indicated. When laser treatment was combined with ultrasound, it was found that the individual therapies obtained better outcomes, and the clinician should choose the most appropriate modality rather than combining them (Gum et al. 1997).

Medications may have an effect on laser efficacy, although more research on this issue is needed. Medications such as nonsteroidal anti-inflammatory drugs, steroids, and calcium channel blockers, to list a few, are thought to block membrane channels and pigment receptors (Meersman 1999), which are important for laser actions, and therefore reduce laser effectiveness. Other medications such as procaine, certain antibiotics, and copper-based local substances may enhance the effectiveness of laser energy by enhancing the receptor sites. Researchers should be sensitive to the presence of medications when selecting subjects for laser studies.

SAFETY CONSIDERATIONS

As with the application of any modality, it is important to be sure the diagnosis is correct. Make sure you know what condition you are treating.

• **Eye safety.** Never look into the aperture of the laser. Eye protection is only effective for indirect exposure. The cornea transmits light energy, and the eye focuses the light on the retina. Wavelengths over 700 nm are invisible; therefore, the light reflex response will be absent. This could result in retinal damage. Eye protection should be provided for both the clinician and the patient, depending on whether the classification of the laser is 3b or higher. Laser warning signs should be present. The laser probe should also be kept in contact with the skin whenever possible. Safety keys and automatic shutdowns are provided with many laser units to help prevent indiscriminate activation of the laser.

• **Training.** With the potential safety concerns about Class 3b and 4 lasers that are becoming more common in sports medicine clinics, the ANSI (Z136.1-2007 and Z136.3-2007) recommends clinicians receive proper training for laser use, documentation of annual surveys, location, and response to accidents or incidents.

• **Cell proliferation.** There was a decrease in mitotic activity with very high doses of laser energy but a proliferation with low doses of 0.5 to 1.5 J/cm^2 in open wounds and up to 4 J/cm^2 in closed wounds. These energy levels will also vary with different types of lasers (lower doses were more effective with the GaAs lasers; higher energies were needed with the HeNe) (Mester, Mester, and Mester 1985). Adult doses should not exceed 50 J, and the maximum dosage for children under 14 years of age is 25 J (Tume and Tume 1994).

• **Fatigue reactions.** Fatigue has been reported after laser treatments (Tunér and Hode 1998). This was short-term and was more common with chronic pain conditions.

• **Pain response.** The patient may complain of a pain response the day after treatment. This is believed to be due to an activation of tissue healing mechanisms that had become dormant (Tunér and Hode 1998). This should be a positive response sign, especially for chronic injuries.

CONTRAINDICATIONS AND PRECAUTIONS

Because low-level laser therapy can inhibit cell function when applied in high doses, laser therapy should be applied at appropriate dosages. A number of contraindications warrant special considerations.

• **Pregnancy.** There is no published research that addresses the effect of laser therapy on the unborn child. As a precautionary measure, laser therapy should be avoided in pregnant women, especially with application to certain acupuncture points and over the lower abdomen.

- **Cancer.** No mutagenic effects have been reported with the use of LLLT. Cancerous cells in vitro have been stimulated to grow, but in vivo studies resulted in a reduction in tumor size that was attributed to an enhanced immunological system (Wohlgemuth et al. 2001). Only oncologists should treat cancer patients.

- **Thyroid gland.** Thyroid gland activity has been modified by laser energy; therefore treating over this area should be avoided (Hernandez, Santistaban, and del Valle Soto 1989).

- **Children.** No studies have identified any impact on open growth plates. Since there are limited studies on the use of LLLT in children, the treatment should not be done unless the benefits clearly outweigh the potential for risk when there are open growth plates. Generally the maximum recommended dosage for children is less than 25 J (Tume and Tume 1994).

- **Steroid usage.** Clinicians should be aware of possible interactions between steroid use and laser treatment. Cortisol antagonists have been found to inhibit the receptors responsible for the anti-inflammatory effects of a laser treatment (Lopes-Martins et al. 2006). Research is being conducted on other common steroids, with some focus being placed on the concern that glucocorticoid steroid usage may decrease cellular responses, decreasing the effectiveness of this modality (Lopes-Martins et al. 2006).

Low-level laser therapy is still under scrutiny using evidence-based research standards. Laser therapy is making gains as research is more controlled and as multicenter studies and contemporary diagnostic measures are being used. Low-level laser therapy has been used for the treatment of many neuromusculoskeletal conditions in many countries, and no adverse effects have been reported in over 1,700 publications. Additional research is required to obtain data about success rates in treating specific conditions, length of exposure, frequency of treatments, and related therapeutic protocols.

SUMMARY

The application of laser is relatively simple because the clinician typically only controls the total area to be treated and how long each area is treated. The machine controls all other parameters. It is important to understand and to be able to compare various manufacturers' devices so that treatment outcomes can be assessed more systematically. For example, it is often difficult to determine whether a laser unit has a power or intensity of 100 or 500 W, even though there is a vast difference in the energy that they produce. Likewise, some companies add supraluminous bulbs or light-emitting diodes (LEDs), which give the illusion that the laser energy is being delivered over a broader area. Although both are still considered to be light therapy, they are not laser energy and would not have the same expected results.

In general, once the clinician knows the power output, then an adjustment in the time that the energy is delivered affects the overall dosage. Applying the same laser for 30 s and 60 s could produce vastly different outcomes. It is often difficult to extract parameters from the literature and apply them in clinical practice. However, it is best to maintain a log of the types of conditions that are treated with LLLT and to measure outcomes from the treatment. That way, the clinician learns how the treatment is influencing patients, and better decisions can be made in the future.

1. *Describe indications, contraindications, and safety considerations of LLLT.*

Low-level laser therapy can inhibit cell function when applied in high doses; therefore laser therapy should be applied at appropriate dosages. LLLT has been used for a plethora of conditions, including pain, wound healing, inflammation, muscle function, and circulation. This form of therapy should not be used in pregnancy, over open epiphyseal plates, in cancer patients, or over the thyroid gland. The clinician should exercise caution when treating around the eyes, since some lasers used in LLLT are invisible, and prolonged exposure can damage the retina.

2. *Describe the application techniques during various phases of healing and the unique characteristics of laser energy.*

The inflammatory process should be outlined (inflammatory phase: days 1-4; proliferative phase: days 5-21; healing phase: days 21-40). The student should determine whether the energy to be added with laser would be helpful in context to the cellular factors that are present. For example, in the inflammatory phase, less energy should be applied as it may disrupt the clotting and perpetuate the inflammatory factors. During later stages, more energy is tolerated.

3. *Perform a laser treatment using a commercially available device.*

The most consistent method for applying LLLT is the use of the grid technique. The laser is applied with the device perpendicular to the target tissue, and direct, light pressure is maintained using the applicator. The laser is applied for the designated duration in each square centimeter of an imaginary grid that covers the treatment area. The dosage is determined by the time during which each area is treated.

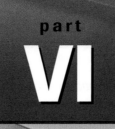
Mechanobiology, Exercise, and Manual Therapies

The effects of mechanical forces on tissue repair are introduced in chapter 4. A great portion of part VI is devoted to providing a much more thorough explanation of the role mechanical forces play in maintaining tissue health and promoting repair. Chapter 16 examines how mechanical signals are transmitted to cells and the effect of mechanical signals on cell function and tissue health. This foundation in mechanobiology is then applied in the context of some common manual therapies in chapter 17. This chapter also covers manual techniques that reduce pain and muscle tension as well as the mobility of joints.

Part VI concludes by examining tissue loading through exercise as a repair stimulus. Although therapeutic exercise is commonly prescribed to treat impairments, restore function, and prepare for a return to participation in sport or work, advances in mechanobiology reveal the effects of loading on repair. With the understanding of mechanobiology provided in chapter 16, the use of exercise in the treatment of conditions affecting tendon, muscle, bone, and cartilage is reviewed. Although it is not possible to describe the optimal exercise regimen for all conditions or patients, the chapter provides guidance for the early integration of exercise into plans of care for patients with musculoskeletal injuries.

Mechanobiology

After reading this chapter, you will be able to

❶ understand the basic principles of mechanobiology and their implications for the clinician;

❷ describe the mechanism of mechanotransduction, in which mechanical force transforms to chemical signals, mediating cell and tissue responses;

❸ describe key components of connective tissue and how they adapt; and

❹ understand tissue-specific mechanobiology.

A lacrosse player presents with recurrence of painful Achilles tendinopathy, with the initial onset approximately 1 year ago. Symptoms include pain during and after running, stiffness in the morning, and intermittent peritendinous swelling. Soft tissue mobilization is begun 10 min per day along with a static and gentle ballistic stretching program for 3 min, 8 to 10 times per day. After 1 week, symptoms have reduced 25%. A heel drop program is begun twice daily. Symptoms subside in 6 weeks. Heel drop and flexibility programs are continued throughout the on and off season with complete resolution of symptoms and unrestricted athletic activity.

Tendinopathy is linked to overuse, so it may seem counterintuitive to select additional loading activities as a means of treatment. In fact, eccentric exercise is very effective at treating "overuse tendinopathy." Manual techniques such as soft tissue mobilization and deep friction massage may also promote repair. The forces imposed on tissues through exercise, manual therapy, and certain modalities result in cell signals that alter gene expression to maintain musculoskeletal tissue health. Clinicians essentially prescribe "units" of stress through exercise instruction, mechanical interventions, and physical modality selection. As clinicians we have a unique skill set in our ability to adjust appropriate stresses delivered during rehabilitation in order to directly influence repair and adaptation. Central to the rehabilitation process is the application of appropriate stress as tissue heals.

The biology of mechanical signals, *mechanobiology*, examines the mechanism in which mechanical energy is transformed to chemical signals, resulting in cell-mediated tissue responses. The ability to adjust mechanical stimuli places clinicians at the front line of musculoskeletal medicine as we learn to dial in physical stimuli to achieve optimal mechanobiologic responses. Mechanical force transduction **(mechanotransduction)** works synergistically with the endocrine system and is affected by a number of endogenous and environmental factors, such as genetics and physical activity. Many of the hormones produced by endocrine glands are also synthesized locally by resident cells in musculoskeletal tissue. A hormone produced within the tissue by resident musculoskeletal cells is called a cytokine. One example would be the anabolic hormone IGF-I, produced by the liver in the endocrine system but also produced by cells in tendon, bone, and cartilage. In this way tissues with limited endocrine access have the ability for local (autocrine and **paracrine**) regulation through the production and action of cytokines.

This chapter explores the mechanobiology of musculoskeletal tissue, beginning with a brief discussion of its influence on and interaction with the endocrine system. An understanding of mechanobiology provides important context for treatment rationale and exercise prescription, essential for optimal outcomes. Therapeutic exercise and interventions are much more than means of restoring motion, strength, and function; they are critical for homeostasis, adaptation, and optimal repair of damaged musculoskeletal tissues. The application of mechanotransduction in clinical practice through the selection of rehabilitation components is presented in chapter 17.

ENDOCRINE INTERACTION

Tight regulation of tissue homeostasis is crucial for musculoskeletal health. Vascular tissues such as skin and muscle are at a tremendous advantage for healing and adaptation due to endocrine access. The endocrine system delivers regulatory hormones and molecules through the bloodstream to peripheral tissues through the sequential activation of glands and organs. For example, a prominent endocrine axis that influences musculoskeletal tissue is the hypothalamic–pituitary–gonadal axis. This axis is responsible for the development and regulation of the immune and reproductive systems, among others; this in turn governs crucial musculoskeletal functions such as healing, remodeling, and adaptation.

Hormones derived from this axis contribute more substantially to the regulation of well-vascularized musculoskeletal tissues such as muscle than to poorly vascularized tissues such as tendon or cartilage. As an example, growth hormone produced in the somatotropic cells of the anterior pituitary stimulates downstream liver-produced insulin-like growth factor (IGF), adrenal produced beta-endorphin, and the gonadotropin testosterone. These hormones result in tissue change through their interaction with transmembrane and intracellular receptors and subsequent activation of intracellular signaling cascades, resulting in gene transcription and protein production. The influence of this process is readily observed in muscular development after puberty.

By definition, the endocrine system works at a distance from effector sites (location of action) and delivers hormones through the bloodstream, leaving tissue with little blood flow (tendon), or no blood flow (cartilage) with very limited or no endocrine support (see figure 16.1). Many of the hormones produced by endocrine glands are also synthesized locally by resident cells in musculoskeletal tissue. A hormone produced within the tissue by resident musculoskeletal cells is called a cytokine. As noted previously, IGF-I is a hormone produced by the liver as well as a cytokine produced by cells in tendon,

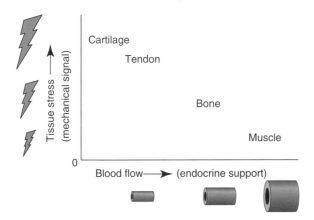

Figure 16.1 Tissues with endocrine access through circulation benefit from systemically produced substances. As access to blood diminishes in tendon, and ultimately disappears in cartilage, reliance on local factors for regulation such as mechanotransduction increases.

bone, and cartilage for local (autocrine and paracrine) regulation.

MECHANICAL SIGNALING

Mechanical signals exert a multitude of effects related to tissue composition and health. Reliance on mechanical signaling is not confined to musculoskeletal tissue by any means; immune cell activation, hearing, and blood pressure control all rely on the physical connection and transmission of force between cells and surrounding tissue.

The link between structure and function can be traced to Wolff's law concerning bony change related to use and disuse (Wolff 1892). The study of mechanobiology at its essence describes the cellular mechanisms underlying Wolff's law, in which adaptation of bone structure in response to imposed stress was described.

Cells create their environment by producing and remodeling extracellular matrix (ECM) components into an optimal configuration to support the development and function of the organism. The organization of multicellular organisms is tightly controlled through distinct structures and characteristics of tissues, which result from specific cellular interactions.

The extracellular matrix (ECM) is the tissue architecture that provides structural and biochemical support to cells. ECM tissue composition influences the nature of the mechanical signal experienced by the cell, as individual ECM components have unique material properties. Since the nature of the mechanical signal influences which ECM components are produced by resident tissue cells, a direct relationship exists between tissue status and cell activity. In other words, cells can create an ECM that best supports their health. Disruption of the symbiotic relationship between cell function and ECM composition results in tissue breakdown, as observed in tendinosis and osteoporosis. The main receptor that cells use to organize and assemble ECM is the integrin receptor.

The manner of converting mechanical force to intracellular chemical signals that affect gene expression and tissue health is similar across tissues. The integrin receptor is central to the transduction of mechanical signals from the extracellular to the intracellular environment (Gillespie and Walker 2001). The integrin is a heterodimer (composed of two similar molecules) with α and β subunits.

Several different forms of α and β subunits exist, and the composition of an integrin determines which ECM components the integrin will bind to.

The integrin has extracellular, transmembrane, and intracellular domains. The extracellular domain binds ECM components. The intracellular domain connects to the **actin cytoskeleton** (figure 16.2). Thus, the integrin physically links the tissue (ECM) with the intracellular environment by a direct connection to the actin cytoskeleton. The actin cytoskeleton is a filament of globular actin that bridges the gap between the integrin receptor and the nuclear membrane. The cytoskeleton organizes signaling pathways and directly links the cell and nuclear membranes, providing a direct line for force transduction. Through this structure, mechanical signals are transmitted to the cell nucleus and affect gene transcription, protein production, and the remodeling of tissue. The integrin is an essential interface for cellular attachment to tissue, which is crucial for cell survival.

The integrin heterodimer is composed of one α and one β subunit that form an extracellular and an intracellular domain. Extracellularly, the combination of different α–β pairings of integrin subunits dictates the binding affinity for various ECM components. Type I collagen is a major structural ECM ligand for integrin binding, along with fibronectin, vitronectin, laminin, and tenascin. ECM components bind to their preferential integrin isomers. For example, α5β1 and αvβ3 integrins bind fibronectin, whereas α6β1 binds laminin (Wang and Thampatty 2006).

EXTRACELLULAR MATRIX COMPOSITION AND FUNCTION

The ECM is the noncellular component of connective tissue (Kjaer 2004). The ECM comprises fibrous proteins and polysaccharides in the space between cells (the interstitial space), along with basement membranes. The basement membrane is a sheet of tissue that separates various structures (such as skin, respiratory and gastrointestinal tracts, body

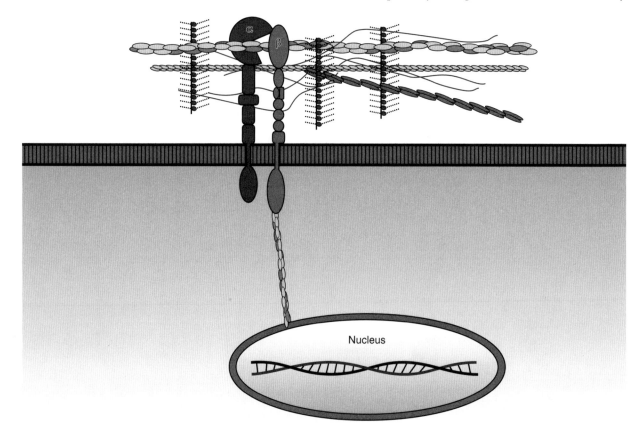

Figure 16.2   The integrin transmembrane receptor binds with tissue components in the extracellular matrix (ECM), traverses the cell membrane and connects intracellularly with the actin cytoskeleton (CSK).

cavities, blood and lymph vessels) from underlying connective tissue.

Connective tissue woven throughout our bodies provides structural support and important biochemicals essential for cell livelihood. The components of connective tissue are fibers, ground substance (proteoglycan, glycosaminoglycan, and water) and cells that function to support, separate, and connect various types of tissues and organs in the body.

Cells are embedded in and attach to this elaborate network of fibrous proteins and polysaccharides, which provides some protection from damaging stresses. In fact, the majority of tissue cells must remain attached to ECM components for survival, and disruption of tissue resulting from injury can lead to cell death. The ECM has other diverse functions such as the regulation of cellular metabolism, proliferation, development, differentiation, and survival. The ECM of the musculoskeletal system is produced locally within the tissue by fibroblastic cell types (tenocytes, osteoblasts, chondroblasts).

The two primary components of the ECM are fibrillary proteins and polysaccharide complexes (see figure 16.3). The fibrillary components include collagen (predominantly), elastin, laminin, and fibronectin. These components of the ECM add strength and resilience to tissue and provide cellular adhesion sites for integrins and other cellular adhesion molecules. Collagen type I is abundant in tendon and bone, forms strong fibers, and is produced and remodeled by fibroblastic cells (Khun 1969). Collagen type III or "reparative collagen" is produced in greater amounts at times of injury or with chronic degenerative conditions such as tendinosis. Collagen III forms a weblike structure that is useful for stabilizing wounds and damaged tissue and provides abundant attachment sites for reparative cells. Collagen III is not nearly as strong as collagen I. Collagen IV is found in basement

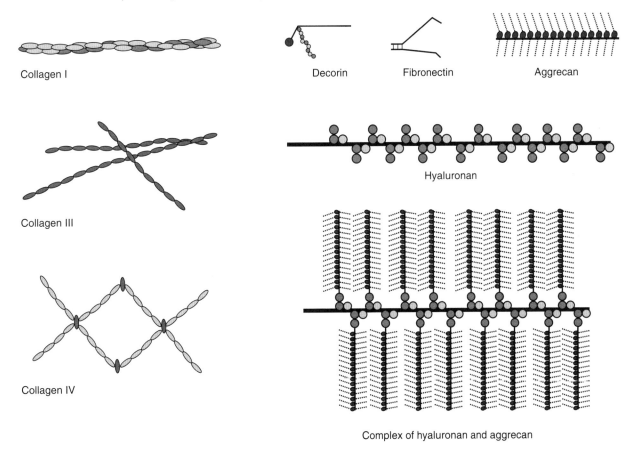

Collagen I

Decorin

Fibronectin

Aggrecan

Collagen III

Hyaluronan

Collagen IV

Complex of hyaluronan and aggrecan

Figure 16.3 The shapes and relative sizes of some of the ECM molecules. Collagens: Type I provides tensile strength; collagen III provides stabilization of wounds and abundant cell attachment sites; collagen IV provides structural support for basement membranes. Proteoglycans: Decorin is abundant in tendon, and aggrecan is abundant in cartilage and forms large complexes when multiple molecules bind hyaluronan, a glycosaminoglycan. Insoluble fibronectin is secreted abundantly in wounds, binds directly to many types of cells, and regulates phagocytosis.

membranes and has a meshlike structure to withstand multidirectional stresses, which is needed for its function in lining vessels and separating body compartments. Fibrillary proteins are interwoven in the hydrogel of polysaccharides, which is comprised of proteoglycan (PG) and glycosaminoglycan (GAG) bound to water (table 16.1).

GAGs are large carbohydrate molecules often attached to ECM proteins to form proteoglycans. Proteoglycans have several essential functions. PGs contribute to the tensile strength of tissue; attract water to keep tissues and cells hydrated; allow diffusion of nutrients, metabolites, and cytokines to support cellular activity; and regulate a variety of cellular functions such as growth, development, and repair.

Proteoglycans play a crucial role during acute repair, as they are produced in abundance and act as a reservoir for chemoattractants. Chemoattraction, the stimulus for attracting cleaning and reparative cells, is discussed in detail in chapter 4. Proteoglycans also protect newly secreted proteins from degradation and help in the aggregation and orientation of collagen as it is secreted from the fibroblast, thereby assisting with the formation of new tissue post-injury. In injured or degenerative tissue, proteoglycans are produced in abundance.

Proteoglycans can also function as a cell membrane coreceptor (a molecule that aids receptor function), spanning the cell membrane and connecting intracellularly with the actin cytoskeleton. An example of transmembrane proteoglycans is the syndecans that are located at focal adhesions and affect integrin function.

Hyaluronan, also called hyaluronic acid, is a massive GAG molecule and a chief component of the ECM. Hyaluronan can bind many proteoglycans and water, forming a large, gelatinous network of force-resistant material. Articular cartilage consists of abundant hyaluronan bound to multiple aggrecan molecules in which collagen type II is dispersed to resist force from multiple vectors.

INTEGRIN ACTIVATION AND FOCAL ADHESION FORMATION

As previously discussed, the integrin receptor is responsible for transmitting mechanical signals from the ECM into the cell. The integrin's direct attachment to the cytoskeleton (CSK), and therefore the nucleus, results in changes in gene expression when activated. The cytoskeleton of the cell is essential for survival and is involved in the regulation of most cellular activities. Similar to any receptor, the integrin must be activated in order to exert its effects.

Integrins on the cell membrane that are not bound to ECM are in an inactive form. The extracellular domain of the integrin is in a "bent" conformation that prohibits ECM binding. Integrins in an inactive form allow the cell to move through vasculature or tissues. The inactive conformation

Table 16.1 Common Forms of Proteoglycans

Proteoglycan	Approximate molecular weight of core protein	Type of GAG chains	Number of GAG chains	Location	Functions
Aggrecan	210 kD	Chondroitin sulfate + keratin sulfate	~130	Cartilage	Mechanical support; forms large aggregates with hyaluronan
Betaglycan	36 kD	Chrondroitin sulfate/ dermatan sulfate	1	Cell surface and matrix	Binds TGF-β
Decorin	40 kD	Chondroitin sulfate/ dermatan sulfate	1	Widespread in connective tissues	Binds type I collagen fibrils and TGF-β
Perlecan	60 kD	Heparin sulfate	2–15	Basal laminae	Structural and filtering function in basal lamina
Syndecan-1	32 kD	Chondroitin sulfate + heparin sulfate	1–3	Epithelial cell surface	Cell adhesion; binds FGF and other growth factors

of the integrin is maintained by extracellular and intracellular receptor stabilizing molecules that are removed during activation, allowing the integrin to assume an active ECM binding conformation (figure 16.4).

The integrin is unique in that signaling occurs bidirectionally. Most receptor information flow is from the outside in (extracellular action elicits intracellular response); however, the integrin also transmits intracellular signals that affect extracellular change. Integrins can be activated outside-in when bound to ECM in response to tissue stress, and inside-out due to cross-activation from neighboring cytokine receptor signaling cascades (figure 16.5). Specific cytokine activation

of nearby receptors and the resulting intracellular signal can activate the integrin. Inside-out activation promotes ECM binding and mechanotransduction.

The result of integrin activation is **focal adhesion complex** (FAC) formation. Activation increases the binding affinity of integrins for specific ECM molecules, but for a strong focal adhesion, hundreds or thousands of integrins cluster and bind ECM. Focal adhesion strength is therefore derived from the avidity of integrin attachments.

The FAC anchors the integrin intracellularly to the CSK. The FAC consists of several proteins and adaptor molecules that sequentially combine upon integrin activation. Focal adhesion proteins

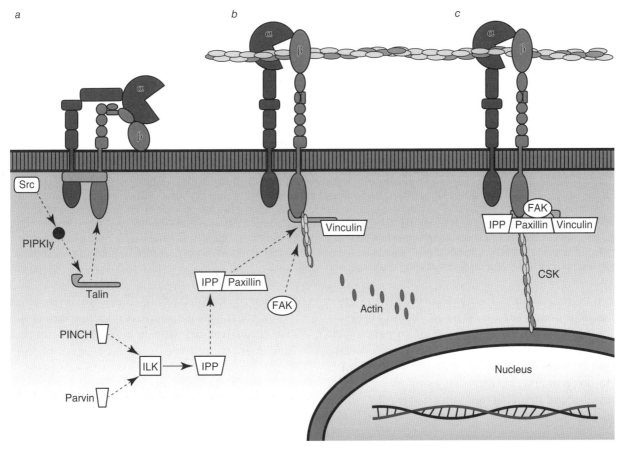

Figure 16.4 Inside-out activation of integrins begins as a result of cytokine receptor activation of Src (Zhang et al. 2002). Src (pronounced "sarc") is a tyrosine kinase located just inside the cell membrane. Tyrosine kinases relay messages by adding phosphate groups to tyrosine amino acids within proteins. (a) Phosphatidylinositol phosphate kinase type-I γ (PIP1Kγ) is an enzyme activated by Src to recruit the cytoskeletal protein talin to bind to the cytoplasmic β-subunit of the integrin. Binding of the cytoskeletal protein talin separates the intracellular domains, and this "primes" the integrin, which allows binding of ECM (b) along with intracellular recruitment of several proteins that comprise the FAC (c). Proteins comprising the FAC are recruited sequentially (b). The IPP complex is composed of the proteins integrin-linked kinase (ILK), parvin, and PINCH, which bind in the cytoplasm and are recruited to the FAC through interaction with the protein paxillin. ILK binds to the cytoplasmic tail of the integrin, connecting the IPP complex (Hannigan et al. 1996). Along with vinculin and focal adhesion kinase, the IPP complex creates a mature FAC, binding at multiple sites to the actin cytoskeleton and resulting in a resilient complex capable of force transmission (c).

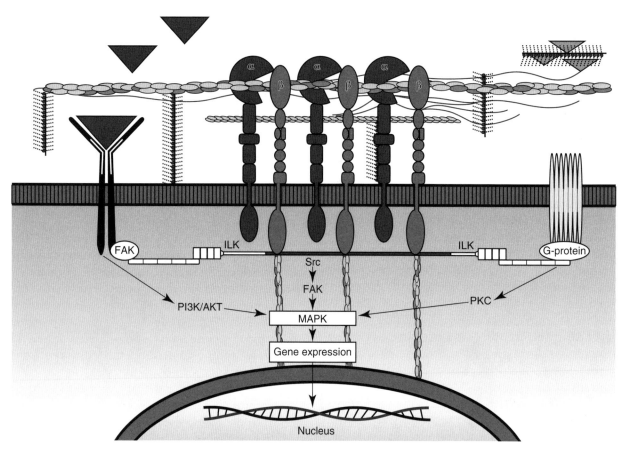

Figure 16.5 The integrin-linked kinase (ILK) can connect intracellular domains of these various receptors, providing a mechanism for coactivation and leading to dramatic cellular responses. For example, focal adhesion kinase (FAK), while associated with ILK, can activate the IGF-I receptor intracellularly. Multiple prominent cell signaling pathways interact with integrin signaling: phosphoinositide 3-kinase (PI3K)–AKT cascades, protein kinase C (PKC), and the mitogen-activated protein kinase (MAPK) cascade, ultimately leading to regulation of essential cell activities and gene expression of ECM molecules, remodeling enzymes, and cytokines.

can be divided into four categories: (1) integrin-bound proteins, such as talin and filamin, that bind directly to actin; (2) integrin-bound proteins, such as FAK, ILK, and paxillin, that indirectly associate and regulate actin; (3) actin-bound proteins with no integrin attachment, such as vinculin; and (4) adaptor and signaling molecules that regulate those just mentioned.

Integrin Clustering and Associated Receptors

There is considerable cross talk between cell receptors. Integrins cluster with various other membrane receptors, including receptor tyrosine kinases (RTKs), G-proteins, syndecan, and CD44 receptor proteins in response to stress activation. The **integrin-linked kinase** (ILK) communicates with and can activate these receptors intracellularly, in the

absence of ligand binding (figure 16.5). In other words, the ILK protein activity resulting from integrin activation can turn on a variety of receptors from inside the cell, even when they have not bound to their ligand, which is the classic mechanism of receptor activation (Legate et al. 2006). In fact, cell membrane stresses proximate to many cytokine receptors can also lead to their activation in the absence of ligand binding (Wang 2006; White and Frangos 2007).

Syndecan and the coreceptor molecule CD44 strengthen the FAC. Integrin activation leads to the mobilization of syndecan to the focal adhesion site. Syndecan is a family of similar transmembrane proteoglycans that act as coreceptors for fibronectin, growth factors, and cytokines. CD44 is a receptor for the glycosaminoglycan hyaluronan, and it has an intracellular binding site for actin, adding further FAC stabilization.

Movement of FACs in response to cell membrane stress activates nearby mechanically sensitive ion channels (calcium, sodium, potassium). Ion channel activity is intimately involved in cellular response to mechanical stress. For example, cell membrane stretch-induced influx of calcium activates nuclear transcription factor CREB, resulting in cytoskeletal contractility and organization (Wang et al. 2007; Matthews et al. 2006). Upon entering the cell, calcium ions feed back and regulate integrin binding to the cytoskeleton, thereby further increasing the mechanical responsiveness of the cell.

The FAC of proteins and coreceptors allows for mechanotransduction through the cell membrane and ultimately to the genetic material residing within. This is accomplished through direct force transmission from the FAC through the cytoskeleton to its attachment on the nuclear membrane. In addition to providing a physical link to the nucleus, the CSK associates with and organizes signaling cascades, resulting in cell and tissue effects. The cytoskeleton is a crucial component of the mechanotransduction network.

The CSK is a collection of fibers and membrane-enclosed organelles in the cytoplasm. The CSK has three distinct roles: (1) to maintain cell shape and structural support, (2) to allow for cell movement as a result of rapid reorganization of cytoskeletal shape, and (3) to provide tracts for intracellular signaling pathways. Mechanotransduction is accomplished through perturbation of cell shape and the transmission of that signal by the cytoskeleton.

Mechanical signaling, integrin activation, and focal adhesion formation lead to the rapid reorganization of the actin cytoskeleton. The cytoskeleton of the cell is essential for survival, and it is involved in the regulation of most cellular activities. A change in cell shape alters cell function (Ingber 1997). In tissue, extracellular and intracellular components work symbiotically. The intracellular cytoskeleton helps organize matrix components, and stimuli received through the matrix affect intracellular activity. The CSK is the intracellular force transducer.

The CSK provides cell structure and can reorganize rapidly to allow motility and phagocytosis in leukocytes. The CSK also provides pathways for intracellular secondary messengers and sig-

naling cascades to and from the nucleus. Signaling enzymes organize around the actin CSK, facilitating phosphorylation cascades (Ingber 1997).

Cell-to-Cell Mechanotransduction

If our discussion of mechanotransduction stopped here, we would have only examined the response of a single cell. For a response to be tissue wide, mechanical signals must be propagated throughout the cellular network within the ECM. This is achieved through cellular interconnectivity.

The cells of a tissue form an interconnected network through which chemical and mechanical signals are transduced through cell junctions. **Gap junctions** are intercellular membrane channels that facilitate the passage of ions and small molecules from the cytosol of adjacent cells (figure 16.6). The principal proteins comprising gap junctions are the connexins. Several connexins form a connexon, and connexons from neighboring cells form a gap junction.

Our physical link to the environment results in extraordinarily complex tissue and cellular interactions. Appreciating the impact mechanical signaling has on tissues and contextualizing its use will continue to advance physical medicine. Perhaps the most obvious musculoskeletal tissue susceptible to mechanical regulation is skeletal muscle. Skeletal muscle also imposes force on the musculoskeletal system.

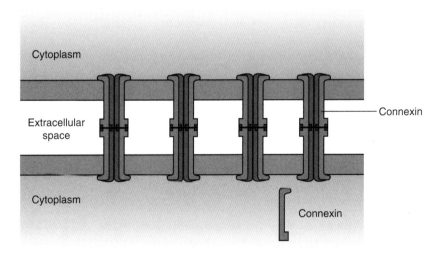

Figure 16.6 Gap junctions connect adjacent cells and allow signals to spread throughout a network of cells.

MAPK Signaling Cascade

The mitogen-activated protein kinase (MAPK) cascade is a prominent signaling junction downstream of multiple stimuli. Its name implies cytokine-activated signaling mechanisms; however, the MAPK cascade is accessed from multiple upstream signals that originate from a variety of stimuli, including mechanical force. In a sequence of phosphorylation events, MAP3K (a.k.a. RAF) activates MAP2K (a.k.a. MEK), which activates MAPK. MAPK is the terminal kinase that, once activated, will travel to the nucleus to initiate translation. MAPKs activate downstream transcription factors such as AP-1, Egr-1, and NF-κB, leading to a multitude of cellular regulatory events that preside over tissue production, cell differentiation, and survival.

MECHANOBIOLOGY IN MUSCLE

Muscle generates force through the stimulation and contraction of muscle cells. The connective tissue architecture of muscle (figure 16.7) facilitates load transmission across the tissue and to the tendon. Inherent and imposed forces on muscle are experienced by the muscle cells (myoblasts and progenitors) as well as fibroblasts residing in muscle connective tissue.

Protein synthesis is essential for tissue health and adaptation. Muscle's ability to adapt to functional demand is well documented, and adaptation is a direct result of protein synthesis. Muscle releases a variety of factors in response to activity, both locally and into systemic circulation. Early research demonstrated the synthesis and release of insulin-like growth factor-I in response to mechanical stimuli and damage. IGF-I in muscle is a potent hormone that regulates protein synthesis and anabolism. The AKT-mTOR pathway is a prominent anabolic signaling cascade activated by the IGF-I receptor.

ILK activity resulting from integrin activation can phosphorylate the IGF-I receptor (IGFR) and activate the AKT-mTOR pathway. Therefore there is considerable synergy between the IGF system and integrin-mediated signal transduction (see figure 16.5). Just as integrin activation stimulates the

IGFR, activation of the IGFR is a likely candidate for the coactivation of integrin receptors and FAC formation. The result is a robust anabolic response resulting in muscle development and repair.

Integrins in muscle are predominantly located at the myotendinous junction, connecting the myofiber with the basal lamina and surrounding endomysium. FAC's formation associated with integrin activation occurs predominantly in this location. Overstretch injury often occurs at the myotendinous junction and involves mechanical disruption of FAC-integrin attachment to the ECM. Immobilization-induced atrophy is associated with decreased phosphorylation of focal adhesion kinase in the absence of increased remodeling enzyme synthesis, further evidence of the predominant regulatory nature of mechanical signals.

Passive stretch of skeletal myotubes in culture has many of the growth-promoting characteristics of insulin stimulation of muscle growth. Stretch activation of sarcolemmal calcium and sodium channels results in mechanotransduction. Calcium influx results in a cascade of events responsible for the activation of quiescent **muscle satellite cells**, necessary for repair and adaptation (Tidball 2005).

Satellite cells are progenitor (immature) cells that have the capacity to differentiate into mature skeletal muscle cells. Muscle satellite cells reside in the basal lamina of skeletal muscle. The basal lamina exists between the muscle cell membrane and the endomysium (see figure 16.7) and contains

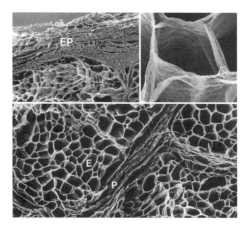

Figure 16.7 Intramuscular connective tissue. Composed of endomysium (E), perimysium (P), and epimysium (EP), the connective tissue architecture is crucial for several functions, including force transmission, cellular attachment, and muscle satellite cell residence.

Reprinted, by permission, from M. Kjaer, 2004, "Role of extracellular matrix in adaptation of tendon and skeletal muscle to mechanical loading," *Physiological Review* 84(2): 649-98.

the muscle progenitor cells. Muscle stretch, exercise, and damage contribute to the activation of satellite cells, which migrate to areas of microdamage, divide, differentiate, and fuse with the adjacent myofiber, providing additional myonuclei for protein synthesis, hypertrophy, and repair (Tidball 2005).

Mechanotransduction contributes to the regulatory control of skeletal muscle at every level. Muscle protein synthesis, healing and repair of muscle injury, and homeostasis are all highly influenced by mechanotransduction. Muscle imposes tremendous force on tendons. It should be no surprise how crucial this stimulus is to the well-being of muscle's attachment to bone, the tendon.

MECHANOBIOLOGY IN TENDON

The success of eccentric exercise for the treatment of tendinopathy is an excellent example of mechanotransduction at work. The tendon fibroblast (tenocyte) is the predominant cell found in tendon and is responsible for producing the components of the ECM and maintaining tissue homeostasis. Tendon is relatively avascular and therefore relies largely on autocrine and paracrine responses for tissue remodeling, repair, and adaptation. In addition to tenocytes, progenitor cells exist in tendon, and they are extremely mechanosensitive. Inappropriate mechanical load pushes these progenitors toward alternate phenotypes (chondrocytes, adipocytes, osteocytes), which results in the pathologic changes characteristic of tendinosis. Tendinosis is a common histologic finding in overuse tendon injuries that is characterized by noninflammatory degenerative changes of the ECM and aberrant cellular responses.

Tendon attaches muscle to bone, transmitting forces to the skeleton and resulting in joint stabilization and movement. As a result, tendons are subjected to high mechanical loads that predispose them to injury. Tendon's reaction to overuse injury has been described as a failed healing response (Maffulli, Sharma, and Luscombe 2004) due to the ineffective and insufficient inflammatory response generated after injury.

Tendon pathology may be classified as either tendonitis: inflammation, pain, and swelling of the peritenon; tendinosis: degeneration of the ECM and absence of inflammation upon histologic examination; or tendinopathy. Tendinopathy is the contemporary clinical term for tendon overuse injuries, as it does not imply an active inflammatory process, which is often the case.

While the etiologic factors of tendinopathy are not fully understood, a failure in the mechanobiologic response of the tenocyte has been implicated. Tendon structure, composition, and mechanical properties are modified in response to altered mechanical loading conditions. Disruption in the mechanobiologic response of the tenocyte creates a vicious cycle of suboptimal ECM production, in turn leading to further changes in mechanical signals transmitted to the tenocyte and propagating degenerative tissue production throughout the tendon (figure 16.8). Many hypothesize that mechanical overload initiates a degenerative signaling cascade that leads to tendinopathy, while some believe tendinopathy is a result of focal disruption of ECM and accompanying mechanobiologic understimulation of locally adherent tenocytes and progenitor cells.

Signaling cascades leading to tendinosis probably result from understimulation of FACs and downstream MAPK-mediated events. The activation of stress-activated protein kinase (SAPK), a member of the MAPK family, is associated with matrix-degrading enzyme production. As mentioned, load affects progenitor cell survival and differentiation. Tendon progenitor cells exposed to 4% strain assume tenocyte function and express collagen type I. However, loads of 8% resulted in the expression of markers for bone, fat, and cartilage differentiation.

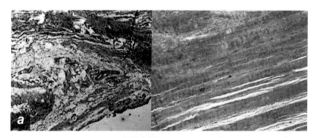
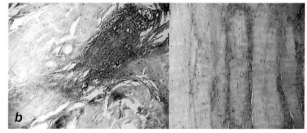

Figure 16.8   Pathologic changes in tendinopathy. *(a)* Collagen organization: H&E. *(b)* Increased proteoglycan.

Reprinted, by permission, from M. Joseph et al., 2009, "Histological and molecular analysis of the biceps tendon long head post-tenotomy," *The Journal of Orthopedic Research* 27:1379-1385.

The presence of these cells and their functional products is destructive to tendon ECM and health (Wang et al. 2007).

An alternative paradigm for the pathophysiology of tendinopathy is emerging and involves tenocyte-produced neuropeptides. Chemical messengers thought to be confined to neurons are produced in abundance in tendinopathic tissue. Substance P and its receptor (neurokinin-1 receptor [NK-1 R]), glutamate (Scott, Alfredson, and Forsgren 2008), acetylcholine (ACTH), and catecholamines are produced by local tendon fibroblasts. Tenocytes produce these neurochemicals in response to mechanical load. Substance P increases cellular proliferation in culture, which corresponds with observations of hypercellularity in early tendinosis. Pain in tendinopathic tissue has been traced to neurovascular ingrowth containing substance P positive nerve fibers, and the ablation of these fibers often results in relief. The NK-1 R is a G-protein coupled receptor that is responsive to mechanical signals. There is likely cross talk between integrin-linked kinase production resulting from integrin stimulation and cross-activation of the G-protein via ILK activation (see figure 16.5). Substance P signals through the MAPK cascade and results in gene expression.

Tendon cell networks communicate throughout the tissue via cytoplasmic extensions and cell junction zones. A signal that is sent in one area propagates through these channels, effecting a tissue-wide response. Intercellular connectivity is achieved through gap junctions, where connexins are the principal protein. In healthy tendon, tenocytes are arranged longitudinally between collagen fibers. Connexins 32 and 34 form communications between longitudinally arranged tenocytes, whereas connexin 43 links cells in all directions (Ragsdale, Phelps, and Luby-Phelps 1997).

MECHANOBIOLOGY IN ARTICULAR CARTILAGE

Articular cartilage is the major load-bearing tissue in synovial joints. Cartilage is unique in that it is avascular, aneural, alymphatic, and sparsely populated with cells. The cartilage cell (chondrocyte) is responsible for the remodeling of cartilage ECM, and it does so in response to mechanical force. Cartilage in relatively unloaded areas such as the medial patellar facet is softer and less resilient. Articular cartilage responds favorably to pulsatile doses of load, while static loading results in up-regulation of a host of inflammatory cytokines, matrix-degrading enzymes, and degeneration.

Chondrocytes are extremely responsive to compressive loads, as their location and function would indicate. A pericellular matrix composed of collagen VI and proteoglycan surrounds the chondrocyte and is an independent unit of force transduction. The pericellular matrix is analogous to the basal lamina in skeletal muscle, bridging the gap between cell membrane and ECM.

Membrane stretch–activated ion channels exist, are proximate to integrins, and likely have overlapping downstream signaling cascades. Stimulation of the integrin $\alpha_5\beta_1$ pathway results in the production of aggrecan, the predominant proteoglycan in cartilage, along with the down-regulation of MMP3, the predominant degrading enzyme of PG. Higher levels of aggrecan and collagen II production are associated with dynamic compressive force, whereas static forces result in MMP production and ECM destruction. Chondrocytes from arthritic cartilage are unresponsive to mechanical stimulation, indicating cellular dysfunction and mechanoinsensitivity in osteoarthritis (Raizman 2010).

Inappropriate mechanical loading is the primary risk factor for the development of osteoarthritis (OA) (figure 16.9). OA is characterized by a loss of tissue homeostasis and the prevalence of catabolism. Molecular components of mechanotransduction in chondrocytes consist of integrin activation and downstream MAPK signaling, as well as stress-activated calcium channel signaling. The $\alpha_5\beta_1$ integrin binds pericellular matrix fibronectin and associates with calcium channels in the surrounding cell membrane. In response to mechanical stimuli, integrin and calcium signaling pathways converge on MAPK cascade, where Ca^{2+} regulation of integrin activity through Src occurs (Raizman et al. 2010).

The Cbp/p300-interacting transactivator 2 (CITED2) is a transcription regulator that is thought to balance catabolic and anticatabolic cascades and is thus centrally implicated in the pathogenesis of OA (Leong et al. 2011). CITED2 binds with and modulates a host of transcription factors. The ability to activate anabolic pathways and to inhibit inflammatory and catabolic pathways in response to mechanical signals suggests a central role in mechanical regulation. CITED2 is downstream of MAPK. Moderate-intensity intermittent loads activate CITED2, whereas high-intensity loads do not

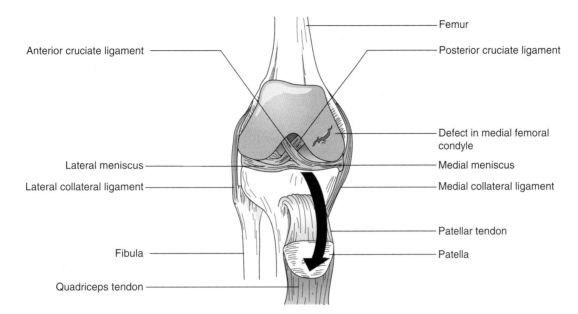

Figure 16.9 Damaged articular cartilage. Large defect in the medial femoral condyle.

(Leong et al. 2011). Increased CITED2 expression correlates with the production of collagen II, maintenance of ECM, and suppression of MMPs. Integrin and associated receptors, downstream MAPK, and CITED2 represent a loading-specific pathway that has direct effects on tissue. Thus, loading of cartilage is essential to tissue health while overload leads to degeneration and OA. Exercise can play an important role in the treatment of OA, but excessive loading may accelerate the disease process.

In summary, the chondrocyte is dependent upon mechanical signals for survival. The aneural, avascular nature of articular cartilage accounts for its susceptibility to damage. Enhanced maintenance and repair of articular cartilage is possible through mechanobiologic manipulation. Chondrocyte preference for dynamic, pulsatile delivery of force will continue to be explored both in exercise prescription and modality delivery.

MECHANOBIOLOGY IN BONE

Metabolic demands on the skeleton are managed largely through calciotropic hormones, but the ability of the skeleton to adapt to its loading environment is essential for bone health. Wolff's law first proposed skeletal change in response to functional demands. We now understand that it is the cells of the skeleton—the osteoblasts, osteocytes, and osteoclasts—that remodel bone in response to stress. An example of bone's sensitivity to mechanical demand

is demonstrated in cortical bone of the dominant arm in elite tennis players, which can be up to 35% thicker than the cortical bone of the non-dominant arm Rapid bone loss during periods of immobility and in microgravity exemplifies the homeostatic necessity of mechanotransduction.

Bone is certainly not as deformable as connective tissue, at least elastically. Bone can experience up to 0.3% strain, much less than ligament or tendon (5%–20%). Bone experiences a wide variety of mechanical stimuli that produce slight deformation in the bone tissue, pressure in the intramedullary cavity and within the cortices, transient pressure waves, and fluid shear forces through the canaliculi.

Osteoblasts at the surface of bone respond to deformation of the cell membrane from strain experienced on the surface of the bone from imposed forces. Osteocytes located deeper in the bone tissue respond to shear stress of fluid flow through the canaliculi (figure 16.10). An externally applied load forces fluid out of regions of high compressive strains. This fluid returns when the load is removed. This results in bone cell exposure to an oscillating fluid flow. The osteocyte population, through its interconnectedness via gap junctions, comprises a three-dimensional sensing system in which amplification of mechanical signals propagates throughout the tissue.

As in tendon, integrins are important conductors of mechanical signals in bone cells (Salter, Robb, and Wright 1997). In bone, the β subunit of the integrin extracellular domain mediates binding

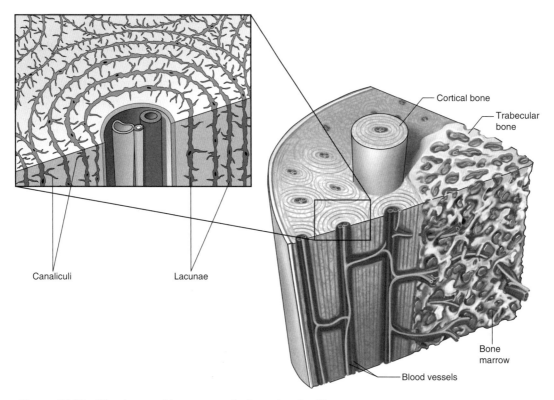

Figure 16.10   Structure and lacuna canalicular network of bone.

to matrix components. Prominent matrix ligands for integrin in bone include collagen I and III and fibronectin. The formation of FAC in response to integrin activation is critical to cell adhesion, survival, and production. Mechanical signals activate the MAPK cascade, leading to down-regulation of RANK ligand (RANKL expression and the formation of osteoclasts.

Strain, shear, and pressure result in the mobilization of intracellular calcium. This rapid increase in intracellular calcium concentration appears to occur due to phospholipase-C activity and IP3 signaling, which results in the release of calcium from intracellular stores (calcium-mediated calcium release).

SUMMARY

Musculoskeletal cells are exposed to forces transmitted through tissue. Mechanotransduction pathways modulate diverse cellular functions. Physiologic effects result from intracellular signaling of membrane receptors and ion channels. The integrin receptor, bound to the tissue and stimulated by stress, can coactivate cytokine receptors and ion channels, resulting in a coordinated cell response. The musculoskeletal system provides a link to the physical environment. The encompassing nature of mechanical signaling likely represents the primary means by which adaptation to force exposure occurs. For clinicians this is exciting, as much of what we do involves modulating force through exercise and physical interventions. The obvious hurdle in fully accessing this tool is the difficulty of quantifying in vivo human forces, both those that result in injury and those produced by specific mechanical interventions. Future research and technology will be essential for identifying optimal mechanical interventions and their specific prescription. This chapter outlines the biology underpinning mechanical intervention. Harnessing the power of mechanotransduction is our most powerful tool for affecting musculoskeletal health and adaptation.

1. *Understand the basic principles of mechanobiology and their implications for the clinician.*

The forces or stresses imposed on our tissues through exercise, manual therapy, and certain modalities result in cell signals that alter gene expression to maintain musculoskeletal tissue health. Mechanobiology examines the interactions and effects of mechanical stimuli such as tissue stress on cells and tissues. Mechanotransduction is the conversion of physical signals to chemical responses that produce changes in gene expression that regulate cell function and tissue status. Appropriate load throughout the day and during training promotes tissue homeostasis and desired adaptations. Inappropriate load over time or with trauma results in tissue breakdown and injury. Adjustments in exercise and physical intervention result in tissue responses; therefore the clinician is positioned to profoundly affect musculoskeletal health. An understanding of mechanobiology provides important context for treatment rationale and exercise prescription, essential for optimal outcomes. Therapeutic exercise and interventions are much more than a means of restoring motion, strength, and function; they are critical for homeostasis, adaptation, and optimal repair of damaged musculoskeletal tissues.

2. *Describe the mechanism of mechanotransduction, in which mechanical force transforms to chemical signals, mediating cell and tissue responses.*

The main receptor that cells use to organize and assemble surrounding tissue is the integrin. The integrin provides a direct mechanical link from the tissue to the nucleus of the cell. The extracellular domain of the integrin receptor binds extracellular matrix components. The intracellular domain attaches to the cell's cytoskeleton, which directly transmits force and organizes signal pathways that alter gene expression. Integrin signaling is essential for cell survival and for the production of tissue components and regulatory cytokines. Considerable cross talk between integrins and a host of cytokine receptors produces unified cellular responses. Integrins cluster with various membrane receptors, including RTKs and G-proteins. Cytokine receptor activation can lead to integrin activation, which is called inside-out activation. Reciprocally, the integrin receptor (through integrin-linked kinase [ILK]) can activate a host of cytokine receptors. The cellular response to tissue stress via receptor activation results in ECM synthesis and secretion, tissue remodeling, and the formation of new tissue during healing and adaptation. Conversely, the extracellular matrix composition affects mechanical signaling in that individual ECM components possess unique material properties that directly influence the stress experienced by the cell.

3. *Describe key components of connective tissue and how they adapt.*

The ECM comprises fibrous proteins and polysaccharides in the space between cells (interstitial space), along with basement membranes. Connective tissue woven throughout our bodies provides structural support and important biochemicals essential for cell livelihood. The components of connective tissue are fibers, ground substance (proteoglycan, glycosaminoglycan, and water) and cells functioning to support, separate, and connect various types of tissues and organs in the body. Cells are embedded in and attach to this elaborate network of fibrous proteins and polysaccharides, which provides some protection from damaging stresses. In fact, most tissue cells must remain attached to ECM components for survival, and disruption of tissue resulting from injury can lead to cell death.

Collagen and proteoglycan are the predominant constituents of ECM, each with various subtypes related to function. Hyaluronan is a giant, nonprotein-bound glycan (glycosaminoglycan) that binds neighboring GAGs, forming a network of matrix.

During the process of healing from an injury, cells make abundant amounts of proteoglycan. Proteoglycan binds growth factors and chemotactic cytokines, creating a reservoir of essential molecules at the site of the injury. Overuse injuries such as tendinopathy can be characterized by both the abundance and size of proteoglycans produced. Collagen provides the structural integrity for connective tissue and blood vessels. Parallel fibril-forming collagen type I is found in tendon and bone, whereas network-forming collagen type IV is found in the connective tissue layer of blood vessels and basal lamina. In the healing process, type III collagen synthesis increases. Type III collagen, with its multiple binding sites, provides structure for cell attachment and wound organization early on in healing. Tenocytes from tendinopathic tendon tissues produce collagen III in culture, demonstrating a shift in cell function and deleterious matrix alterations.

4. *Understand tissue-specific mechanobiology.*

The success of eccentric exercise for the treatment of tendinopathy is an excellent example of mechanotransduction at work. ECM disruption may occur traumatically at first through overuse or due to systemic factors such as insulin insensitivity. Altered mechanical signaling due to the disruption of ECM leads to degenerative tendinosis. Due to the intimate relationship between ECM composition and the transmission of stress to the integrin, eccentric exercise and other physical interventions can positively affect tissue repair through the delivery of appropriate stress.

Bone remodeling occurs through a combination of endocrine and mechanical factors. Integrins in the canaliculi of the osteon are subject to fluid stress and physical strain, leading to activation and signaling for remodeling. Conditions such as osteoporosis, which relates to endocrine function, directly influence integrin signaling through the blunting of inside-out integrin activation from hormone receptors.

Articular cartilage has restricted endocrine access due to its avascular nature. Mechanical signals are important for tissue homeostasis. Osteoarthritis exemplifies the deleterious effects of a disruption of tissue-to-cell communication.

Skeletal muscle relies heavily on mechanical signaling for healing and adaptation. Most integrins in skeletal muscle are located at the myotendinous junction. Due to muscle's vascular nature, integrin activation and cooperation with anabolic endocrine signals results in hypertrophy and satellite cell activation, essential for both healing and adaptation.

chapter 17

Applications of Exercise and Manual Therapy to Promote Repair

OBJECTIVES

After reading this chapter, you will be able to

1 discuss the application of mechanobiology (chapter 16) to the treatment of tendinopathy, muscle strain, and fracture;

2 describe how tendon, muscle, and bone respond to stress on the tissues; and

3 discuss how the pain response can assist in guiding exercise progression.

A freshman collegiate volleyball player complains of tenderness well localized to the mid-portion of the patellar tendon prior to the beginning of preseason practices. Quadriceps contraction reproduces symptoms at this site. Diagnostic ultrasound performed during consultation with the team physician reveals a small hypoechoic lesion and some fiber disorganization. A program of resisted incline squats as described by Biernat et al. (2014) is instituted, and the player is permitted to continue training and participation as tolerated with regular reevaluation by the sports medicine staff. Substantial improvement is noted after 3 weeks, and complete resolution is confirmed at 16 weeks despite increasing volleyball activities and game competition. How has the sports medicine team used mechanical forces to encourage tissue repair and guide levels of activity to maximize participation in sport?

The connections between mechanical stimuli and cell activity are complex, but the evolution of mechanobiology provides the clinician with new uses for an old tool, namely exercise. Historically, therapeutic exercise, including stretching and resistance training, has been recommended to restore motion and increase the force developed by muscles to complete specific tasks. These treatment goals and the need for a plan of care that progresses resistance and functional exercise, and thus sets the stage for a return to demanding physical activity, remain critical to clinical care. Movement, however, generates forces that are transmitted to cells and regulate their activity. The mechanisms through which cell function is controlled are detailed in chapter 16. This chapter offers guidance on progressive mechanical loading to facilitate healing and repair.

Tendinopathy is a common condition that provides a context for the discussion of exercise as a repair modality. Tendon is relatively avascular and thus depends on mechanical signaling to maintain homeostasis and stimulate repair to a greater extent than tissue with more exposure to endocrine regulation. The treatment of damaged tendon has been recognized as a challenge for generations. The benefits of eccentric loading in the management of what was referred to as "tendinitis" were reported in the 1980s (Stanish, Rubinovich, and Curwin 1986). Since that time, eccentric loading has become recognized as the most effective treatment for tendinopathy. The

mechanisms that explain how eccentric loading, and mechanical loading of all tissues, affects tissue health and repair have only recently become better understood.

Eccentric and heavy resistance loading protocols for the Achilles, patellar, and wrist extensor tendons are reviewed and pictured in the next section. Muscle is highly vascular, but it requires mechanical loading to maintain tissue health and stimulate growth. Bone health is also highly dependent on the transmission of force. Consider the loss of bone mass associated with prolonged space flights. The absence of gravity leads to osteopenia. Conversely, heavy resistance training leads to increased bone diameter. Specific protocols that exist for the treatment of tendinopathy do not exist for the management of muscle strains or bone fractures. This chapter provides guidance in the frequency, intensity, and duration of resistance training that promotes muscle tissue repair and the resumption of high-intensity training. Like tendon and muscle, healing bone may benefit from appropriate and progressive loading. As with other tissues the repair process can be disrupted by excessive loading.

This chapter includes guidelines to help clinicians and patients choose appropriate levels of loading. Passive interventions can also deliver a mechanical stimulus. Massage, transverse friction massage, and compression garments may promote repair, and we review the use of these techniques.

EXERCISE FOR REPAIR IN TENDINOPATHY

Much of the evidence for the effectiveness of eccentric exercise programs in the treatment of Achilles and patellar tendinopathy comes from the works of Alfredson and Lorentzon (2000). Before we outline these treatment protocols it is important to recognize key features. First, the exercise programs position the body to isolate force on the affected muscle-tendon unit. The clinician needs to instruct the patient in proper technique and periodically reassess the patient's performance. The programs are progressive, with a gradually increasing load as tolerated. The eccentric exercises often cause pain at the affected tendon. The patient should understand that some pain is normal. Pain that causes aberrant movement patterns or results in greater pain following exercise signifies excessive load on the tissues. Lastly, tendon repairs and adapts slowly. Regardless of the parameters of the exercise program, 6 to 12 weeks is needed to determine if more aggressive intervention is warranted (Alfredson and Cook 2007).

The persistence and patience required is not a message that active people are always receptive to. The recovery period, however, does not mean complete restriction from participation. There are no precise guidelines as to how much patients with tendinopathy should restrict activity. The greatest concern related to being active with a painful, swollen tendon is tissue overload and tendon rupture. These events are more common in older (>age 30) patients, more common in men, and more often associated with sports that require extensive jumping and cutting, such as basketball and tennis. Pain is likely not a good indicator of the degree of risk in these sports; it is not uncommon for patients to report being asymptomatic before experiencing a rupture of the Achilles or patellar tendon.

The extent to which an athlete with tendinopathy participates requires careful examination, evaluation, and guidance from the medical team. Participation in low-risk activities such as cycling, swimming, and running may be permitted as long as the pain does not limit the quality of the motion and is not made worse with activity. The patient and the health care team must monitor progress and balance therapeutic exercise and activity in light of the rate and magnitude of improvement. Steady improvement suggests that the patient's level of activity is appropriate and may be progressed depending on individual circumstances.

Achilles Tendinopathy

Video 17.1 demonstrates eccentric loading on the Achilles tendon.

Eccentric loading of the Achilles tendon is accomplished through heel drops. Heel drops are performed unilaterally off a step or a box or with a calf raise machine if available. Heel drops are performed with the knee straight to target the gastrocnemius component, and with the knee bent to target the soleus contribution to the Achilles. The contralateral limb rather than a concentric contraction is used to return to the starting position. Frequently prescribed exercise parameters proven successful are three sets of 15 repetitions, knee straight and knee bent, twice daily (figure 17.1). Stevens and Tan (2014) suggested that completing two sessions of the exercises daily as tolerated resulted in similar improvements at 6 weeks when compared to patients who completed all 180 repetitions daily. Regardless of the protocol, the frequency of eccentric exercise for tendon rehabilitation is much different than that used for muscle; with tendon, the goal is to provide a frequent dose of mechanical stimulus to the tendon cell. External resistance as tolerated may be added by the use of a weighted backpack if a calf raise machine is not available (figure 17.2).

Along with external resistance, progressive loading is achieved through the rate of eccentric contraction. Based upon force-velocity characteristics, increases in force accompany increased speed of contraction (figure 17.3). A static hold at the bottom of the heel drop for 15 to 30 s may be beneficial, particularly when initiating a heel drop protocol. Pain or discomfort is allowed during the activity, but pain that persists after heel drops indicates a slower progression. This may be accomplished by decreasing external resistance, decreasing the speed of the exercise, or both. While three times 15 reps, knees straight and bent, twice daily has good evidence for beneficial effects, other parameters have not been explored. Patient reports and objective improvement should inform adjustments in program variables. Tendon responds much more slowly to loading than skeletal muscle, and therefore increasing the frequency of loading beyond twice daily may be indicated along with adjustments to the volume of activity.

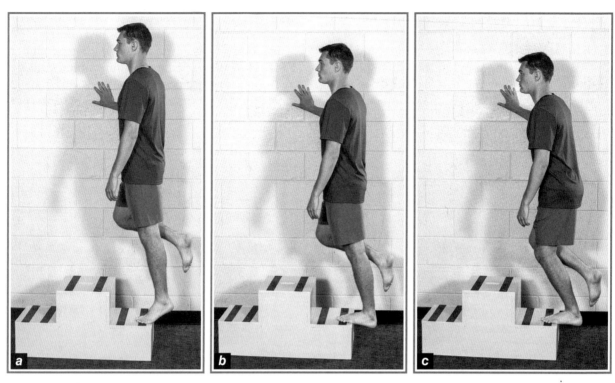

Figure 17.1 The starting position *(a)* of the heel drop. Rapid heel drops are performed with the knee straight *(b)* and bent *(c)*. The contralateral limb rather than a concentric contraction is used to return to the starting position.

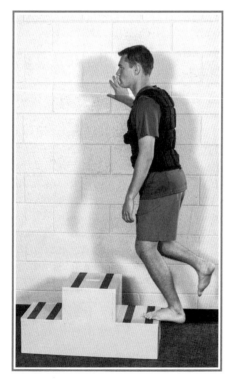

Figure 17.2 External resistance may be added with a calf raise machine or weighted backpack.

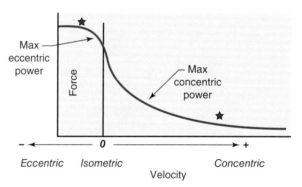

Figure 17.3 The force-velocity relationship describes the decline in force production with faster concentric velocities and the increase of force production with eccentric contractions. During eccentric contractions, while the total muscle length is increasing, the muscle fibers may in fact be contracting concentrically (shortening), with lengthening occurring primarily in the connective tissue elements of the musculotendinous complex. This provides the fundamental rationale for the response of connective tissue to eccentric exercise.

Success has also been demonstrated with an exercise program proposed by Silbernagel et al. (2001), which incorporates a warmup, stretching, and progressive loading. This program has three phases. The initial phase is similar to a warmup, designed to increase blood flow, ankle range of motion, and tissue compliance. Included are toe extension and flexion and ankle dorsi and plantar flexion; three sets of 20 s of gastrocnemius and soleus stretching, single leg balance, heel and toe walking, and concentric and eccentric heel raises, all performed three times per day. Phase 1 lasts two weeks.

Phase 2 includes all exercises in phase 1 with a progression to unilateral eccentric toe raises. Phase 2 lasts two weeks. Phase 3 from weeks 4 through 12 continues to progress the toe raise exercises and introduces a plyometric component of quick rebounding toe raises, 20 to 100 reps performed three times per day. Instructions to patients included allowing pain to reach 5 out of 10 on a visual analog scale (VAS) during and after exercise. Pain and stiffness were not allowed to increase on a daily basis. If pain and stiffness exceed these limits, patients are told to return to an earlier phase of the program.

A recent systematic review (SR) (Malliaras et al. 2013) compared loading programs and concluded greater satisfaction and return to function for eccentric than concentric exercise, greater patient satisfaction and VAS pain outcomes with the Silbernagel combined loading program when compared to concentric and eccentric calf raises and stretching, and better VAS pain and return to play outcomes with eccentric and concentric loading than with isotonic loading. The study of optimal program variables for treating Achilles tendinopathy will evolve with expanding evidence-based treatment options. The application of eccentric loading will likely remain an effective component in treating the Achilles tendon.

Patellar Tendinopathy

Video 17.2 demonstrates eccentric loading for patellar tendinopathy.

Success has been demonstrated with both eccentric decline squats and heavy slow resistance training for patellar tendinopathy (Kongsgaard et al. 2010). Parameters for decline squats are similar to those described for the Achilles: three sets of 15 repetitions, twice daily. Squats are performed on an incline board to preferentially load the quadriceps (figure 17.4a). Heavy slow resistance training mimics a more traditional strength training routine. Squats, hack squats, and leg presses are performed three times per week (figures 17.4b-17.4d). Both eccentric and concentric contractions occur over 3 s. Four sets of each exercise with increasing loads are progressed across 12 weeks. Exercise progresses as follows: week 1—15 repetition maximum (RM); weeks 2 to 3—12RM; weeks 4 to 5—10RM; weeks 6 to 8—8RM; weeks 9 to 12—6RM. Repetition maximum is described as the maximum weight that is used to complete the prescribed number of repetitions. For example, if a patient can leg press 180 lb 15 times but fails in attempting the 16th repetition, the RM is 180 lb. As patients progress, the RM will increase if the number of repetitions is held constant. Progression of the protocol leads to using greater resistance for fewer repetitions.

HSR Training Progression

- 3×/week for 12 weeks.
- Exercises: squat, leg press, and hack squat.
- 3 s concentric, 3 s eccentric.
- 4 sets of each exercise, 2 to 3 min rest period.
  - 15RM, week 1; 12RM, weeks 2 to 3;
  - 10RM, weeks 4 to 5;
  - 8RM, weeks 6 to 8;
  - 6RM, weeks 9 to 12.
- Pain during exercises OK, pain after training was not.
- Allowed to perform sporting activities if these could be performed with only light discomfort (maximal pain on VAS, score of 30).
- Control subjects were asked to maintain their normal activity levels.

The patellofemoral joint is important to consider in the treatment of patellar tendinopathy. All of the exercises described exert tremendous force on the patellofemoral joint. If the patient is a novice to squatting, irritation of the patellofemoral joint related to poor technique can easily occur. As with instruction in exercise for Achilles tendinopathy, attention to technique throughout the treatment period is warranted.

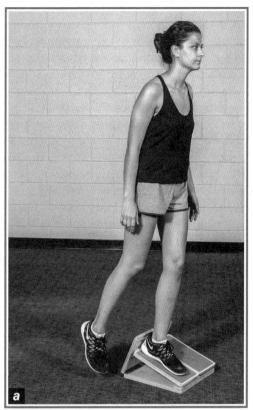

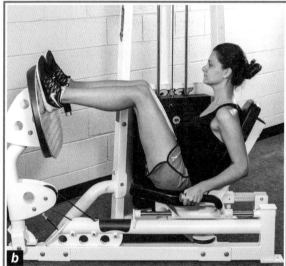

Figure 17.4 Heavy slow resistance (HSR) for patellar tendinopathy. *(a)* Eccentric decline squat, 3 × 15 2×/day. HSR: *(b)* Leg press, *(c)* squat, *(d)* hack squat. 90° knee angle. *(b)*, *(c)*, and *(d)* performed bilateral.

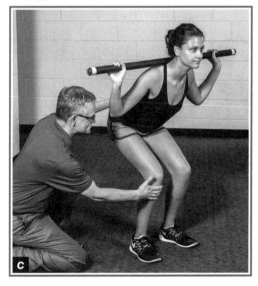

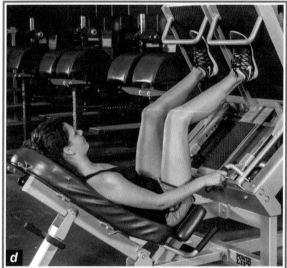

Extensor Carpi Radialis Brevis Tendinopathy

Tendinopathy of the extensor carpi radialis brevis (ECRB) is often called lateral epicondylalgia or tennis elbow. Careful examination is needed to differentiate tendinopathy from other causes of elbow pain, including radial nerve irritation. When ECRB tendinopathy is the source of pain, the benefit of eccentric training is well established (Cullinane, Boocock, and Trevelyan 2014). During the first week of treatment, eccentric wrist extension exercise with a dumbbell is initiated, three sets of 10 repetitions progressing from slow to fast (days 1 and 2, slow; days 3 to 5, moderate; days 6 and 7, fast) (figure 17.5). Resistance is increased on day 7, and the repetition cycle repeats. Resistance is progressed by maintaining load during painful contractions and increasing resistance when exercise becomes pain-free. Resistance tubing (figure 17.6) can also be used to generate an eccentric load. Rapid, forceful wrist extension is followed by an effort to hold the wrist in extension. The pull of the band results in a sudden eccentric impulse. It is more difficult to guide progression when resistance bands are used, but the use of a band can be more convenient in a home exercise program. It is important to encourage maximal effort in each set and to periodically monitor performance and progress.

These programs encourage the patient to exercise through pain as long as the symptoms do not change the quality of motion or persist after exercise. The pain associated with the degenerative changes of tendinopathy is a bit of an enigma. Although it is not considered an inflammatory condition, some chemical mediators of pain such as prostaglandins may be present. Additionally, the ingrowth of new capillaries may be accompanied by nerve tissue, resulting in sensitization. Conversely, patients with substantial tendon degeneration might not experience pain. The progression of exercise is accomplished by adding external resistance and increasing the speed of contractions in a manner that promotes gradual, long-term improvement. Determining the extent to which patients should refrain from exercise requires a comprehensive assessment of their symptoms, desired activity, and risk of rupture. Many patients, however, can continue with most or all of their physical activities while recovering from tendinopathy.

EXERCISE FOR REPAIR IN MUSCLE TISSUE

The management of muscle strain is more complex than that of tendinopathy. First, muscle strain is an acute injury that produces an inflammatory response, as detailed in chapter 4. Muscle is also highly vascularized. Muscle homeostasis and growth are strongly influenced by endocrine regulation and the interaction of mechanical stimuli and humoral factors. Muscle is also active tissue under the control of the nervous system. Chapter 9 reviews the impact of pain, swelling, and joint damage on the ability of the body to recruit muscle to generate force. Appropriate mechanical loading is crucial for muscle repair. Muscle at rest will atrophy.

How can clinicians balance all of these factors in developing a plan of care? Here some parallels can be found in the treatment of tendinopathy and strain injuries. The initial stimulus must be low intensity. Since pain inhibits neuromuscular control, early activity should be minimally painful. Gentle isometric contractions provide a mechanical stimulus, encourage lymphatic drainage, and facilitate neuromuscular control. Active range of motion can begin in a limited range and progress to full range of motion as tolerated. With full range of motion established, low levels of resistance can be added. At this stage of repair, the goal is to complete sets of 20 or more repetitions without pain. The number of sets and the frequency of exercise must be based on individual responses. However, since the resistance is well below maximum effort, extensive recovery between exercise sessions is not needed.

As repair progresses, the focus of resistance training shifts toward restoring neuromuscular control and muscle force generation. Achieving these goals requires heavier resistance. When resistance is increased, the number of repetitions someone can

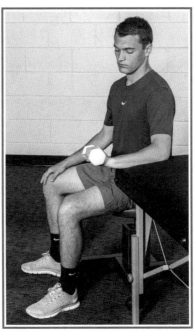

Figure 17.5 Dumbbell exercise for the treatment of extensor carpi radialis brevis tendinopathy.

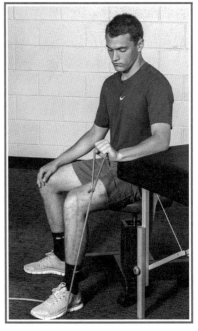

Figure 17.6 Resistance tubing can also be used to generate an eccentric load.

complete diminishes. Heavy resistance causes some muscle damage, which the body responds to through repair and building of new muscle. The recovery period needed between sessions that target specific muscles increases to 48 hours or more.

Restoring the force-generating capacity of muscle is central to any rehabilitation plan of care following musculoskeletal injury. Retraining neuromuscular control is central to this process. However, clinicians should not lose sight of the fact that adaptation of the tissue is the result of the mechanical forces transmitted to cells and that when muscle is damaged, mechanical signaling is central to the repair process.

Neuromuscular interaction between the alpha motor neurons and the muscle fibers governs force production. Neural firing frequency and the number and types of muscle fibers activated will determine force production. If muscle fibers are not activated, there is no stimulus for adaptation. Low-load exercise primarily recruits small motor units composed of slow-twitch, fatigue-resistant type I fibers. As load increases, motor unit recruitment of larger high-threshold type II units occurs, with maximal loads recruiting the full spectrum of motor units. High velocity and fatiguing activities of submaximal loads also recruit high-threshold motor units.

As the healing process progresses through remodeling and repair and greater activity is tolerated, resistance exercise focuses not only on neuromuscular adaptations but also on muscle tissue growth and recovery. The clinician's role in exercise prescription is to safely optimize fiber activation through the modulation of exercise program variables. Program variables include exercise choice, load (resistance), volume (sets × repetitions × load), exercise order, and rest between sets and exercises (Kraemer and Ratamess 2004).

Exercise choice will determine the muscles activated and the types of contractions. Exercises involving large muscle groups and eccentric contractions result in a prolific hormonal and metabolic response, necessary for adaptation. Load is expressed as percent of repetition maximum. Strength, hypertrophy, and endurance adaptations occur specifically with the amount of resistance (load). For instance, low-load, high-repetition exercise (30RM) improves muscular endurance but does not promote hypertrophy. Heavy-load, low-repetition exercise (1–12RM) promotes strength and hypertrophy. Early in the healing process, excessive load will disrupt repair, but as healing commences, if load is not increased, improvements

in strength will not occur. This is directly related to motor unit recruitment as discussed.

There is an obvious interaction between load and exercise volume. As the amount of load increases, the number of repetitions one can complete decreases. Volume of exercise can be adjusted through the number of repetitions, the amount of resistance, and the number of exercises. Up to a point, higher-volume programs result in superior adaptation, but if exercise volume is excessive and rest insufficient, the amount of damage incurred will exceed repair potential. During healing, this is particularly important to keep in mind. Low-load activity performed with excessive sets and repetitions will lead to detriments in performance, swelling, and pain.

Exercise to return strength and performance after muscle injury must be closely monitored. In the early acute phase, activity is limited to gentle passive and active assisted motions within patient tolerance. As inflammation subsides, isometric contractions provide force without tremendous stress to healing tissues. Isotonic strength exercises are progressed according to tolerance and begin with low load and high repetitions. Neuromuscular recruitment patterns are promoted. Adequate load is required to activate the full spectrum of motor units to promote the recovery of all involved muscle fibers.

EXERCISE FOR REPAIR IN BONE

The health of bone depends on exposure to mechanical forces. Bone at rest atrophies and becomes osteoporotic. The osteocyte is central to the mechanoregulation of bone. Mechanical forces imparted on the osteocyte result in the production of chemoelectric signals and the production of extracellular matrix that maintains or builds bone. In fact, the contribution of mechanical signaling to the ultimate strength of bone through modeling and remodeling is approximately 40%, whereas hormones, calcium, vitamin D, and genetics contribute less than 10% (Frost 2001).

The ultimate architecture and mass of bone are influenced by maximal stress, whereas the rate at which new bone is formed relates to the frequency of stimulation. Bone models its size and shape in response to imposed loads and removes damage while preserving strength. Remodeling occurs in response to microfracture, leading to apoptosis and cell signaling between progenitor and mature cells that are involved in removing and rebuilding bone. Bone models in response to strains of elastic deformation caused by muscle contraction and gravity. The largest voluntary bone strains come from momentary muscle contractions, not body weight. In fact, it is said that strong muscles make strong bones. The rate of bone remodeling is influenced largely by the magnitude, frequency, and duration of loading.

Injury to bone has similarities to injury of both muscle and tendon. An acute fracture is similar to a muscle strain. Tissue damage is immediate, and inflammation results (figure 17.7). Unlike strain, there is great variety in the extent of tissue injury and separation between fracture lines. The repair of many fractures is facilitated by efforts to approximate pieces of bone and the use of external or internal fixation. As with other tissue injuries that result in inflammation, early repair is stimulated by the chemical mediators of inflammation discussed in chapter 4. However, this repair stimulus is not enough to fully restore the ability of bone to resist external forces. Left at rest, areas of a bone not affected by the fracture will become weaker, and the strength of the repair will be compromised.

The potential to influence bone repair with external stimuli is apparent from the research into the effects of LIPUS and PEMF therapy reviewed in chapters 12 and 13. Progressive loading occurs as patients improve and are allowed to progress activity. What may be missing, however, is a planned progression of loading to facilitate fracture repair. There is little to guide the appropriateness of loading. The forces directed at healing bone should not pose a risk of further damage. The range of strain that may promote healing of fracture is thought to be very small (about 1%-4% of fracture strain).

The periosteum is well innervated, and pain signals excessive loading. Some discomfort during activity, however, is common, and if transient it is likely not concerning. Clinicians may use strategies such as pool activity or the use of antigravity or unloading treadmills to stress healing lower extremity bone in patients who cannot tolerate the full forces of walking, running, or jumping. Loading of fractures in the upper extremities is also guided by the ability to control forces in a safe but progressive exercise regimen. The extent to which earlier loading accelerates repair and return to full participation warrants additional study. Healing is affected by many factors, including the extent of the injury, the general health of the patient, and age. Diagnostic imaging and patient reports of symptoms can guide progression and decisions about return to sport and work activities. Loading of injured bone, however, should not be simply viewed as a progression of function but rather a potential facilitator of repair.

Stress fractures are more similar to tendinopathy than they are to acute fractures. Both stress fractures and tendinopathy represent an imbalance between anabolic (tissue building) and catabolic (tissue damaging) pathways. The endocrine role in health and metabolism is more significant in bone than in tendon, but the goal in the treatment

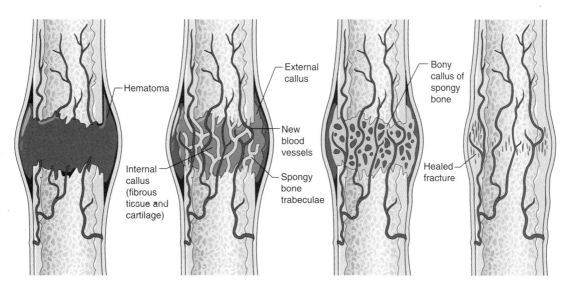

Figure 17.7   Bone healing. Like other vascular tissue, clotted blood in the area of injury forms a provisional matrix (callus) that is remodeled over time by bone cells.

of both conditions is to stimulate repair processes. Once nonloading sources of bone compromise (e.g., endocrine disorders and conditions) are considered, the management of stress fractures requires a controlled introduction of mechanical load until repair is realized and the patient can resume participation. Tenforde and colleagues (2012) described the successful management of a collegiate distance runner through a gradual increase in running load using an antigravity treadmill (figure 17.8).

In summary, rest is not the cure in the management of fractures. Rest may be necessary to manage symptoms before a program of progressive loading is initiated. As with the care of patients recovering from acute fracture, self-report and imaging can guide efficient recovery and minimize the risk of setbacks and complications. Parameters of treatments to optimize fracture repair, perhaps in concert with LIPUS or PEMF, will emerge as new technologies and research emerge.

MASSAGE THERAPY AS REPAIR STIMULUS

Massage may be the first therapeutic modality used in treating disorders of the body. With new understanding of the effects of mechanical signals on cellular

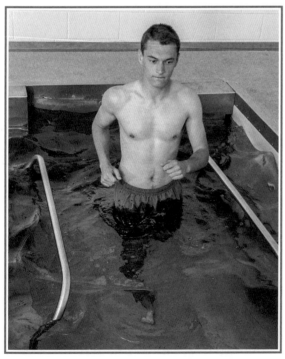

Figure 17.8 An aquatic treadmill allows earlier return of functional movement while reducing imposed forces.

activity, this treatment warrants consideration from a different perspective—repair. Clinical trials suggest that techniques such as massage, self-massage with the use of a foam roller, and compression garments affect recovery from intense exercise-induced muscle injury (Macdonald et al. 2014; Zainuddin et al. 2005; Kraemer et al. 2001). While the mechanisms of these effects are not fully known, it appears that the mechanical stimuli reduce levels of inflammatory cytokines and increase some markers found in tissue repair pathways (Crane et al. 2012).

Considering massage as a stimulus for repair changes the perspective on which to base treatment recommendations. Like many therapeutic modalities, massage has been used to reduce pain, muscle tone, and guarding and in some cases to help restore range of motion. The technique, duration, and frequency of treatment can be based on patient response, access to treatment, and the patient's preferences. When administering any stimulus to affect tissue repair, the parameters (e.g., frequency of ultrasound, duration of treatment, frequency of treatment) of the treatment must be considered. As with the optimal mechanical exercise stimulus, research is needed to identify optimal loading across the tissue repair process. More is not necessarily better.

DEEP FRICTION MASSAGE AS A REPAIR STIMULUS

Treatment of tendinopathy using transverse friction massage was described by Dr. James Cyriax (Cyriax

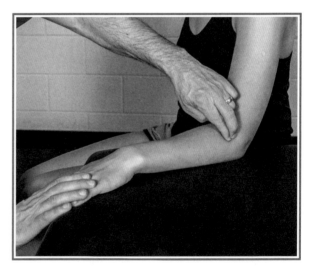

Figure 17.9 Soft tissue and deep friction massage may stimulate tissue to enhance repair and recovery. Anecdotal evidence supports its use for tendinopathy.

A Few Words About Ligaments

You may have been puzzled by the conspicuous absence of ligament injuries in this chapter. Ligaments do respond to mechanical stresses and become thicker and stronger. Unlike tendon, however, it is not possible to isolate loading on these tissues through therapeutic exercise. Thus there are no specific guidelines that can guide the progression of loading after a sprain. Moreover, the repair capacity of ligaments may differ, depending on whether the ligament was exposed to repetitive overloading, such as that which occurs at the ulnar collateral ligament of baseball pitchers and other throwing athletes, or a single excessive load. For example, when the tibial collateral ligament is injured because the knee was exposed to high valgus loading, the tissue damage occurs during a very brief period of extreme stress.

Recovery of ligament strength during healing depends upon appropriate exposure to force. Ligaments such as the tibial collateral ligament often have good tissue approximation after injury and undergo an acute inflammatory process. As inflammation subsides and healing begins, the introduction and progression of force through exercise and soft tissue mobilization techniques may provide an important repair stimulus. Strengthening activities requiring incremental increases in frontal plane stress to the knee will encourage newly synthesized ligament to align and respond to increasing valgus loads. In this way, ligament, like trained tendon, can probably increase tissue strength in response to imposed stress.

1984) at a time when tendon pain was considered primarily an inflammatory disorder (figure 17.9). As new understanding of the effects of mechanical stimuli on repair processes has emerged, the effectiveness of the technique has garnered new attention. Joseph et al. (2012) completed a systematic review of clinical trials involving deep friction message. Heterogeneity of the target conditions (e.g., Achilles vs. supraspinatus), treatment technique, and parameters of treatment along with study methodologies precluded recommending or not recommending treatment. These authors concluded that anecdotal evidence, advances in mechanobiology, and the current understanding of tendinopathy serve as a foundation for further investigation into the role of deep friction massage as a treatment or adjunct treatment in patients suffering from tendinopathy.

SUMMARY

Musculoskeletal tissue responds to mechanical loading by stimulating cellular functions that govern homeostasis, remodeling, and repair. The processes affected by mechanical forces are presented in detail in chapter 16. Appropriate exercise and the application of physical modalities such as LIPUS and PEMF can promote tissue repair and improve the outcome of treatment. Musculoskeletal tissues have specific force requirements for maintenance, repair, and enhanced performance. Tendon responds well to frequent bouts of eccentric stress. Muscle, capable of a prolific inflammatory response, must be slowly reintroduced to gradually increasing stress after injury. Bone is very responsive to pulses of force as seen with dynamic weight-bearing activities and repeated muscle contractions. The cellular basis of mechanobiology offers new perspectives on the role of exercise in tissue repair. The progression of stress directed at healing tissue must be carefully controlled to avoid disrupting the repair process. The sports medicine team must adjust the plan of care according to the state of repair throughout the healing process.

KEY CONCEPTS AND REVIEW

1. *Discuss the application of mechanobiology (chapter 16) to the treatment of tendinopathy, muscle strain, and fracture.*

   As described in chapter 16, mechanical signaling that results from exercise and physical modalities leads to altered tissue composition and can greatly enhance repair. Mechanotransduction pathways are activated by stress experienced in the tissue, resulting in cellular perturbation and activity. Much is still unknown about true in vivo forces experienced during specific rehabilitation activities. The clinician must apply current knowledge of preferred tissue stress and force progression to optimize healing, recovery, and performance.

2. *Describe how tendon, muscle, and bone respond to stress on the tissues.*

   Tissues respond specifically to stress. Tendon responds to axial tension delivered through eccentric exercise and passive lengthening. Tendon responds better than muscle to frequent loading, as can be seen by the success of twice-daily eccentric exercises. Healthy muscle responds to high resistance with maximal recruitment and activation. Adequate recovery is necessary for the repair of microdamage, and therefore 48 hours of recovery is typically required between similar exercise bouts. Healing muscle must be progressed slowly and is prone to overabundant inflammation. The healing processes for bone and muscle are similar. Bone is very responsive to pulses of force, such as those seen with dynamic weight-bearing activities and repeated muscle contractions.

3. *Discuss how the pain response can assist in guiding exercise progression.*

   Close monitoring of patient progress throughout rehabilitation will help avoid poor outcomes. Pain can guide progression but must be interpreted in the context of an injury. Pain during eccentric loading of injured tendons can be expected and is not believed to signal excessive stress. In fact, patients can be encouraged to stress the tissue to the point that mild to moderate discomfort is reported. It is important, however, to monitor patients regularly to make sure that they are not experiencing increases in pain at rest or during daily activities; these are symptoms of further damage, not repair. Some pain can be expected in the treatment of muscle strains, but pain is known to alter neuromuscular control. Monitor patients carefully to make sure that pain is not compromising movement quality or exercise technique and that it does not persist after exercise. The pain of a fracture is distinct and localized. Sharp pain is indicative of excessive loading of healing tissues. Mild discomfort with loading is likely safe and indicative of loads that stimulate repair.

Mechanical Energy and Manual Therapies

OBJECTIVES

After reading this chapter, you will be able to

1 discuss the potential benefits of using manual therapy techniques in rehabilitation;

2 describe massage, myofascial release, strain–counterstrain, muscle energy, and joint mobilization;

3 describe the afferent and efferent innervation of intrafusal and extrafusal muscle fibers and the relationship between the gamma and alpha motor neurons;

4 apply the convex–concave rule in performing joint mobilization;

5 describe the manual and mechanical traction techniques used to treat cervical spine dysfunction;

6 identify contraindications for manual therapies and mechanical traction;

7 describe the mechanical traction techniques used to treat lumbar spine dysfunction;

8 describe the application of, and contraindications for, intermittent compression therapy; and

9 describe how the principles of mechanobiology might apply to manual therapies.

A field hockey player is referred for care of her injured right ankle. She injured the ankle about 2 months ago and was diagnosed as having suffered a sprain. She complains of mild pain and swelling at the ankle, primarily associated with running, and new pain at the midportion of the Achilles tendon. Evaluation of the ankle reveals restrictions in dorsiflexion and posterior glide of the talus. Grade III and IV joint mobilization result in improved dorsiflexion after three treatments, and a daily regimen of eccentric exercises of the plantar flexor muscles alleviates Achilles tendon pain after several weeks. How did the new treatment make a difference? Joint mobilization and other manual therapy techniques can speed recovery from a variety of musculoskeletal injuries. Mechanical loading or the application of mechanobiology in rehabilitation is increasingly being recognized as a stimulus to tissue repair. This chapter introduces manual therapies and other modality applications that deliver mechanical energy to the body.

Physical activity and some therapeutic modalities, such as mechanical traction and intermittent compression, exert mechanical forces on the body. However, the most common "devices" used in the treatment to impart a mechanical force on the body are the hands of the clinician. The hands are powerful assessment and treatment tools. At one time, manual therapy in the form of massage and manual resistance was commonly practiced by athletic trainers and physical therapists. These practices, to a large degree, were abandoned because of demands on their time and the development of devices such as transcutaneous electrical nerve stimulation (TENS) and isokinetic dynamometers. Now, manual therapy techniques developed in osteopathic medicine, chiropractic medicine, and physical therapy are broadly applied in the treatment of musculoskeletal conditions.

This chapter covers the topics of mechanical traction, intermittent compression, and manual therapy, and introduces exercise as a stimulus for tissue repair. Much of the chapter is devoted to introducing several manual therapy approaches. This chapter is intended only to introduce manual therapy. A detailed discussion of manual therapy techniques is available in texts devoted to one or more of the techniques described. Issues of treatment efficacy are, however, discussed as in the previous three chapters.

Much of this text is devoted to understanding how therapeutic modalities affect the nervous system and connective tissues. Although manual therapies can be considered procedures as opposed to applications, the clinician's hands affect the connective tissues and alter neural input. Some clinicians shun the use of therapeutic modalities such as ultrasound and TENS for newer manual techniques, whereas others view manual therapies as a subspecialty separate from contemporary care of musculoskeletal injuries. A treatment that combines modalities like ultrasound or TENS and manual techniques may provide the greatest relief of symptoms. For example, when treating a person with myofascial pain, you may find TENS, superficial heat, or occasionally cold combined with massage, strain–counterstrain, or release techniques to be effective. These all change neural activity at the spinal level and relieve pain and muscle spasm. Also, because heated tissues are more pliable, ultrasound or diathermy may be useful before treatments such as joint mobilization in which the goal is to stretch connective tissues and restore normal joint function. The use of low-level laser therapy, when combined with exercises that eccentrically load tendon, may be more effective than exercise alone in the treatment of tendinopathy, although additional study is needed to confirm the benefits of adding laser to plan of care.

Unlike cold therapy or TENS, manual treatment cannot be learned from a book but must be learned through laboratory instruction and hands-on practice. Both students and experienced clinicians will continually refine their manual therapy skills and add variations and new techniques. Over the years, proprioceptive neuromuscular facilitation, joint mobilization, myofascial release, and strain–counterstrain techniques have been used to treat physically active people. These skills have largely been developed from clinical observation and passed from teacher to student. Often various techniques are recommended for treating the same condition. For example, patients with neck pain may respond to myofascial release, joint mobilization, or strain–counterstrain. No single manual therapy approach has been shown to be universally superior to another. Controlled clinical trials are needed to assess the short- and long-term effectiveness of many applications of manual therapy. Developing skill in the manual therapy techniques offers a greater number of options when developing a plan of care and improves the clinician's ability to evaluate the musculoskeletal system. Manual therapy techniques can be applied in any setting; these skills require time and practice rather than a large budget and an athletic training room. Practice, experience, and attention to the clinical literature will guide your development of manual therapy skills and your ability to integrate traditional therapeutic modalities with manual therapy. This chapter provides a foundation on which you can build your skills in the hope that you will pursue further training in manual therapy.

MANUAL THERAPY

Unfortunately, the scientific foundation for manual therapy has evolved more slowly than the art. There is relatively little evidence of cause-and-effect relationships between manual therapy and recovery from injury. However, there is scientific support for much of the theory behind many forms of manual therapy, and the following sections include important components of the theoretical foundation for manual therapy. Before discussing individual therapies, we will address one additional aspect of manual therapy that is neither anatomical nor clearly neurological: the power of touch and human interaction.

Clinicians who care for patients with musculoskeletal injuries encounter a variety of circumstances. Some patients are entering the medical system on an emergency basis, perhaps for the first time. The high school athlete injured for the first time, the university freshman far from home, or the older person whose work and family life have been disrupted present with more than an injured body part to be treated. These people come for care with anxiety, unanswered questions, and a sense of being lost in the health care system. Our increasingly bureaucratic and technology-driven health care system often leaves people wondering if anyone really cares about them. Manual therapy requires hands-on time with the patient. A caring touch and opportunity for conversation can ease anxiety and foster confidence that the person is being cared for and will recover. A sense of being in good hands promotes compliance with a plan of care and a positive outlook, which in turn promote recovery. Some of the benefits of manual therapy are due to the psychological-affective responses to treatment rather than the anatomical-neurological responses. Some may call this a placebo response; however, improvement is improvement, and perhaps much of the failure of our medical system stems from the loss of the personal touch. Certainly, medical technology has advanced medical care, but at a price. The skilled manual therapist who provides a personal touch will help some patients whom others cannot.

Massage

Massage, the rubbing or kneading of a part of the body, is one of the earliest recorded treatments for human suffering. Massage developed in many early cultures. The terminology and techniques of massage, as well as its acceptance as a therapy, have changed over time. Today, massage techniques are applied by several allied medical professionals as well as massage therapists.

Physical therapists and athletic trainers have used massage since the beginnings of the professions. Massage has been purported to relieve pain, increase blood flow, enhance lymphatic drainage, and stretch connective tissues. Experience and observation provide evidence of the effects of massage on pain and muscle spasm. Certainly relief of spasm may enhance lymphatic drainage, and mechanical energy can stretch connective tissues. However, blood flow to deep tissues is regulated by metabolic demand. The effect of massage on blood flow has not been extensively studied, but an understanding of circulatory regulation suggests that massage has little impact on blood flow to deeper tissues.

Pain relief, reduced muscle spasm, and increased tissue extensibility are traditionally thought to be the primary benefits of massage. But how does massage relieve pain and muscle spasm? Contact with the skin exerts a mechanical force that stimulates the cutaneous receptors and increases input along large-diameter afferent pathways. The gate control theory of spinal-level pain modulation (figure 18.1) offers a plausible explanation for the analgesic benefits of massage techniques that employ gentle stroking motions (**effleurage**) and kneading (**petrissage**) of muscle. Because muscle guarding and spasm are the result of pain, massage alleviates the trigger for muscle spasm and mobilizes the muscle and surrounding connective tissues.

Video 18.1 demonstrates cross-friction massage.

Deeper massage techniques over trigger points may result in a deep sensation of pain during massage yet provide extended relief. Painful stimulation activates the descending analgesic pathways described in chapter 6. Thus, the response to deep, kneading massage techniques also has a plausible explanation.

Relief of pain and muscle spasm and mobilization of connective tissues are important treatment goals. In theory, achieving these goals enhances lymphatic drainage. Certainly, pain relief and muscle relaxation promote free, active contraction of muscle, which is the primary means by which lymph is pumped through the body.

More recently, massage is being considered as a stimulus for muscle repair. A massage is part of routine training and preparation for many endurance athletes. This is particularly true in professional cycling; all of the European professional teams employ one or more *sorvoiners*, or massage therapists, and postrace massage is also a regular practice.

Deep friction massage (DFM) is a technique popularized by James Cyriax (1984) for the treatment of tendon disorders (now called tendinopathy). Cyriax proposed that deep friction perpendicular to the collagen fiber alignment of the tendon increases blood flow to the tissue and disrupts adhesions in the extracellular matrix. Advances in the study of mechanobiology offer another plausible explanation, the up-regulation of tenocyte activity and progenitor cell differentiation resulting from mechanical signals transmitted through the tissues to the cell nuclei, as described in chapter 16. More research is needed to enable us to fully understand the effects of deep friction massage on the outcomes of care. Joseph et al. (2012) completed a systematic review of the clinical literature and concluded that "the examination of DFM as a single modality of treatment in comparison with other methods and control has not been undertaken, so its isolated efficacy has not been established. Excellent anecdotal evidence remains along with a rationale for its use that fits the current understanding of tendinopathy."

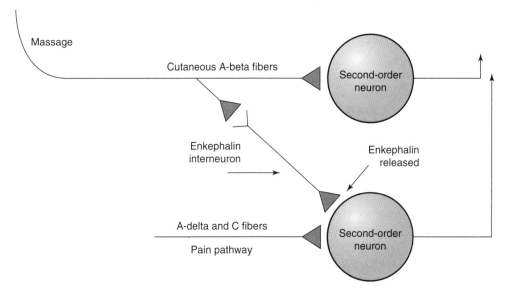

Figure 18.1   Massage stimulates cutaneous receptors, increasing large-diameter afferent input and resulting in enkephalin release and inhibition of pain pathways.

Myofascial Release

Myofascial release (MFR) is similar to massage in that the clinician uses his or her hands to influence the connective tissues and neural input. There are multiple release techniques. The techniques and terminology of MFR overlap with those of other manual therapies. However, MFR, as a component of manual therapies, has a much more elaborate theoretical basis, which has resulted in a greater understanding of somatic dysfunction.

Video 18.2 demonstrates myofascial release.

Myo refers to muscle and *fascia* to the system of supporting connective tissue that maintains the integrity of the human body. Injury, illness, stress, repetitive movements, poor posture, and fatigue can contribute to changes in the length–tension relationship of the fascia and muscles over time. For example, extensive swimming can strengthen and shorten the chest muscles while stretching and weakening the muscles of the upper back. The surrounding fascia adapts accordingly, setting the stage for a myofascial pain pattern.

Injuries such as whiplash can cause a pattern of guarding that in turn results in fascial adaptations. Psychological stress also results in tension and can contribute to the development of a myofascial pain pattern.

At the center of myofascial pain is gamma gain. When muscle is in spasm or protective guarding, it becomes hypersensitive to stretch due to increased input along gamma efferent nerves to the muscle spindles (figure 18.2). The cycles of pain, protective guarding, and fascial shortening gradually escalate until the athlete experiences myofascial pain.

The role of the clinician is to break the cycle and address the physically active person's symptoms. Many modalities can be used to treat physically active people, and all treatment plans for myofascial pain should include active therapeutic exercises. However, these interventions do not directly address the problem of fascial restrictions and gamma gain.

Myofascial release techniques can be divided into direct and indirect techniques. In applying indirect techniques, the athletic trainer tries to place muscle and fascia in positions that remove stress from the tissues, resulting in decreased noxious input from the fascia, which in turn diminishes activity in gamma efferent nerves. These techniques are gentle but require practice to master. Direct techniques are aimed at stretching bound fascia to decrease the stress on and afferent input from the tissue. Both types of techniques can be used to treat a myofascial pain pattern. Practice and experience will improve your manual skills as well as your ability to integrate traditional modalities, manual therapy, and exercise into a comprehensive plan of care.

Myofascial pain patterns are common in the neck, upper back, and shoulder. Poor posture, several hours spent driving or sitting in front of a computer, stress, and general fatigue slowly take a toll. Gentle release techniques often dramatically relieve pain, spasm, and accompanying headaches.

Strain–Counterstrain

Strain–counterstrain, another type of manual therapy, was originated by Dr. Lawrence Jones (Jones, Kusunose, and Goering 1995). Like MFR, strain–counterstrain relieves pain and dysfunction by altering neural activity. Strain–counterstrain is a technique in which a body segment is passively moved into a position of greatest comfort, thereby relieving pain by reducing or arresting inappropriate proprioceptive activity that is responsible for the dysfunction.

Jones provided a holistic view of somatic dysfunction, recognizing that injury to one structure, such as a ligament, affects other tissues including muscle, fascia, blood vessels, lymphatic vessels, and neural elements. Strain–counterstrain techniques are directed toward treating not the primary lesion, such as the sprained ligament, but rather the resulting dysfunctions.

Strain–counterstrain techniques can increase pain-free range of motion after musculoskeletal injury. As with MFR, direct and indirect techniques of strain–counterstrain are described. Direct techniques involve applying force against a restrictive barrier to improve motion, whereas indirect techniques involve moving the body away from a motion-restricting barrier to a position of comfort and relaxation.

By placing a body segment in a position of comfort, the indirect techniques inhibit the cycle of pain and increased muscle guarding due to increased gamma efferent outflow (figure 18.3). One key element of indirect techniques is slowly moving the treated body segment back to a resting position after a period (90–120 s) of passive positioning. The

Muscle is made up of two types of fibers. Extrafusal fibers are the contractile fibers that allow muscle to generate force. The extrafusal fibers are innervated by alpha motor neurons. Interspersed within the extrafusal fibers, which make up most of the substance of muscle, are intrafusal fibers. Intrafusal fibers house muscle spindles that are specialized mechanoreceptors; these send information about changes in muscle length, and therefore movement, to the central nervous system.

Intrafusal fibers receive neural stimulation from gamma efferent neurons. The efferent input allows for continual adjustment of the length of the spindle so that it is maintained at an optimum length to detect changes within the muscle.

In some circumstances, there may be excessive activity in the gamma efferent neurons to a particular muscle or portion of a muscle, which is referred to as **gamma gain**. The effect of gamma gain is to maintain the spindles in a hypersensitive state, resulting in normal movements causing reflexive contraction throughout a muscle via the reflex arc depicted in figure 18.2. The increased tension **(hypertonicity)** in a muscle will ultimately result in adaptive shortening in surrounding fascial tissues. The taut bands of tissues and hypersensitive trigger points associated with myofascial pain syndrome (MFPS) are thought to result from gamma gain.

The question of what causes gamma gain has not been fully answered. The likely trigger is pain. Acute pain results in muscle spasm and guarding. Rapid movement of muscle in spasm results in a reflexive contraction of the affected muscle, suggesting that muscle spindles are in a hypersensitive state due to increased gamma efferent activity. The increase in gamma activity is the result of input from nociceptors. This explanation makes sense when applied to the response to acute injuries, but how does it relate to persistent pain problems such as MFPS?

The increased tone and resulting fascial adaptations found in MFPS are an insidious process. When fascia becomes shortened, it too becomes hypersensitive to stretch. Stretch of fascial tissue is painful; free nerve endings are being stimulated. Noxious input from the fascia triggers an increase in gamma efferent activity, perpetuating a cycle of spindle hypersensitivity, increased tone in muscle, fascial adaptations, and painful movement when the tight fascia is stretched. The cycle builds from mild discomfort into a pain pattern that can include referred pain and frequent headaches. Effective treatment of MFPS requires that the causes, which may include combinations of stress responses, muscle imbalance and poor posture, injury, and illness, must begin with breaking this cycle.

Breaking the cycle just described by arresting gamma gain is the focus of two manual therapy techniques, strain–counterstrain and indirect myofascial release. These techniques place muscles and fascia in shortened positions of comfort. Such positioning decreases gamma efferent activity and interrupts the cycle that is maintaining the body in a dysfunctional state.

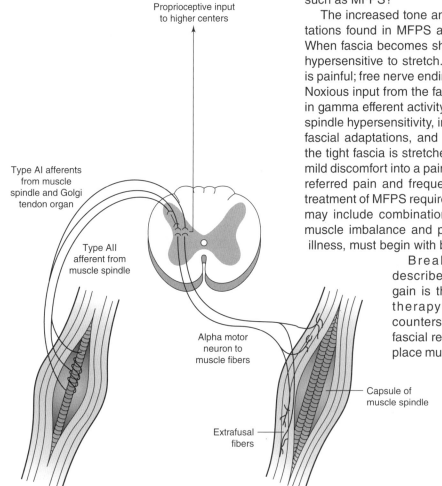

Proprioceptive input to higher centers

Type AI afferents from muscle spindle and Golgi tendon organ

Type AII afferent from muscle spindle

Alpha motor neuron to muscle fibers

Capsule of muscle spindle

Extrafusal fibers

Figure 18.2 Sensory input from the muscle spindles and Golgi tendon organs affects motor function of same muscle via synapses at the spinal cord level.

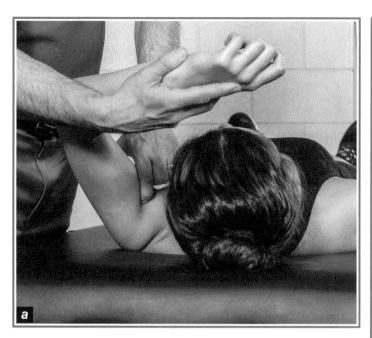

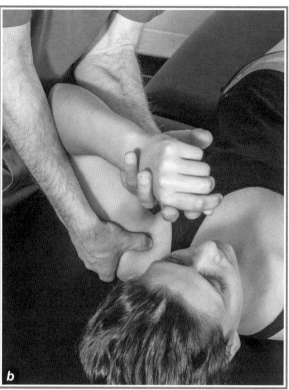

Figure 18.3 Strain–counterstrain for the *(a)* short and *(b)* long heads of biceps brachii dysfunction.

slow, painless movement prevents a surge of input from spindles and reestablishment of the movement dysfunction.

Video 18.3 demonstrates the strain–counterstrain technique.

You need laboratory instruction and practice in order to become proficient at both MFR and strain–counterstrain techniques. Over the years, clinicians have become increasingly interested in these manual therapies, probably because they address the notion of a pain–spasm cycle. Clinicians understand that modality applications do not repair injured tissue but are used to treat the signs and symptoms of injury, including loss of function. Strain–counterstrain techniques are most useful in short-duration pain patterns and during tissue repair and early maturation. Myofascial techniques, although similar, seem to be most effective in treating more long-standing pain patterns, especially those related to the spine.

Pain results in muscle guarding and spasm, which in turn cause more pain. Sometimes this cycle persists despite adequate time for tissue repair. Strain–counterstrain can be used to place a body segment in a position of comfort and break the cycle. A slow return to anatomical or resting position prevents a recurrence of pain, often leading to prolonged relief.

Joint Mobilization

Muscle energy and joint mobilization are manual therapies primarily directed at restoring joint function. Joint mobilization is used to restore intrinsic joint motion or arthrokinetics in synovial joints. Joint mobilization also stimulates joint receptors and increases afferent input across large-diameter afferent fibers. Thus, joint mobilization may also ease pain and improve the person's willingness to move a joint.

To appreciate the value of joint mobilization techniques, you must fully understand how joint movement occurs. Joints are formed by the articulating surfaces of bones. Muscles, through the attachments of tendons, cause bones to move upon one another at the joint. Outwardly, the articulating surface of one bone appears to pivot about a single, fixed axis, but few joint motions actually occur about a single axis. During most joint movements, the articulating surfaces slide and glide upon one another while the rolling or pivoting occurs about a moving axis.

The subtle slides and glides are referred to as **arthrokinematics**, whereas the observed motion created by movement of one bone upon another is referred to as **osteokinematics**. Joint mobilization involves the assessment and treatment of arthrokinematics. The convex-concave rule, illustrated in figure 18.4, will help you assess and treat restricted arthrokinematic movements.

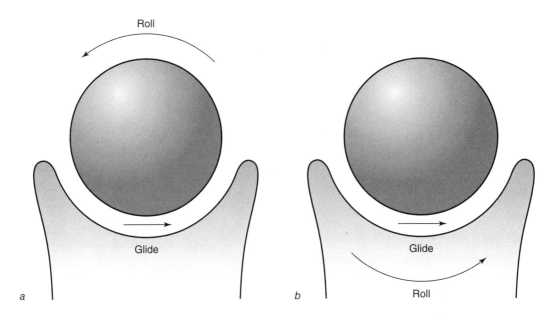

Figure 18.4 *(a)* When a convex surface moves on a concave surface, roll and glide are in opposite directions. *(b)* When a concave surface moves on a convex surface, roll and glide occur in the same direction.

Video 18.4 demonstrates joint mobilization.

When arthrokinematic movement is limited, range of motion is limited, and the joint is often painful. From the perspective of modality application and pain management, joint mobilization addresses the first two priorities in an injured person's plan of care: pain relief and restoration of range of motion. In fact, when pain and loss of motion are due to arthrokinematic dysfunction, joint mobilization is the treatment of choice. Moreover, restricted joint motion impairs neuromuscular control. Thus, joint mobilization and the restoration of arthrokinematic motion can be essential to address impairment in volitional control over muscle and restore balance and postural control during functional movements.

Optimal techniques for performing joint mobilization vary by the joint being treated. A thorough understanding of the structure of a joint and appropriate instruction and practice are needed to develop proficiency in joint mobilization. However, this technique is introduced in the context of therapeutic modalities because of its application in managing joint pain and loss of motion as well as linking impairments in joint motion to control during functional movements.

Consider a loss of range of motion after a sprain of the lateral ankle ligaments. A loss of dorsiflexion affects balance and the ability to walk and run. Stretching of the gastrocnemius and soleus can help restore motion, but often the problem is related to a restriction of posterior glide of the talus in the mortise. In these cases, joint mobilization techniques in which the talus is manually moved posteriorly will be far more effective at restoring motion than stretching. Moreover, when normal glide is lost, efforts to improve motion through activities such as stretching create focal compression of articular cartilage. Normal arthrokinematic motion is essential for normal distribution of loading of joint surfaces and thus should be the first priority in efforts to restore range of motion following injury.

Muscle Energy

Muscle energy techniques are manual procedures in which the injured person's muscles are actively contracted against a counterforce in a specific treatment position. These techniques may be used, for example, in the treatment of sacroiliac (figure 18.5) and lumbar facet dysfunction.

Video 18.5 demonstrates the muscle energy technique on the sacroiliac joint.

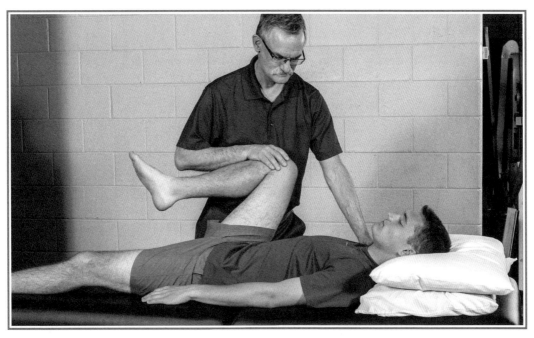

Figure 18.5 Muscle energy technique for an anterior innominate rotation, a common source of sacroiliac dysfunction.

Like joint mobilization, a muscle energy technique can be considered a procedure rather than a modality application. However, when restricted joint movement causes pain and movement dysfunction, a therapeutic modality usually fails to relieve symptoms and allow pain-free, functional movement. Muscle energy and joint mobilization techniques address the cause of the injured person's complaints and often speed the recovery of normal movement and function. Modalities such as TENS and moist heat can be combined with most manual techniques, including MFR, muscle energy, and joint mobilization. TENS and heat can relieve pain and reduce muscle spasm. Relief of pain and reduction in muscle tension and guarding may allow for more effective manual therapy in some cases.

Like all modalities, manual therapy techniques are contraindicated in the treatment of some injured athletes. These contraindications are summarized in table 18.1. Injuries to ligaments and bone are the most common contraindications for manual therapies. However, these contraindications are not absolute, and they require sound clinical decision making. For example, if an athlete suffered a fracture and dislocation at the ankle, this injury would initially contraindicate all manual therapies. However, once the tissues have healed and the leg is removed from immobilization, massage, MFR, and joint mobilization could be used to restore range of motion in the foot-ankle complex. It is also possible that the prolonged use of crutches could result in sacroiliac dysfunction that may respond to muscle energy techniques.

As emphasized elsewhere in this text, the patient's medical history, history of the current concern, and a physical examination lead to the diagnosis from a medical and rehabilitative perspective. Plans of care are developed based on the assessment of all of the information gathered. Patient assessment can also reveal medical conditions that contraindicate the interventions described in this chapter and often warrant referral to a physician for further evaluation. Practicing clinicians must be able to recognize signs and symptoms of infections and diseases in patients seeking care. If the nature or etiology of musculoskeletal pain is unclear, further evaluation must be conducted before any manual therapy is attempted.

In addition to the specific precautions and contraindications discussed previously and in *Therapeutic Exercise for Musculoskeletal Injuries, Third Edition* (Houglum 2010), there are additional contraindications for joint mobilization and muscle energy procedures because of the greater force applied to the body during those procedures. Joint mobilization and muscle energy procedures should not be used in the presence of joint or bony instability or when degenerative changes result in a bony block to motion. Joint mobilization and muscle energy

Table 18.1 Indications and Contraindications for Manual Therapies, Traction, and Intermittent Compression*

	Indications	Contraindications
MANUAL THERAPIES		
Massage	Pain Muscle spasm Edema	Infection Skin breakdown or disease
Myofascial release	Persistent pain with fascial restrictions; taut bands or trigger points	Acute inflammation, recent fracture, or surgery Caution with joint instability or joint prosthesis Caution if pregnant
Strain–counterstrain	Persistent pain with well-localized tender points	Increased pain during treatment Caution after fracture or if joint instability present
Muscle energy	Subluxation or malpositioning of a bony element	Recent fracture Joint instability Joint fusion Bony instability Severe osteoporosis
Joint mobilization	Loss of range of motion due to arthrokinematic restriction	Infection Joint instability Bone-on-bone end-feel Recent fracture Bony instability Advanced osteoporosis Mobilization of cervical spine in the presence of advanced rheumatoid arthritis
TRACTION		
Cervical	Pain Muscle spasm Hypomobile facet Disc herniation	Positive vertebral artery test Positive alar ligament test Acute neck injury (fractures, sprains with joint instability) Advanced rheumatoid arthritis Bone cancer Increased pain or radicular symptoms with treatment Advanced osteoporosis
Lumbar	Pain Muscle spasm Disc herniation Hypomobile facet Nerve root impingement	Pregnancy Claustrophobia Internal disc derangement Fractures, sprains with joint instability Bone cancer Increased pain or radicular symptoms with treatment Advanced osteoporosis Hiatal hernia
Intermittent compression	Swelling and edema	Thrombophlebitis Infection Acute fracture Pulmonary edema and congestive heart failure

* General: Symptoms of organic disease or cancer must be followed up before a modality, including a manual procedure, is administered.

procedures also should not be used in the presence of malignancies or advanced osteoporosis; mobilization of the cervical spine should not be performed in the presence of advanced rheumatoid arthritis.

There is considerable debate about whether dysfunction at the sacroiliac joint is a common cause of low back pain. Identification and treatment of asymmetry with muscle energy techniques dramatically relieves pain and spasm for some people. Muscle energy techniques incorporated into a comprehensive plan of care can be the key to relief from weeks or months of pain and dysfunction.

IS MANUAL THERAPY EFFECTIVE?

Unlike the modalities discussed in previous chapters, manual therapy is a collection of treatment techniques used for a broad spectrum of musculoskeletal problems. A search for evidence of the effectiveness of manual techniques reveals that most studies have involved manipulative procedures (grade V mobilization) in the treatment of spine-related conditions. A selection from results of a search of the Physiotherapy Evidence Database is found in table 18.2. These references illustrate the array of conditions and techniques that continue to be investigated to identify safe and effective interventions for conditions that often present a clinical challenge. Manual therapy techniques require formal instruction and practice that are well beyond the scope of this text. There is relatively less information on the effects of grades I through IV mobilization; thus grade V or manipulative procedures were included in this review.

There is evidence that early posterior mobilization of the talus on the calcaneus (Green et al. 2002) speeds recovery from lateral ankle sprains and may prevent residual loss of normal arthrokinematic motion at the ankle (Denegar, Hertel, and Fonseca 2002). Restrictions of distal tibiofibular mobility have also been identified, but results from clinical trials of mobilization of this articulation have not been reported. Lin et al. (2008), however, reported that talocrural joint mobilization provided no additional benefit in terms of activity restriction or quality of life over a standard regimen of physical therapy at 4 to 24 weeks after cast removal following ankle fracture. Conroy and Hayes (1998) reported some benefit of joint mobilization in a small group of patients with glenohumeral impingement syn-

drome. While pain reduction was found at 24 h after treatment, a larger, longer-term study is needed to better assess the efficacy of this intervention.

Searches of PubMed and the Physiotherapy Evidence Database using search terms "myofascial release," "muscle-energy," and "strain–counterstrain" identified few reports from clinical trials. Sucher (1993) reported on four patients with carpal tunnel syndrome who did not respond to conservative care. All improved and carpal tunnel dimensions changed following a regimen of "manipulative myofascial release" and self-stretching.

While much has been written about massage, clinical trials are sparse. Furlan et al. (2002, 2009) completed systematic reviews of massage in the treatment of low back pain. These authors concluded that "massage might be beneficial for patients with subacute and chronic, non-specific low-back pain, especially when combined with exercises and education" (Furlan et al. 2009). This conclusion is supported by the results reported by Preyde (2000), who found that patients with subacute low back pain treated by experienced massage therapists had less pain and greater functional improvement at the conclusion of treatment and 1-month follow-up and by Mitchinson et al. (2007), who reported that massage reduced pain intensity, unpleasantness, and anxiety in patients recovering from major surgical interventions. In a smaller study, Hernandez-Reif et al. (2001) reported that two 30 min massages per week were effective in decreasing pain and improving motion in women with at least 6-month histories of back pain. Low back pain is a complex syndrome, and no single treatment is completely effective. Massage offers a low-cost, low-risk adjunct to a comprehensive plan of care for many physically active individuals with back pain.

Moraska et al. (2008) reported that massage reduced symptoms associated with carpal tunnel syndrome in a randomized trial of general versus targeted intervention. Perlman et al. (2006) found massage to be an effective adjunct treatment in the management of osteoarthritis of the knee. Blackburn, Simons, and Crossley (1998) studied the effects of massage and stretching in a group of young athletes. Subjects received six sessions of massage over 5 weeks and performed a regimen of stretching. The authors reported an increase in work performed by the dorsiflexor muscles before symptoms of exertional compartment syndrome occurred. Measures of functional performance were not included in this study. Massage has been reported to decrease the

Table 18.2 Assessing the Efficacy of Manual Therapies: Main Conclusions From Recent Studies

Author	Type of report	Nature of problem	Main conclusion
CERVICAL SPINE AND HEADACHE			
Vincent et al. 2013	Systematic review	Nonspecific neck pain	Manual therapies contribute effective management, but in the long run exercise or exercise plus manual therapy is more effective than manual therapy alone
Hurwitz et al. 2009	Systematic review	Neck pain and associated disorders	Treatments involving manual therapy and exercise are more effective than alternative treatments
Bronfort et al. (2001)	Systematic review	Chronic headache	Spinal manipulative therapy better than massage; lack of data to draw strong conclusions
Gonzales-Iglesias et al. (2009)	Clinical trial	Headache	Manual therapy more effective than general care for chronic tension headache
Escortell-Mayor et al. (2011)	Clinical trial	Acute neck pain	Thoracic spine manipulation plus electro- or thermo therapy more effective than modalities alone
Escortell-Mayor et al. (2011)	Clinical trial	Subacute and chronic neck pain	Manual therapy similar to a regimen of TENS use. >50% of patients had meaningful improvement after 10 treatments. Improvement was found in only 33% of patients at 6 months
Castin et al. (2011)	Clinical trial	Chronic tension-type headache	Greater reduction in headache frequency, duration, and intensity when compared to patients receiving standard care from primary physician
THORACIC SPINE			
Schiller (2001)	Clinical trial	Mechanical thoracic spine pain	Greater decrease in pain and improved lateral flexion immediately and 1 month after six treatments (included control group comparison)
LUMBAR SPINE			
Hsieh et al. (2002)	Clinical trial	Subacute low back pain	No difference in amount of improvement between manipulation, myofascial therapy, combined treatments, or completion of back school
Assendelft et al. (2003)	Meta-analysis	Acute/chronic low back pain	Manipulation not found to be superior to other treatment approaches
Hurwitz et al. (2002)	Clinical trial	Low back pain	Chiropractic care and medical care resulted in similar 6-month outcome assessment; physical therapy provided somewhat greater benefit than medical care alone
Ferreira et al. (2002)	Systematic review	Chronic low back pain	Manipulation superior to sham treatment, response similar to that with NSAIDs
Aure, Hoel Nilsen, and Vasseljen (2003)	Clinical trial	Chronic low back pain	16 treatments of manual therapy superior to exercise therapy on several outcome measures at 0-, 1-, 6-, 12-month follow-up
Kumar, Beaton, and Hughes (2013)	Systematic review	Nonspecific low back pain	Emerging body of evidence of effectiveness of massage therapy for the treatment of nonspecific low back pain

frequency and duration, but not severity, of tension headaches, although control group comparison was not made (Quinn, Chandler, and Moraska 2002).

Clinical trials addressing the efficacy of manual therapy techniques in the treatment of specific musculoskeletal conditions, as well as cost analyses, are needed to maximize health care resources and improve treatment outcomes. At present the clinician must rely heavily on personal experience and preferences in deciding if and when to include a manual technique in a plan of care and if so, which one.

TRACTION

Machines can also be used to exert a manual force on the body. Mechanical traction involves using a machine or apparatus to apply a traction force to the body (figure 18.6), whereas with manual traction the force is applied by the hands of the certified athletic trainer. Most traction treatments are administered to distract or separate segments of the cervical or lumbar spine. Research has demonstrated that vertebral separation occurs (Colachis and Strohan 1965, 1969). However, gravity reduces the separation as soon as the individual sits or stands. Thus, the efficacy of traction in the management of spinal dysfunction is questionable. The use of mechanical traction, in particular, has declined in all allied medical fields and has never been extensive in athletic training.

Although the use of mechanical traction in rehabilitation is limited, an understanding of the principles and applications of manual and mechanical traction is useful. Some cervical manual traction is necessary during joint mobilization. Traction, joint mobilization, and MFR techniques can be combined to treat cervical facet dysfunction and myofascial pain patterns. Some people with acute low back pain respond well to traction, especially when placed in a position of comfort.

Cervical Traction

Distraction of the cervical spine can benefit those with cervical facet dysfunction or cervical disc pathology, degenerative changes that narrow the intervertebral foramen and cause myofascial pain. Manual traction should be performed before mechanical traction is considered. Manual traction allows you to carefully control head position and the application of force to maximize the relief of symptoms. Manual traction also allows you to combine manual techniques. If manual traction relieves pain or radicular symptoms, you can move to mechanical traction for longer treatments that require less of your time. Take care to reproduce the position and traction force that provided the greatest relief. You cannot precisely quantify the traction force that you apply through your hands. However, a force of 15 to 25 lb will result in a perceived elongation of the cervical spine. The best approach to adjusting the mechanical force is to gradually increase it until the patient reports relief similar to that experienced with manual traction.

Manual Traction Technique

To apply cervical traction manually, place the patient in a supine position. Place your hands in a position

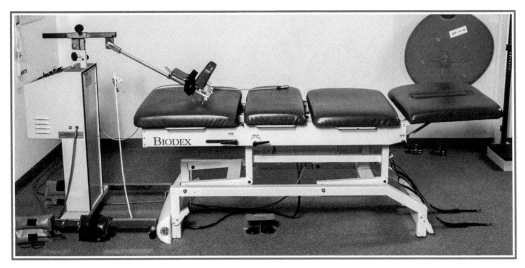

Figure 18.6 A split traction table.

that allows distraction of the cervical spine without causing discomfort (figure 18.7). Relax your hands as much as possible, because tension in your hands will result in tension and guarding by the person being treated. When this occurs, the traction forces are resisted by the muscles, defeating the purpose of the treatment. Massage or release techniques can be used first to minimize tension in and guarding by the paraspinal muscles.

Video 18.6 demonstrates manual cervical traction.

As traction is applied, the head can be positioned for greatest comfort. In neutral position, the greatest separation occurs in the upper cervical spine. As the neck is flexed to 30°, the traction forces are directed to the lower cervical spine. You can also carefully side-bend and rotate the head and neck to find the position of greatest relief. Side-bending is especially useful in relieving pressure on spinal nerves in people with degenerative changes that result in radicular symptoms.

Traction treatment does not structurally change the spine. However, the treatment can break the cycle of pain, muscle spasm, and guarded movement. Postural training and upper body reconditioning can result in long-term management of symptoms in some individuals.

Mechanical Traction Technique

In people who respond well to manual traction, mechanical traction is an option that requires less of your time. The physically active person should be positioned supine, with the neck flexed and side-bent to a position of greatest comfort. A halter or Saunder's traction device (figure 18.8) can be used to transmit the traction forces. A Saunder's device is easier to set up than the halter, especially for those who rarely apply cervical traction. To apply the device, position the person's head so that the pads align with the base of the occiput; then adjust the pads securely at the base of the occiput. If the pads are too tight, the person will complain of pain. If they are too loose, the pads will slide and pinch the ears, and little traction force will be transferred to the spine.

You can select continuous or intermittent traction. With intermittent traction, the maximum traction force is applied for a set time period (typically 30 s) and then a reduced force is applied; this is more comfortable and better tolerated in most cases. The period of reduced force, or rest period, is usually about the same duration as the length of time the maximum force is applied. The traction force during rest is usually 50% of the maximum traction force.

The amount of traction force should be gradually increased to provide a tolerable distraction. Begin with 15 lb on smaller patients and those with more pain and 25 lb on larger patients with more long-standing pain. Treatment time can be adjusted up to 20 to 30 min, depending on the patient's response. Traction can be combined with moist heat to control pain and promote muscle relaxation.

Irritation of a nerve root due to herniation of an intervertebral disc or stenosis causes pain that

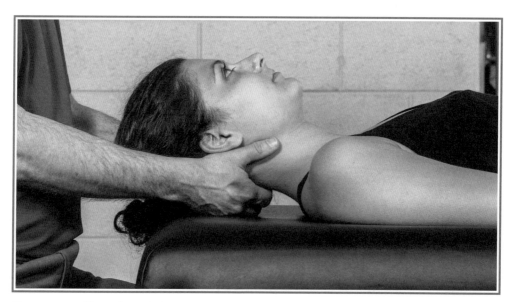

Figure 18.7   Manual cervical traction.

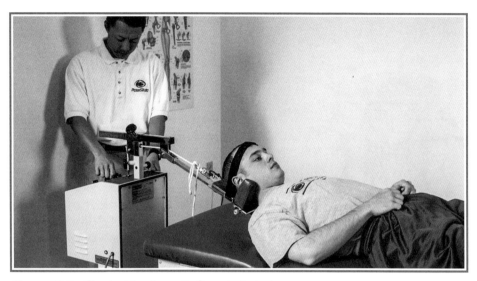

Figure 18.8 Cervical traction with Saunder's device.

radiates along the course of the nerve. This pain, referred to as radicular pain, can be excruciating. Manual and mechanical traction can relieve radicular symptoms. Often relief is temporary at first; however, short-term relief offers hope. A combination of appropriate positioning, exercise, and the frequent use of cold or superficial heat at home can reduce stress on damaged and irritated tissues and result in long-term resolution.

Precautions and Contraindications

Mechanical cervical traction is not appropriate for everyone, and it could result in catastrophic injury when applied inappropriately. In general, mechanical or manual traction is contraindicated after acute injury to the neck, the term *acute* implying that trauma caused the symptoms. Trauma to the head and neck may damage bone, ligament, and musculotendinous structures, resulting in laxity or instability. Fracture and injury to the stabilizing soft tissues must be ruled out or allowed to heal before you use traction. If traction is applied too early, the result may be greater permanent laxity and instability or, in the worst case, subluxation and injury to the spinal cord. As a rule, use manual traction rather than mechanical traction for patients with a history of traumatic injury to the cervical spine.

One extremely important consideration is the possible existence of a fracture of the dens or odontoid process of the second cervical vertebra (axis) (figure 18.9). Trauma, especially with a whiplash mechanism, can fracture the dens. Unfortunately, this fracture is not always recognized and may not be particularly painful. If traction is applied in the presence of a dens fracture, dislocation of the first or second cervical vertebra could result, an often fatal injury. The alar ligament test allows you to evaluate the integrity of the dens. The alar ligament attaches to the occiput and the dens (figure 18.10). When the head is rotated or side-bent, the pull through the alar ligament causes a palpable rotation of C2. If the dens is fractured, the leverage to rotate C2 is lost. Thus, to assess the integrity of the dens, you can palpate the spinous process of C2 and passively side-bend or rotate the person's head. If the spinous process does not move, the individual should be evaluated for fracture of the dens by the team or referring physician. You should perform the alar ligament test before using cervical traction when treating someone with a history of

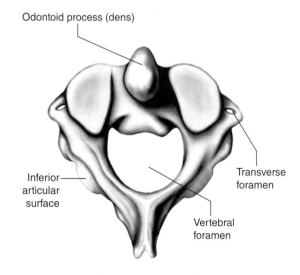

Figure 18.9 Odontoid process (dens).

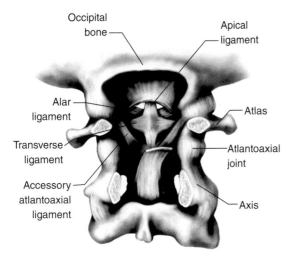

Figure 18.10   Alar ligament.

traumatic injury to the neck, especially if a whiplash mechanism was involved.

Another concern related to cervical traction involves the potential to place the head in a position that compromises the vertebral arteries. The vertebral arteries pass through the foramen in the transverse processes of the fifth to second cervical vertebrae. These vessels ascend to the circle of Willis, which distributes blood supply to a large area of the brain (figure 18.11). Rotation and extension of the head will diminish blood flow through the vertebral artery on the side to which the head is rotated. Normally this does not pose a problem, because the vertebral arteries are paired and sufficient blood supply is provided through the contralateral side. However, some people present with a compromised vertebral artery on one side. Prolonged positioning of the head can lead to an insufficient blood supply to the brain and pose the risk of stroke. To test the integrity of the vertebral arteries, extend and rotate the head (figure 18.12). If the person notes dizziness or blurred vision, or you note nystagmus or slurred speech, the vertebral artery on the opposite side may be compromised. The situation can be quickly reversed by repositioning the head in neutral and restoring flow through the vertebral artery system. A positive vertebral test is not common, yet you should always perform a vertebral test before you administer mechanical cervical traction. A positive vertebral artery test contraindicates mechanical traction where long-term positioning of the head poses a risk.

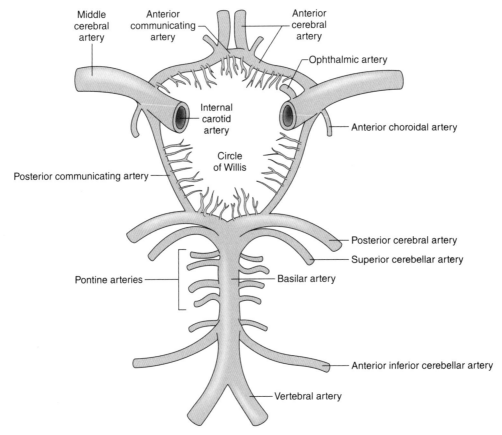

Figure 18.11   The vertebral arteries and their intracranial branches.

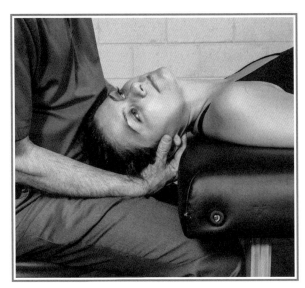

Figure 18.12 The vertebral artery test.

Traction is also contraindicated in some patients with osteoporosis and rheumatoid arthritis, conditions that may render the bone or connective soft tissues of the cervical spine unable to withstand traction forces. If you have any concerns when treating people with these conditions, consult with the referring physician. It is much better to err on the side of caution than to risk injury to the cervical region. The contraindications to cervical traction are summarized in table 18.1.

Lumbar Traction

Distraction of the lumbar spine can also be accomplished with mechanical traction. The traction forces can separate or distract the facet joints and relieve pressure on spinal nerves caused by disc injury. Most facet dysfunction, or mechanical low back pain, responds better to manual techniques such as mobilization and muscle energy.

Most physically active people with disc pathology need help to find a resting position that alleviates symptoms. Most disc injuries involve the posterior lateral aspect of the disc. Lumbar extension is believed to encourage the nucleus to migrate anteriorly, away from the spinal nerves. Thus, lying prone with a tolerable extension of the lumbar spine often alleviates the radicular symptoms associated with disc injury. The advantage of finding positional relief is that the person can control symptoms at home.

Because of the nature of managed care and success in treating low back problems without mechanical lumbar traction, it is not used often. However, it may be very useful in the management of acute conditions when manual techniques and positioning fail to bring relief.

Setup

Setting up a physically active person for lumbar traction is somewhat involved. Two wide harnesses must be applied, one above the iliac crests and one over the lower ribs. The belts must be snug or the traction force will cause the belts to slide, diminishing the traction forces at the lumbar spine. The belts can be applied with the person supine but might be much easier to apply with the person standing (figure 18.13). Once the belts are in place, you can position the individual on the traction table. Those whose symptoms are worse in sitting or improved with lying or lumbar extension should be positioned prone (figure 18.14*a*). If sitting is more comfortable or lying and lumbar extension more painful, position the patient supine with the hips and knees flexed (figure 18.14*b*).

Once the person is positioned, traction forces are administered in either a continuous or an intermittent mode. Intermittent traction (30–45 s on, 15–30 s rest) is better tolerated. Shorter "on" times (15 s) have been suggested for treating facet dysfunction and longer "on" times (60 s) for disc

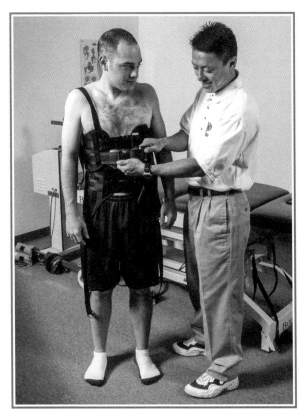

Figure 18.13 Placing lumbar traction harnesses.

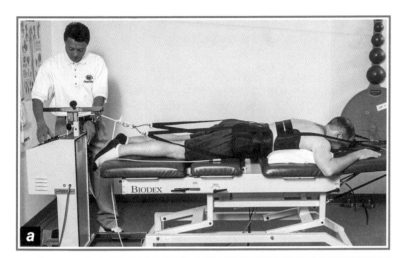

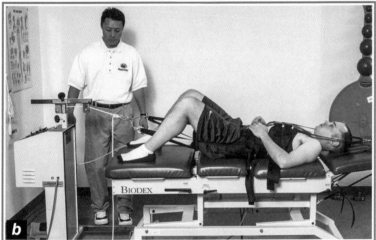

Figure 18.14 Mechanical lumbar traction: *(a)* an individual in the prone position with a pillow under the abdomen to help control lumbar spine extension, and *(b)* an individual in the supine position with hip flexed to approximately 90°.

injury. Unfortunately, little research supports the efficacy of mechanical lumbar traction or provides well-substantiated treatment parameters.

An initial traction force of 25% of body weight is a reasonable starting force. If the initial force is tolerated, increase the traction force up to 50% of body weight. Treatment times usually range from 10 to 20 min, depending upon the nature of the problem and the response to treatment.

Precautions and Contraindications

There are fewer contraindications for lumbar traction (summarized in table 18.1) than for cervical traction. Pregnancy, hiatal hernia, and advanced osteoporosis are absolute contraindications. Fractures and medical conditions, such as cancer, that affect the integrity of the connective

tissues also contraindicate mechanical traction. Occasionally patients experience a significant increase in pain during traction, in which case traction must be terminated. This is particularly common in persons suffering from internal disc derangement.

In daily practice, practical considerations such as belt adjustment and an inability to tolerate treatment affect decisions about the application of mechanical lumbar traction more often than do absolute contraindications.

The harness used to apply lumbar traction is adjustable; however, it is often difficult to fasten the belts snugly on very thin patients, and often the belts cannot be fitted on obese individuals. Furthermore, some people experience claustrophobia when the belts are tightened to prevent sliding.

INTERMITTENT COMPRESSION

Intermittent compression involves the use of a pneumatic device that intermittently inflates a sleeve around an injured joint or limb. Intermittent compression devices are used to reduce edema and posttraumatic swelling. In athletic training, the primary cause of fluid accumulation in the tissues is trauma. Chapter 4 reviewed the mechanism for posttraumatic swelling and covered the role of the lymphatic system in resolving swelling. Elevation of an injured extremity and contraction of the skeletal muscles can reduce swelling. Intermittent compression may speed the resolution of posttraumatic swelling in some situations. The limited evidence, as discussed further on, does not support the use of intermittent compression in the management of some common musculoskeletal injuries.

Therapeutic modalities that relieve pain and muscle spasm—followed by active exercise—reduce swelling more effectively than does intermittent compression. The exercise activity must be well tolerated and must not cause further tissue damage. However, simple active range of motion exercises within the limits of pain are sufficient to increase lymphatic drainage over that in a resting state. Thus, intermittent compression is better reserved for treating complicated problems such as persistent swelling and wounds caused by venous insufficiency.

Setup

Intermittent compression is easy to administer. A compression stocking is applied to the limb to be treated (figure 18.15). Once the stocking is in place, the intermittent compression unit is adjusted for duty cycle and maximum pressure. No single duty cycle has been established as the most effective. Inflation times of 30 to 40 s are well tolerated when interspersed with 20 to 30 s off or deflation periods.

There is some disagreement about the optimal inflation pressure. Manufacturers have developed guidelines for various conditions (Fond and Hecox 1994). The maximum pressure recommended in treating posttraumatic edema is 50 to 90 mmHg (Fond and Hecox 1994; Hooker 1998). A setting just below diastolic blood pressure is well tolerated by physically active people and appears to reduce edema. Once the duty cycle and pressure have been

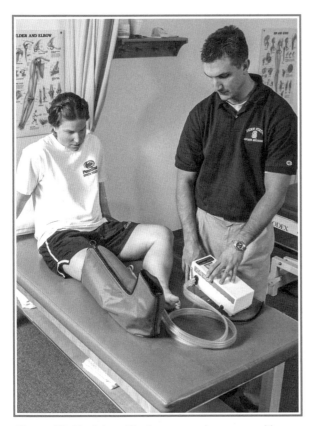

Figure 18.15 Intermittent compression pump with sequential air filling.

set, the injured person remains with the affected limb elevated throughout a 20 to 30 min treatment.

Contraindications

There are few contraindications for intermittent compression (table 18.1). Certainly all situations in which tissue movement is restricted, such as healing fractures and gross joint instability, would contraindicate intermittent compression. Infection, thrombophlebitis, pulmonary edema, and congestive heart failure also contraindicate intermittent compression.

Intermittent compression is a relatively safe, passive approach to reducing posttraumatic edema. However, setup is somewhat time-consuming, and the patient is not actively engaged in the rehabilitation process. Thus, the injured person will likely improve more quickly by performing pain-free active exercises to encourage lymphatic drainage during treatment in the clinic or athletic training room, and three to four times daily at home, as long as the swelling persists.

ARE TRACTION AND INTERMITTENT COMPRESSION EFFECTIVE THERAPIES?

Clinical trials of traction have involved patients with pain in the lumbar and cervical regions. Clarke et al. (2005), Beurskens et al. (1995, 1997), and Pal et al. (1986) concluded that traction was ineffective in the treatment of patients with low back pain. These investigators had follow-up as long as 6 months posttreatment. Not all the evidence is unsupportive of the use of traction. Fritz et al. (2007) presented data indicating that there is a subgroup of patients likely to benefit from traction. These patients present with leg symptoms, signs of nerve root compression, and peripheralization of symptoms with lumbar spine extension or a crossed straight leg raise. Van der Heijden et al. (1995) reported that high-dose traction (44% of body weight) was more effective in reducing back pain and improving function than low-dose (19% of body weight) continuous lumbar traction at 5 and 9 weeks posttreatment. The sample size for the study was small (12 and 13 subjects per group), and the differences reported did not reach statistical significance. Furthermore, the treatments were not compared to rest or active interventions.

Similarly, Meszaros et al. (2000) reported that 5 min of static lumbar traction applied in supine at 30% and 60% body weight increased the pain-free range of a straight leg raise immediately after treatment in patients with back pain. However, the duration of this change in motion was not established.

Cervical traction may be effective in the management of patients with radicular symptoms associated with cervical dysfunction. Moeti and Marchetti's (2001) case series on patients with radicular symptoms reported complete resolution of pain in 7 of 11 patients with symptom duration of less than 12 weeks but in only 1 of 4 with longer-duration symptoms. Constantoyannis et al. (2002) came to similar conclusions in a series of four patients. Swezey, Swezey, and Warner (1999) reported that home over-the-door traction devices were effective in helping a large percentage of patients classified on the Quebec Task Force of Whiplash Associated Disorders Cohort Study scale. None of these studies involved comparison to control groups. Two reports comparing cervical traction to no-treatment controls provide conflicting results. Zylbergold and Piper (1985) reported that treatment with intermittent traction over 6 weeks was more effective than no traction in reducing pain and improving motion in patients with cervical spine disorders. Klaber-Moffett, Hughes, and Griffiths (1990) found that similar patients treated with traction "improved slightly more" than no-traction controls. While the design of this study was of high quality, traction forces were limited to 6 to 15 lb. The use of greater traction forces might have yielded different results.

The use of intermittent compression has been studied in a variety of patients, including those with lymphedema after mastectomy and venous insufficiency. However, few studies could be located that addressed the efficacy of intermittent compression in the management of musculoskeletal conditions. Stockle et al. (1997) reported that intermittent compression reduced postoperative swelling more effectively than a cold compression unit or periodic ice bag application in patients suffering foot and ankle trauma. Airaksinen et al. (1991) reported that intermittent compression decreased lower limb edema after 6 to 12 weeks of cast immobilization in patients with leg fractures. However, this intervention was not compared with active exercise. Griffin et al. (1990) reported decreases in hand edema immediately after intermittent compression in patients suffering from trauma to the hand. Measurements were obtained only immediately after 30 min of treatment.

The timing of measurements is important. Tsang et al. (2001; Tsang, Hertel, and Denegar 2003) reported that intermittent compression decreased effusion at the ankle after ankle sprains. The reduction in effusion, however, was very brief. Within 5 min of weight bearing, limb volumes had returned to pretreatment levels. Rucinski et al. (1991) found that intermittent compression increased effusion after ankle sprain.

At this time there is a lack of evidence to recommend the routine use of either lumbar traction or intermittent compression in the treatment of musculoskeletal conditions. When contraindications and precautions are observed, these interventions might be beneficial adjuncts to a comprehensive plan of care in selected circumstances. The certified athletic trainer should, however, consider the time required and the cost of treatment before applying these and other interventions for which much of the evidence suggests that treatment outcomes do not improve. The evidence for management of radicular symptoms of cervical origins is somewhat more favorable. Certainly when treatments can be safely rendered through low-cost home devices, the use of cervical traction may be an important component of a comprehensive treatment strategy.

SUMMARY

This chapter covers a range of topics that are related to applying mechanical forces on the body for therapeutic effects. Much of the chapter is devoted to various manual therapy techniques, including massage, myofascial release, strain–counterstrain, muscle energy, and joint mobilization. The neurological response, a review of afferent and efferent innervation of intrafusal and extrafusal muscle fibers, and the convex–concave rule (which guides joint mobilization) are presented. The application of manual and mechanical traction techniques used to treat dysfunction in the cervical and lumbar spine is discussed as well as the role of intermittent compression in the treatment of musculoskeletal injuries. The chapter concludes with a discussion of exercise as a repair stimulus. The concepts of mechanobiology and tissue repair introduced in chapters 4 and 16 are reinforced with specific reference to the treatment of Achilles tendinopathy. Safety (especially in the application of traction to the spine) and contraindications for all treatments are emphasized.

KEY CONCEPTS AND REVIEW

1. *Discuss the potential benefits of using manual therapy techniques in rehabilitation.*

Because manual therapies require hands-on treatments, they offer time for conversation and an opportunity to develop open communication and mutual understanding. Manual therapies offer additional approaches to relieving pain and muscle spasm and restoring range of motion.

2. *Describe massage, myofascial release, strain–counterstrain, muscle energy, and joint mobilization.*

Massage is a collection of techniques that involve rubbing or kneading part of the body. Myofascial release (MFR) is similar to massage in that the certified athletic trainer uses the hands to influence the connective tissues and neural input. However, MFR is directed at specific trigger points and areas of fascial tension and restriction. Strain–counterstrain involves placing the body into a position of greatest comfort, thus relieving pain by reducing or arresting inappropriate proprioceptive activity. Joint mobilization is used to restore intrinsic joint motion or arthrokinetics. Using the convex–concave rule, you can apply joint mobilization techniques to identify and treat motion restriction resulting from the loss of normal gliding between bones during rotation at a joint. Muscle energy techniques are manual procedures that involve active contraction of the individual's muscles against a counterforce in a specific treatment position. Muscle energy techniques can be used to stretch tight muscles and fascia, strengthen weakened muscle, or mobilize restricted joints.

3. *Describe the afferent and efferent innervation of intrafusal and extrafusal muscle fibers and the relationship between the gamma and alpha motor neurons.*

Muscle is made up of contractile, extrafusal fibers and sensory, intrafusal fibers called muscle spindles. The contractile fibers are innervated by alpha motor neurons. When an impulse is transmitted down an alpha motor neuron, all of the extrafusal muscle fibers it innervates contract. When many alpha motor neurons are stimulated, many extrafusal fibers contract, and the muscle generates force. The length and tension of a muscle are perceived by the muscle spindles. Gamma afferent fibers send information from the spindle to the central nervous system. The length of a muscle spindle must be constantly adjusted in order for it to optimally sense changes in muscle length and tension. The gamma efferent motor nerves innervate the spindle to adjust the resting length.

4. *Apply the convex–concave rule in performing joint mobilization.*

Joint mobilization is used to restore normal joint arthrokinematics. In normal joint function, when a convex surface, such as the head of the humerus, moves on a concave surface, such as the glenoid, the convex surface glides in the direction opposite to the direction of roll. For example, during abduction of the arm, the head of the humerus rolls upward but glides downward. If a concave surface such as the tibial plateau moves on a convex surface, such as the femoral condyles, roll and glide occur in the same direction. For example, during knee flexion, the tibia rolls and glides posteriorly.

5. *Describe the manual and mechanical traction techniques used to treat cervical spine dysfunction.*

The cervical spine can be distracted manually or with the use of a traction device. Manual traction offers the advantage of finding the position and traction force that provide the greatest relief. Mechanical traction, with the recipient lying supine, can be accomplished with a traction harness or a Saunder's traction device.

6. *Identify contraindications for manual therapies and mechanical traction.*

Symptoms of organic diseases such as cancer must be followed up before treatment with any modality, including manual therapies. Massage is contraindicated if infection or skin breakdown or disease is present. Release techniques should not be used during acute inflammation or shortly after a fracture or surgery. Caution is advised if the recipient is pregnant or has a joint replacement or joint instability. Strain–counterstrain should be discontinued if pain increases, and it should be used with caution after a fracture or if a joint is unstable. Muscle energy is contraindicated in those with a recent fracture or when there is joint instability or a joint fusion. Infection, joint instability, recent fracture, and a "bone-on-bone" end-feel contraindicate joint mobilization; also, mobilization of the cervical spine is contraindicated in the presence of advanced rheumatoid arthritis. Both muscle energy and joint mobilization are contraindicated in the presence of bony instability and advanced osteoporosis. There are several contraindications for cervical traction, including a positive vertebral artery or alar ligament test, acute neck injury including fracture and joint instability, advanced rheumatoid arthritis, bone cancer, and advanced osteoporosis. Cervical traction should be discontinued if pain increases or radicular symptoms are exacerbated by treatment. Lumbar traction is contraindicated by pregnancy, claustrophobia, internal disc derangement, fractures and sprains with joint instability, bone cancer, advanced osteoporosis, and hiatal hernia. Lumbar traction should also be discontinued if pain is increased or radicular symptoms are exacerbated by treatment.

7. *Describe the mechanical traction techniques used to treat lumbar spine dysfunction.*

Traction to the lumbar spine can be administered with the patient in prone or supine position. If symptoms are reduced when the person is sitting, as is often the case with foraminal or spinal stenosis, having the person lie supine with the hip flexed is preferred. If symptoms decrease when the spine is extended, as is the case when the person lies prone, the person should be treated in prone position. A traction force of one-fourth to one-half of body weight with intervals of traction (e.g., 40 s) and rest (e.g., 20 s) is generally recommended.

8. *Describe the application of, and contraindications for, intermittent compression therapy.*

Intermittent compression involves the use of a pneumatic device that intermittently inflates a sleeve around an injured joint or limb. Intermittent compression facilitates lymphatic drainage, which will reduce swelling. Intermittent compression should not be applied in the presence of thrombophlebitis, infection, acute fractures, or in cases in which the person has pulmonary edema or congestive heart failure.

9. *Describe how the principles of mechanobiology might apply to manual therapies.*

Movement results in the transduction of mechanical forces that affect and can help regulate cell function. The mechanical forces exerted through manual techniques such as deep friction massage up-regulate cellular processes that regulate repair. In a similar manner, mechanical signaling triggers depolarization of afferent nerves, which can reduce pain and muscle spasm.

part VIII

Putting It All Together

Our intent in writing this book was to go far beyond the description, application, procedures, and physiological effects of therapeutic modalities included in plans of care for musculoskeletal injuries. Although there are commonalities among patients and health conditions, each case is made unique by the patients' characteristics, medical histories, beliefs, experiences, and goals. Clinicians therefore must consider many factors in developing a recommended plan of care. In part VII, several cases are described to help you to integrate information and recommend treatments that are founded in a knowledge of human physiology and supported to the extent possible by existing clinical research. The rationale underlying the choices of treatments provides a template for making decisions in clinical practice.

Case Scenarios

Throughout this text, we have continually emphasized the importance of adopting an evidence-based approach to clinical health care practice. Gone are the days when clinicians do something "because that's how they were taught," utilizing treatment techniques without consideration of efficacy or purpose. The contemporary health care provider stays current on the best research evidence and combines this knowledge with clinical expertise. Each patient is treated as a whole rather than just the physical injury; patients' emotional and behavioral responses are monitored as they are integrated into the development of the rehabilitation plan.

The task of selecting interventions, whether therapeutic exercises or modalities, is purposeful and goal oriented. Consideration must be given to timing (tissue healing processes), patient values (short- and long-term goals), physiological responses (indications and contraindications), and clinician experience (operational parameters). A therapeutic modality should not be viewed as a stand-alone treatment, but rather as a directed component of the rehabilitation program.

This approach of "thought preceding action" is quintessential *critical thinking* and is essential to the success of the modern clinician. The purpose of the following modules is to stimulate thought by presenting various challenges in different patient injury scenarios. There is no one absolute or correct answer, and therefore no answer key is provided. In addition, we will challenge you to demonstrate proficiency in the clinical application of varying modalities.

Neck Pain

A 28-year-old female tennis coach and player is referred for care, complaining of neck pain following a motor vehicle accident 6 days ago. She was at a complete stop when her car was hit from behind. She was transported to the emergency department at a local hospital. She was discharged after being evaluated for injuries. A neurological screen was normal, and concussion assessment and diagnostic imaging were negative. She complains of pain (6 on a scale of 10 with walking and standing) and muscle spasm in her neck and upper back, and intermittent headaches made worse with prolonged sitting and exercise and relieved by oral over-the-counter medication and lying down. She states at times she gets pain that radiates down her right arm.

She states that she is married and has no children. She works as a college tennis coach and director of the campus tennis center. Her medical history is unremarkable other than having sustained a right sprained ankle in high school and having wisdom teeth removed.

On presentation she denies lightheadedness, concentration and memory deficits, tinnitus or vision disturbances, and a history of neck injuries. On examination, the patient's head is slightly tilted to the left side. The patient has limited active and passive rotation and side-bending to the right side and painful end-range extension. She has tenderness to palpation along the right cervical paraspinal muscles. Upper quarter scan for sensory, strength, and reflex deficits is normal. Physical examination reveals restricted left side-glide at C5-C6, and the patient is evaluated as suffering from a flexed, left rotated, and side-bent facet with soft tissue pain and muscle spasm.

The patient complains that she has difficulty raising her right arm overhead and that her neck and upper back pain increase with prolonged sitting, driving, and lifting and carrying.

The forces involved in motor vehicle accidents can cause catastrophic injuries. The whiplash mechanism of injury may result in fracture, sprain, and muscle strain. The medical history, history of the current condition, and medical and physical examinations conducted in this case provide assurance that serious structural damage has been avoided. A thorough examination and evaluation of all pertinent information is needed before proceeding with a rehabilitation plan of care, especially in conditions involving the spine.

The first step in developing a rehabilitation plan of care is the development of a problem list. It is usually best to build a problem list around the impairments, functional limitations, and participation restrictions identified in the evaluation of the case. From the problem list, mutually agreeable short-term goals can be developed and a goal-directed application of therapeutic modalities, manual therapy, and exercise developed.

What are the problems identified in this case?

Impairments

Pain

Loss of cervical range of motion

Headache

Functional limitations

Reaching overhead and prolonged sitting/driving

Participation restrictions

Unable to play tennis or coach effectively due to pain and loss of motion

Has difficulty with management responsibilities due to poor tolerance of sitting

The clinician has several options to recommend for the problems listed. Pain and muscle spasm could be treated with periodic cold or superficial heat. TENS could be used as needed for the same purposes.

What would you do?

A decision on the treatment needs to be based on any contraindications for an intervention, the current condition, the patient's preferences, the clinician's experiences, and existing clinical research. After ruling out contraindications to the treatment options and conferring with the patient about the ability to control pain with oral medications, it is decided to treat her with massage to decrease pain and muscle spasm before performing joint mobilization to restore range of motion. The patient states that a hot shower is soothing and that she has access to superficial heat. She demonstrates a substantial increase in cervical range of motion after the initial treatment. She is instructed in active range of motion exercises and agrees with a plan of 20 to 30 min of superficial heating as needed for relief of pain and spasm and a four-times-per-day regimen of active range of motion, which is also to be performed after heat application. Over two subsequent visits she reports the resolution of pain at rest other than mild aching and stiffness upon rising, and she demonstrates full cervical range of motion. Postural and functional exercises are introduced to increase tolerance to daily activities and return to coaching. Three and a half weeks after her accident she is able to work a normal day, drive, and play tennis for up to an hour without limitations. She is discharged to continue with a postural and tennis function exercise program.

This case illustrates some of the complexities of developing a plan of care. There is not a single correct approach to meeting the needs of many patients. The first mandate is to do no harm. The clinician and patient must then decide which problems are most concerning, discuss the options, and agree on a plan. Once short-term goals are achieved, the intervention progresses. Modalities used to relieve pain and muscle spasm are replaced by exercises aimed at addressing functional limitations and participation restrictions.

Case Scenario 2

Elbow Injury

A 23-year-old graduate student and avid golfer is referred for care due to a lingering loss of elbow range of motion and aching (graded 1 to 2 on a scale of 10) after exercise, especially golf, in his left elbow. He sustained a radial head fracture/dislocation while in a bicycling accident 5 months ago. He reports that the fracture was considered stable and he wore an elbow brace for a few weeks after the injury. He initiated therapy to restore motion and strength while at school but did not continue after graduating 1 month after the injury.

The patient is a physically fit young man. His medical history is unremarkable beyond seasonal allergies and two left ankle sprains sustained while playing high school basketball. Physical examination reveals normal sensation and strength throughout the upper extremities except for weakness secondary to pain at the end range of active left elbow extension. The patient lacks 17° of elbow extension and 5° of flexion on the left in comparison to his dominant right side.

The patient's primary concern is the impact of his injury on his ability to perform resistance exercises and play golf. He states that he has not quit participation but feels limited.

What are the problems identified in this case?

Impairments

Pain

Loss of elbow range of motion

Mild postexercise pain (1–2/10)

Functional limitations

Reaching and actively extending left elbow

Participation restrictions

Perceived limitations with participating in golf and resistance training

Injuries to the elbow are often challenging to manage. Some patients will require surgery in order to stabilize fractures but rarely to repair ligaments, which heal through the mechanisms described in chapter 4. Many patients, however, will experience a loss of range of motion with functional limitations. Participation restrictions are variable and depend on the extent of functional loss and the demands of the activity. Restoring motion after injury or surgery at the elbow is often challenging due to the robust repair of the capsular ligaments.

The problem list in these cases is usually short. The primary goal is restoration of motion followed by activity-specific therapeutic exercises. What is the most effective means of restoring motion?

The clinician has options that include manual therapy and active range of motion exercises. These interventions may be combined with superficial heating, although these treatments may prove ineffective. Are there treatments that offer more promise of effectiveness? A search of PubMed with the terms "elbow" AND "range of motion" AND "mobilization" identifies a case series report (Draper 2014) that suggests a combination of deep heating with pulsed short wave diathermy (PSWD) and joint mobilization is often effective in restoring elbow range of motion, even in very difficult cases. Since ultrasound is also a deep heating modality, might that be an option? A search with the terms "ultrasound" AND "range of motion" AND "mobilization" identifies another report by Draper (2010) that involved addressing wrist motion restrictions using therapeutic ultrasound and joint mobilization. The parameters of the treatments are described in both reports.

What would you do?

As noted in Case Scenario 1, a decision on the treatment needs to be first based on any contraindications for an intervention. No contraindications to modality application, manual therapy, or exercise exist in this case. Clinical experience suggests that manual therapy and exercise alone may not yield the desired results. The best available literature offers evidence that the addition of a deep heating modality may facilitate success. The patient is available to receive two or three treatments per week over the next 3 weeks and agrees with the plan of care. If PSWD is available, that would likely be the treatment of choice, as the device heats a larger area of involved tissue, and there is evidence for success in managing the elbow. If PSWD is not available, therapeutic ultrasound offers an alternative. Care must be taken to use a large enough sound head to heat the anterior elbow joint capsule. Since tissue cools fairly quickly, especially following ultrasound, joint mobilization is initiated immediately after heating. Finally, the elbow is positioned in extension and an ice bag is applied as suggested by Draper (2014). The patient is instructed in a regimen of active range of motion and stretching to be completed four times daily and scheduled for five additional treatments.

This case illustrates some of the additional complexities of developing a plan of care. Clinical experience with managing lost elbow extension after injury or surgery is integrated with available research to recommend a combination of deep tissue heating with PSWD or ultrasound, manual therapy, ice application, and a home exercise program. Based on the existing literature, reassessment is planned after six treatment sessions. Once range of motion is restored, a gradual return to resistance training and golf activities is completed over 3 weeks, and the patient is discharged to a home program with unrestricted activity.

Case Scenario 3

Ankle Injury

An 18-year-old male basketball athlete comes into the clinic complaining of pain on the right lateral ankle. He reports the injury occurred a few days ago as he was rebounding a ball when he landed on the opponent's foot. Upon landing he states he heard a "pop" and noticed immediate swelling. He states he has localized pain over the lateral malleolus. The athlete states he has trouble weight bearing and walking but is able to walk five steps without assistance. On examination you notice localized ecchymosis and edema over the area of pain. There is no deformity on the ankle. On palpation the patient has tenderness over the anterior talofibular ligament and calcaneofibular ligaments. There is no tenderness to palpation at the base of the fifth metatarsal, at the anterior distal fibula, or over the tarsal navicular. The athlete has increased laxity and pain in his ankle with the anterior drawer test and talar tilt test.

The patient is a freshman on the collegiate basketball team and indicates this is his first injury ever. He is concerned the injury will affect his position on the depth chart and diminish his playing time with the start of the season in a few weeks. He asks if he can be issued a brace or have his ankle taped to allow him to get back to practice. He demonstrates he can walk and jump on the ankle, but upon observing his functional performance you note he has established an antalgic gait by ambulating flat-footed. Upon further examination the patient is guarded and apprehensive with non–weight bearing active range of motion and passive weight-bearing range of motion.

What are the problems identified in this case?

Impairments

Pain

Edema

Ecchymosis

Functional limitations

Altered gait

Non-weight bearing and weight-bearing movements

Participation restrictions

Unable to practice with the team due to pain

This case describes a very common occurrence in the traditional athletic training clinic and illustrates the importance of appreciating the entire patient and not just focusing on the physical injury. The unique circumstances of competitive environments such as organized athletics often lure both the patient and the clinician to seek a quick fix or a cure-all. In addition to adopting evidence-based practices, health care providers should acknowledge the natural course of tissue healing and try to provide the best environments for healing to occur. The use of prophylactic bracing may address the immediate functional limits, but it will not effectively complement the tissue healing process.

After the clinician discusses the situation with the patient and addresses his concerns about his status on the roster, they establish goals that follow the course of tissue healing. Pain is identified as the primary cause of guarding and apprehension and the subsequent limitations in movement.

What would you do?

There is enough evidence to support the use of cold therapy for modulating pain and facilitating functional improvements in an environment of arthrogenic muscle inhibition (AMI). Decreased conductivity of nociceptive fibers will diminish the pain-muscle spasm cycle and allow the introduction of motion to the affected area. Regardless of the form of motion (e.g., massage, passive or active range of motion), movement will better facilitate the reduction of swelling, guide fibroblast activity, and direct appropriate alignment of collagen.

Cryotherapy can be applied by various media and can integrate tissue motion and elevation. Application protocols vary between the different forms of cold; therefore the clinician should be aware of established recommendations for parameters such as temperature and duration.

How often should cold therapy be applied?

While the use of cryotherapy in such cases is common, there is insufficient evidence to support improved treatment outcomes. Available reviews indicate that cryotherapy is effective in reducing pain, and it may influence recovery after ankle sprains and knee surgery, but evidence for its ability to expedite recovery is not compelling. We encourage clinicians to avoid routinely applying cold therapy (or other modalities) based on what they were taught and the practice habits they have developed. Instead, they must evaluate each patient to determine the status of the injury and the healing process at each treatment interaction. For example, if the patient does not report pain, there is no need to use cryotherapy.

Case Scenario 4

Rib Pain

A 19-year-old football player complains of pain over the right sixth and seventh ribs after being involved in a tackle during a game. On-field examination reveals that he is medically stable. There is pain to palpation and to anterior-posterior rib cage compression. He reports more pain with deep inspiration. Diagnostic imaging is performed at the stadium, and the examining physician concludes the player has suffered nondisplaced, stable fractures of the fifth and sixth ribs. Although the athlete is offered medications for pain, he indicates that he prefers not to use any medications.

What are the problems identified in this case?

Impairments

Pain

Functional limitations

Loss of active trunk range of motion secondary to pain

Pain at end of range of deep inspiration

Are there other options for pain management to offer this athlete?

What would you do?

The use of a compression wrap may provide comfort, and cold application may relieve pain, although it can be quite uncomfortable over the trunk. TENS using the parameters described in chapter 8 to stimulate A-beta afferent nerves may be the best option. Oncel et al. (2002) concluded that TENS was more effective than NSAID or placebo in patients with uncomplicated minor rib fractures. The patient agrees to try using the TENS device after learning that there are no known risks or side effects of treatment.

A portable TENS device is adjusted to provide 80 μs pulses at a rate of 100 pulses per second (pps). Four electrodes are placed on the skin over the lateral aspect of the right fifth and sixth ribs. The patient is advised to let the medical team know when he perceives a tingle. He is then asked to adjust the stimulus to the highest comfortable level without eliciting a muscle twitch.

How long should this patient wear the TENS device?

There is no limit for the use of TENS. This patient is instructed in how to adjust the stimulus when the tingling diminishes. He is told he can turn the device off if he is comfortable but to use the device as much as needed. He is instructed not to use the device while bathing but is asked to use it when he goes to bed. It is suggested that he will be more com-fortable if he does not lie flat and that sleeping in a recliner may be the best position in which to rest. He is told to report to the athletic training clinic the following morning.

Upon return, the patient reports aching pain over the fractured ribs rated 3 out of 10 on a visual analog pain scale. He indicates he slept fairly com-fortably, awakening once to use the bathroom, and needed about 15 min to fall back asleep. Pain with deep inspiration persists but has not worsened. A treatment plan of continued use of TENS for pain control will continue as needed. After 3 days the patient reports 1 out of 10 pain at rest and with deep inspiration. TENS is discontinued and a gradual progression of activity is instituted. He is cleared to begin regular upper body resistance training after 2 weeks but misses the final two games of his season.

TENS can be an effective treatment or adjunct to the management of pain associated with fractures and other acute musculoskeletal injuries. The very low risk associated with treatment and moderate evidence of effectiveness are considerations when weighing plan-of-care decisions. In this case, avail-able evidence, the patient's preferences, and the expe-rience of the care team were combined in choosing this plan of care.

Case Scenario 5

ACL Reconstruction Surgery

A recent series of athlete-patients recovering from anterior cruciate ligament reconstruction surgery at a university athletic training clinic sparked dis-cussion of the potential benefit of adding neuro-muscular nerve stimulation of the quadriceps to a standardized rehabilitation plan of care. Loss of neuromuscular control of the quadriceps in patients suffering from knee pain and swelling, especially those recovering from surgery, is well recognized. A review of the available literature suggested potential benefit, so a protocol described by Fitzgerald et al. (2003) was adopted.

One of the patients in the clinic underwent a right hamstring autograft reconstruction 12 days ago. She is comfortable walking without crutches and demonstrates a normal walking gait at a moderate pace. Active knee range of motion is measured at +3° extension, 130° flexion compared to +5° and 140° on the uninvolved knee. She can activate her quadriceps and complete a straight leg raise, complete a resisted knee extension exercise from 70° to 40° flexion with 7 lb of resistance, pedal a stationary bike comfortably, and leg-press 60 lb on a leg press machine.

What are the problems identified in this case?

Impairments

Mild pain with activity (1 to 2 out of 10)

Likely impaired neuromuscular control

Functional limitations

Running

Jumping

Rapid change in direction

Participation restrictions

Unable to participate in or train for skiing

What would you do?

Given this patient's desire to return to high-level athletic activity, it is essential that she be able to rapidly generate large forces. What would you tell the patient about why the treatment is being recommended and what to expect during treatment? Describe how you would position the patient for treatment, place the electrodes on the leg, and adjust the parameters of the TENS device.

The application of neuromuscular stimulation has been suggested to improve quadriceps function and foster progression of activity during the first 12 to 16 weeks of rehabilitation. While the sensation of having muscles contract without volitional effort can be discomforting to some patients, there is a very, very low risk of harm. Injury to the anterior cruciate ligament and surgery to repair it result in arthrogenic inhibition of the quadriceps (see chapter 9). The use of neuromuscular electrical stimulation can reverse the inhibition and accelerate the restoration of normal quadriceps activity.

Thus, the goal of treatment is to restore neuromuscular control of the quadriceps.

After the patient consents to the treatment, she is placed supine on a treatment table with her right leg extended. The available device differs from the one used by Fitzgerald et al. (2003) but allows adjustment of a biphasic square wave to deliver a 200 µs pulse at a rate of 70 pps. A 2 s ramp and a 15 s on, 50 s off duty cycle are selected. With electrodes placed over the vastus medialis and lateralis, the device is turned on and the amplitude adjusted. The initial contractions are not very forceful, but after five cycles the patient can tolerate a strong, visible contraction of the quadriceps. During the first session a total of 15 repetitions are completed. The treatment is completed with 10 strong contractions in conjunction with the rehabilitation plan of care twice each week for 5 weeks. The patient progresses well in her recovery and is cleared to resume running 14 weeks after surgery. She returns to playing lacrosse the following season, approximately 9 months after being injured.

Did the addition of neuromuscular electrical nerve stimulation accelerate this patient's recovery?

A positive (or negative) long-term outcome in a single patient cannot be confidently attributed to any single factor. There are many facets to a rehabilitation plan of care and considerable variation in individual responses to many interventions. In this case, the best available literature suggests that the addition of neuromuscular electrical nerve stimulation is likely to have been beneficial and very unlikely to have been harmful. Thus given the patient's desires, the experience of the clinicians involved, and the best available evidence, the addition of neuromuscular electrical nerve stimulation to the plan was justified.

Case Scenario 6

Achilles Pain

A 30-year-old male recreational basketball player presents to the clinic reporting long-standing (since college) intermittent right Achilles pain. He experienced an acute exacerbation of symptoms since his last pick-up game 7 days ago. Symptoms include posterior ankle stiffness, especially upon rising in the morning, which causes him to limp until he "warms up," as well as pain in the Achilles tendon made worse with walking and stair climbing that he rates 5 out of 10 on a VAS. Examination reveals midportion and insertional Achilles pain and a thick nodular tendon upon palpation. Pain is reproduced upon unilateral heel lifting, and a 5° loss of ankle dorsiflexion is present. Diagnostic ultrasound shows a large, diffuse hypoechoic region in the midportion along with vascular ingrowth in the anterior midportion of the tendon. At the insertion, focal hypoechoic lesions and tissue disorganization are evident. He is currently unable to participate in athletic activities or exercise and has a mildly antalgic gait due to decreased pushoff.

What are the problems identified in this case?

Impairments

Pain

Swelling

Loss of ankle range of motion

Functional limitations

Stair climbing

Walking

Participation restrictions

Unable to participate in athletic activities or exercise

What would you do?

Chronic Achilles tendinopathy represents a degenerative condition that can have acute reactive periods in which peritendinous swelling, pain, and stiffness are exacerbated. During this acute "reactive" period, active rest is advocated in which gentle flexibility exercises and avoidance of pain provocation may be warranted (Cook and Purdam 2009; McCreesh 2013). During this time, active ROM exercises, gentle passive stretching, and soft tissue mobilization (STM) are indicated. Cryotherapy may be applied acutely after pain-provoking activity for symptomatic relief, but the degenerative, noninflammatory nature of tendinopathy typically does not benefit from cold. As tendinopathy has a notoriously poor pain response, the active rest period during an acute reactive period should not last longer than 1 to 2 weeks.

Treatment with eccentric loading is effective and may be performed through pain with the caveat that pain should not persist or get worse after exercise (Alfredson et al. 1998). After 1 week of active rest and STM, eccentric heel drops are initiated twice daily, three sets of 15 reps, straight and bent knee. Progression of external resistance as tolerated is achieved through a weighted vest, backpack, or heel raise machine. An eccentric exercise program has been shown to reduce symptoms in 6 to 12 weeks and often allows for a return to activity (Mafi, Lorentzon, and Alfredson 2001). Eccentric exercise is superior to other modes of exercise. After 12 weeks, 82% reported satisfaction and return to activity compared to 36% of patients training concentrically. That exercise is superior to doing nothing should be no surprise

with a 62% success rate compared to 24% of patients who adopt a wait-and-see approach. Unfortunately, progress is often slow, and roughly 20% of patients report an inability to return to activity on long-term (8-year) follow-up (Rompe, Nafe, and Furia 2007). Although eccentric exercise is effective, not everyone will respond.

Insertional Achilles tendinopathy is not as successfully treated with eccentric exercise as mid-substance tendinopathy (Alfredson et al. 1998). Extracorporeal shock wave therapy (ESWT) and low-level laser therapy (LLLT) have been explored and show some success, primarily with chronic recalcitrant cases and when combined with a loading program (Kearney and Costa 2010; Bjordal, Lopes-Martins, and Iversen 2006). The recommended parameters for ESWT include 1,500 to 2,000 impulses with energy flux density ranging from 0.08 to 0.4 mJ/mm^2. Dosage is typically four sessions spread 1 week apart (van der Worp et al. 2013). ESWT is often suggested when loading alone has failed, prior to surgical intervention. LLLT may be effective when recommended dosages are used. Typically, LLLT is applied in three locations along the tendinopathic Achilles tendon with a wavelength of 830 nm, 3 J per point at a power density ranging from 5 to 100 mW/cm^2 (Bjordal, Lopes-Martins, and Iversen 2006).

Chronic, degenerative Achilles tendinopathy is a frequently occurring pathology that can lead to disability in both active and sedentary people. The incidence of tendinopathy is greater in men and in addition to overuse, is associated with metabolic disorders such as insulin resistance and diabetes (Abate 2014). Success has been achieved primarily through eccentric rehabilitation exercises. Optimal parameters for eccentric exercise as well as effective adjuncts to loading continue to be studied.

Case Scenario 7

Osteoarthritis

A 43-year-old administrator is referred to a university sports medicine clinic for care. His physician has diagnosed grade II medial and lateral compartment osteoarthritis in his left knee. He reports injuring the knee while playing college soccer and undergoing a partial meniscectomy at age 23 and a second arthroscopic surgery to remove loose bodies

at age 33. He complains of persistent aching that is often worse after activity and ranges from 2 to 6 out of 10 on a visual analog pain scale. Examination of the knee reveals mild swelling and a loss of 4° of extension in comparison to the right knee. Isometric quadriceps strength assessment with handheld dynamometry reveals a 15% strength deficit on the left. The patient's BMI is calculated to be 30, suggesting he is overweight. The patient reports that he takes acetaminophen for pain once or twice per day but does not tolerate nonsteroidal anti-inflammatory medications well. The patient wants to manage pain and initiate an exercise regimen to address his weight and strength losses as well as his increasing difficulty with climbing stairs and walking for more than 30 min.

What are the problems identified in this case?

Impairments

Pain

Loss of knee range of motion

Swelling

Functional limitations

Stair climbing

Walking

Participation restrictions

Unable to fully participate in a health-related exercise regimen or recreational activities requiring prolonged walking or running

What would you do?

What are the recommended guidelines for the management of moderate knee osteoarthritis in a middle-aged adult? The goals of management of early and moderate knee osteoarthritis include pain management with medications and/or superficial heating or cooling, exercise, and weight management (Porcheret et al. 2007). The extent of pain relief with heat or cold varies between patients and by patient preferences. Patients with osteoarthritis who prefer cold reported greater relief of knee pain when using cold, and those preferring heat reported greater pain relief with superficial heating. These modalities will not fully alleviate pain, but they can result in meaningful relief (Denegar et al. 2010).

The use of superficial heat or cold as an adjunct to exercise has not been extensively studied. Cetin et al. (2008) found that hot packs, TENS, diathermy, or ultrasound before isokinetic exercise augmented exercise performance, reduced pain, and improved function. Others have reported that low doses of ultrasound are of no benefit in the outcomes of care for patients with knee osteoarthritis (Cakir et al., 2014; Ulus et al. 2012). Given the limited and sometimes conflicting data, there is no single best plan of care to recommend to this patient. A reasonable plan might include the use of a stationary bicycle due to the ease of access and low impact of the activity. Resistance exercise to increase quadriceps and general lower extremity strength can be gradually introduced. Experimentation with superficial heating and cooling before and after exercise is a low-cost and potentially effective means of reducing pain and maximizing the gains achieved through exercise. These treatments can also be self-administered.

While such a plan of care is not guaranteed to alleviate pain or improve function, it is sustainable over a long period. Although osteoarthritis is a progressive disease, early management should address the patient's problem and try to slow the degenerative changes. This case illustrates the need to consider the problem and seek low-risk, convenient, and cost-effective solutions. If these solutions fail to produce enough improvement, referral for further evaluation, more aggressive pharmaceutical management, and ultimately total joint arthroplasty is warranted. However, many patients can obtain pain relief and functional improvement so that more complex care can be delayed for extended periods of time.

SUMMARY

Each of the scenarios identified a different therapeutic modality to integrate into the treatment plan. By no means should the plans of care described in these scenarios be construed as dogma or as the best or only choice of treatment options. In these cases we want to emphasize the discussions that occur in the process of selecting a therapeutic modality. Each patient and each injury or condition is unique; not every inversion ankle sprain produces the same impairments. What is equally important is that the impairments do not create the same functional limitations and participation restrictions in everyone. Integrating therapeutic modalities (and exercise) is purposeful and goal oriented. We encourage you to use these scenarios to further discuss the status of an injury (including the tissue healing process), patient values (short- and long-term goals), expected physiological responses (indications and contraindications), and other intervention options (based on clinician experience and operational parameters).

Chapters 1 and 3 introduced and expounded on the importance of adopting an evidence-based approach to therapeutic modality application and health care practices in general. In fact, the format throughout this text is to present the best available evidence on various therapeutic modalities and to emphasize treating the whole patient. These are two of the three tenets of evidence-based practice (integration of best research evidence with clinical expertise and patient values). In this chapter, we emphasize the significance of the remaining component, clinical expertise. Be aware that expertise is often confused with experience; a colleague once said, "practice does not make perfect, but rather practice makes permanent." The modern clinician must think before acting. To optimize the quality of care we provide to our patients, we can no longer continue to use treatment techniques without considering their efficacy or purpose simply because that is how we were shown. Clinical expertise, then, is built on the practice of seeking and considering the best available evidence and purposefully integrating that knowledge with our health care practices. We encourage athletic trainers (and health care providers) to make this a permanent part of their professional development.

Glossary

A-beta fibers—Large diameter myelinated primary afferent nerve serving touch and vibration sensation.

A-delta fibers—Thinly myelinated primary afferent nerve serving touch, pressure, temperature, and pain sensation.

accommodation—A decrease in the response of a nerve to an electrical impulse.

actin cytoskeleton—Polymer of actin connecting the integrin to the nuclear membrane. Functions include cell motility and mechanotransduction.

afferent—Conducting from the periphery toward the center (as in conduction of nerve impulses to the central nervous system).

alpha motor neuron—Efferent nerve innervating the myofibril.

alternating current (AC)—Continuous current with positive and negative phases.

ampere—A measure of electrical current (abbreviated A).

amplification—To increase in magnitude.

analgesia—Without pain.

anaphylactic reaction—A severe, potentially fatal systemic response to a substance that a person is highly sensitive to.

anesthesia—The loss of physical sensation.

arthrogenic muscle inhibition—A loss of muscle function caused by an injury or condition affecting a joint.

arthrokinematics—Sliding, rolling, and gliding of joint surfaces during motion (e.g., during abduction at the glenohumeral joint, the head of the humerus rolls superiorly and glides inferiorly); also called accessory motion.

atrophy—A wasting away or loss of muscle cell mass.

avascular—Without or having lost blood supply.

average current—The amount of current supplied over a period of time, which takes into consideration both the peak amplitude and the phase duration.

beam nonuniformity ratio (BNR)—A measure of the quality of the ultrasound head.

beta endorphin—A 31-peptide-chain endogenous opioid that is important in the body's pain control system.

bifurcated—Divided.

biomodulation—The stimulation of the normal physiological function of a cell by the administration of energy (either light, electrical, sound, or thermal).

biphasic current—A pulsatile current with positive and negative phases.

canaliculi—Present in bone, a network of interconnecting channels in which osteocytes communicate.

capacitance—Ability to store an electrical charge.

carrier frequency—The frequency of pulsed energy for the period of time that the laser is emitted.

cavitation—The formation of cavities within the body; used in the context of ultrasound, the formation of gas bubbles within cell walls.

C fibers—Non-myelinated primary afferent nerve serving pain, temperature, and pressure sensation.

chemotactic—To chemically attract.

chemotaxis—A chemical attraction.

chondroblasts—A type of fibroblast that forms cartilage.

chondrocytes—Resident cartilage cell.

chronaxie—The phase duration required to depolarize a nerve fiber when the amplitude is two times the rheobase.

clinical trial—A prospective study of treatment efficacy or effectiveness conducted with patients.

coherence—A property of laser light in which all discharged photons are in sync with each other and travel in parallel.

cold urticaria—An allergic reaction to cold exposure.

collagen—Principal protein found in ligament, tendon, and scar tissues.

collimation—A property of laser light in which the light travels in one direction without diverging. Once a medium change is encountered, there is a possibility for reflection, refraction, and absorption of the light.

complex regional pain syndrome (CRPS)—Symptom complex characterized by pain that is disproportional to the injury.

conduction—Transfer of heat through the direct contact between a hotter and a cooler area.

convection—Transfer of heat by the movement of air or liquid between regions of unequal temperature.

conversion—Term implying that energy is changed from one form to another—for example, acoustic energy to thermal energy through the administration of ultrasound.

coulomb—Measure of electrical charge or a quantity of electrons (abbreviated C).

cryokinetics—Use of cryotherapy to facilitate therapeutic exercise.

cryotherapy—Therapeutic use of cold.

denervated—term used to describe a muscle that no longer is stimulated by a peripheral nerve. In denervation, the muscle membrane can be stimulated directly using galvanic current, but only a twitch will result.

depolarization—To change from a polarized state.

depression—State of deep sadness, dejection, and gloom; distinguished from grief, which is an appropriate response to personal loss.

diathermy—Heating of tissue with electromagnetic energy.

dipole—A molecule with areas of opposite electrical charges.

direct current (DC)—Continuous current without alternating positive and negative phases.

disability—All limitations on performance of normal daily tasks, including those related to schoolwork, employment, family responsibilities, and sport participation, due to disease or injury.

disinhibitory TENS—Any physical agent that is applied to either the joint or the muscle in order to excite the motor response or to diminish the inhibitory effect that is present.

dorsal horn—Area of synapse between first- and second-order afferent nerves.

duty cycle—Ratio of "on" to "off" time.

effective radiating area (ERA)—Area of the ultrasound head emitting acoustic energy.

effectiveness—A response to treatment applied during routine clinical practice.

efferent—Conducting from the center toward the periphery (as in conduction of nerve impulses from the central nervous system).

efficacy—A response to treatment administered in a controlled setting or under ideal conditions.

effleurage—A massage technique using long stroking motions.

electromotive force—A potential difference in electrical charges that results in a flow of electrical current.

electromyography (EMG)—A measure of the electrical activity in muscle.

enkephalin—A family of five-peptide chain transmitter substances that inhibit synaptic transmission in nociceptive pathways.

etiological factors—Factors that cause a condition.

evidence-based health care—The integration of the best research evidence with clinical expertise and patient values.

extracellular matrix—The tissue architecture that provides structural and biochemical support to cells.

fibrin—A protein converted from fibrinogen to form the meshlike foundation of a clot.

fibroblasts—Cells that produce collagen and elastin.

focal adhesion complex—Consists of several proteins and adaptor molecules that sequentially combine upon integrin activation, leading to integrin clustering and focal adhesion to extracellular matrix.

free radical—A molecule containing an odd number of electrons, which can injure healthy tissues.

frequency—Number of cycles or sinusoidal waves per second.

functional limitation—Inability to perform physical tasks; in physically active individuals, specific examples could include sport-specific activities such as running and jumping.

galvanic—Direct current.

gap junctions—Intercellular membrane channels that facilitate the passage of ions and small molecules from the cytosol of adjacent cells, allowing cell-to-cell and whole-tissue responses.

gamma gain—An increase in gamma motor neuron discharge.

ground state—The atom in its most stable form with no electrons in an elevated valence level.

hyperemia—An increase in blood flow to a part of the body.

hypertonicity—An increase in the resting tension of muscle.

hypomobility—Less than normal mobility.

hypovolemic—Referring to low blood volume.

hypoxia—Lack of oxygen.

impairment—Anatomical, physiological, psychological, and emotional aftereffects of disease and injury.

impedance—Resistance + inductance + capacitance.

inductance—Opposition to electrical current created by electromagnetic eddy currents that are generated when current passes through a wire.

inflammation—Series of physiological events that occur in vascularized tissue.

integrin—Transmembrane receptor that binds to the extracellular matrix and is responsible for transmitting mechanical signal to the cell.

integrin-linked kinase—Intracellular protein activated by the integrin that signals many downstream cellular events and has the ability to promote cross-activation of several different cytokine receptors.

integrin protein—Transmembrane receptors connecting cells to extracellular matrix.

intensity—Dose of sound energy delivered to the tissue; measured in watts per square centimeter (W/cm^2) of area of sound head transmitting energy.

interstitium—Space between the cells.

iontophoresis—Use of an electrical current to drive medications into the tissues.

labile—Changeable, fluctuating.

lasing chamber—An enclosed area in a laser apparatus where stimulated emissions may take place. This usually has mirrors on either side to reflect the photon energy.

law of Dubois Reymond—Concept of electrophysiology that explains how the nerve responds to electrical stimulus. In order for the nerve to be stimulated, the intensity or amplitude of current must exceed threshold, the duration of the current must exceed the capacitance of the tissue, and the rate of rise of the leading edge of the pulse must be fast enough to prevent accommodation.

leukocytes—White blood cells, of which there are five types: neutrophils, macrophages, basophils, eosinophils, and lymphocytes.

maladaptive behavior—Faulty, self-defeating, or injurious intrapersonal adaptation to stress or change.

mast cell—Type of cell found in connective tissue that releases several chemical mediators of inflammation.

mechanobiology—The study of mechanotransduction and the molecular mechanisms by which cells sense and respond to mechanical signals.

mechanoreceptors—Superficial receptors that respond to stroking, touch, and pressure.

mechanotransduction—The conversion of mechanical stimuli to intracellular chemical signals affecting cell survival, differentiation, and gene expression.

monochromatic—Being only of one color.

monophasic current—Pulsatile current with only positive or negative pulses.

MRI arthrogram—Injection of dye into a joint capsule and a series of x-rays to improve diagnostic capabilities. An MRI-Arthrogram or MRA is the combination of the two tests.

muscle satellite cells—Quiescent muscle progenitor cells that, when stimulated, can differentiate into muscle cells. Important in repair and hypertrophy.

muscle spindle—Sensory receptor of length-tension changes in muscle.

myocyte—Resident muscle cell.

myofascial pain syndrome (MFPS)—Persistent pain of soft tissue, origins characterized by taut fibrous bands and focal areas of hypersensitivity called trigger points.

necrotic—Dead.

negligence—Entails (1) doing something that a similarly qualified person under like circumstances would not have done (a negligent act or act of commission) or (2) failing to do something that a similarly qualified person would have done under similar circumstances (act of omission).

neuromuscular control—Use of sensory neural input and motor output to exert volitional control of skeletal muscle.

neuromuscular stimulation—Use of TENS to cause a muscle contraction.

nociceptive—Pain sensing.

nociceptors—Superficial receptors that are stimulated by potentially damaging mechanical, chemical, and thermal stress.

noxious—Pain producing.

ohm—A measure of resistance to the flow of electrons (abbreviated Ω).

opiates—Substances derived from opium.

opioid—A naturally occurring or synthetic substance having an opiate-like effect.

osteoblast—A type of fibroblast that forms bone.

osteocyte—Resident bone cell.

osteokinematics—Referring to movement of one bony segment on another; for example, glenohumeral abduction results in movement of the humerus on the glenoid.

palliative care—Treatments that relieve symptoms, often temporarily, without curing.

paracrine—regulation of cells by surrounding cellular activity, typically through cytokine interaction.

peak current—The maximum amplitude of the current at any point during the pulse without regard to its duration.

permanent—Unchangeable, as in permanent tissues that last through life but cannot be repaired.

petrissage—A massage technique in which the skin is lifted, squeezed, or kneaded.

phagocyte—A cell that engulfs and digests microorganisms and cellular debris.

phonophoresis—Method of driving medications into tissues with sound waves.

photon—A measurement of electromagnetic energy that lacks mass, lacks an electrical charge, and has an indefinite lifetime. Photons contain a specific amount of energy depending on wavelength.

physical agents—Treatments that cause some change to the body.

physiochemical effect—To alter bodily functions by changing chemical balance (e.g., softening of scar under negative direct current).

physiological effect—To alter bodily functions by changing specific tissue activity (e.g., trigger the release of endogenous opioids through nerve stimulation).

placebo effect—Improvement in a condition not related to the effect of a treatment or medication.

proteoglycans—Components of extracellular matrix composed of polysaccharide complexes linked by proteins.

population inversion—A condition in which the majority of the atoms in a particular environment are in a high-energy state. This allows the creation of a laser.

practice act—State law regulating the practice of a profession.

progenitor cells—Immature cells that differentiate into mature tissue cells.

pulsatile current—Noncontinuous current; the flow of current is broken by intervals between pulses.

pulse train—Method of delivering laser energy so that the energy is pulsed for short periods of time. The end result is packets of pulsed energy to be emitted.

radiation—The emission of energy; radiant energy may be emitted from a source such as a heat lamp and absorbed by the body.

resistance—Opposition to the flow of electrical current by a material (measured in ohms).

rest–reinjury cycle—Pattern of injury in which physically active people return to activity only to aggravate a condition from which they have not fully recovered.

reactive oxygen species—Chemically reactive, oxygen containing molecules.

rheobase—The minimum amplitude required to depolarize a nerve fiber.

root mean square (RMS)—A means of determining phase charge or the effective area contained in the waveform that results in the physiochemical effects.

signs—Indicators of illness or injury that the clinician measures, for example, fever.

somatization—A somatic (bodily) manifestation of psychological dysfunction.

somatosensory information—Neural input that allows for sensation such as temperature, pressure, and pain as well as allowing for awareness of how the body is oriented in relation to time and space.

spontaneous emissions—Random discharge of a light wave that occurs naturally. An atom absorbs energy to raise its valence level and the same amount of energy is emitted spontaneously when the atom releases a photon.

stable—Slowly changing or resistant to change; opposite of labile.

stimulated emission—A discharge of a light wave is stimulated by another light wave. When the photon strikes another excited atom, two identical photons are released.

substance P—A facilitatory transmitter substance in the nociceptive pathways.

symptoms—Indicators of injury or illness that the patient discloses, for example, "My shoulder hurts."

synapse—Junction between nerves.

tendinopathy—A term used to describe disease of a tendon, including reactive tendinitis through tendinosis.

tendinosis—Degenerative tendon injury with damage to the extracellular matrix and cell death.

tenocyte—Resident tendon cell.

tetanic muscle contraction—A sustained contraction of a muscle.

therapeutic modality—Literally, a device or apparatus having curative powers.

thermoreceptors—Superficial receptors that respond to temperature and temperature change.

tort—Private, civil legal action brought by an injured party, or the party's representative, to redress an injury caused by another person.

transcutaneous electrical nerve stimulation (TENS)—The use of a therapeutic device that stimulates peripheral nerves by passing an electrical current through the skin.

transmitter substance—Chemical that influences the transmission of neural impulses across a synapse; the substance may facilitate or inhibit transmission.

trigger point—A hypersensitive fibrous band of tissue.

ultrasound—High-frequency acoustic energy.

vascularized—Having a blood supply; perfused.

vasodilation—An opening of the capillary beds.

viscera—Thoracic, abdominal, and pelvic organs.

voltage—Measure of electromotive force (abbreviated V).

Wedenski's inhibition—An action potential failure in a nerve caused by a medium-frequency electrical current.

References

Chapter 1

Board of Certification. 2010. *Role delineation study/practice analysis*. 6th ed. Omaha: BOC.

National Athletic Trainers' Association. 2005. *Code of ethics*. Dallas: NATA, www.nata.org/codeofethics/code_of_ethics.pdf

National Athletic Trainers' Association. 2011. *Athletic training education competencies*. 5th ed. Dallas: NATA.

Ray, R., and J. Konin. 2011. *Management strategies in athletic training*. 4th ed. Champaign, IL: Human Kinetics.

Sackett, D.L., S.E. Straus, W.S. Richardson, W. Rosenberg, and R.B. Haynes. 2000. *Evidence-based medicine: How to practice and teach EBM*. 2nd ed. Philadelphia: Churchill Livingstone.

Scott, R.W. 1990. *Health care malpractice*. Thorofare, NJ: Slack.

Chapter 2

American Psychiatric Association. 1994. *Diagnostic and statistical manual of mental disorders*. 4th ed. Washington, D.C.: American Psychiatric Association.

Andersen, M.B., and J.M. Williams. 1999. Athletic injury, psychosocial factors and perceptual changes during stress. *Journal of Sports Sciences*. 17 (9): 735-41.

Bianco, T., S. Malo, and T. Orlick. 1999. Sport injury and illness: Elite skiers describe their experiences. *Research Quarterly for Exercise and Sport*. 70: 157-69.

Brewer, B.W. 1999. Adherence to sport injury rehabilitation regimens. In S.J. Bull (ed.), *Adherence issues in sport and exercise*. Chichester, UK: Wiley, pp. 145-68.

Brewer, B.W. 2001. Psychology of sport injury rehabilitation. In R.N. Singer, H.A. Hausenblas, and C.M. Janelle (eds.), *Handbook of sport psychology*. New York: Wiley, pp. 787-809.

Brewer, B.W., D.E. Linder, and C.M. Phelps. 1995. Situational correlates of emotional adjustment to athletic injury. *Clinical Journal of Sports Medicine*. 5: 241-45.

Brewer, B.W., J.L. Van Raalte, A.E. Cornelius, A.J. Petitpas, J.H. Sklar, M.H. Pohlman et al. 2000. Psychological factors, rehabilitation adherence, and rehabilitation outcome following anterior cruciate ligament reconstruction. *Rehabilitation Psychology*. 45: 20-37.

Byerly, P.N., T. Worrell, J. Gahimer, and E. Domholdt. 1994. Rehabilitation compliance in an athletic training environment. *Journal of Athletic Training*. 29: 352-55.

Depression Guidelines Panel. 1993. *Depression in primary care: vol 1. Detection and diagnosis. Clinical Practice Guidelines*, Number 5. Rockville, MD: U.S. Department of Health and Human Services, Public Health Services, Agency for Health Care Policy and Research.

Duda, J.L., A.E. Smart, and M.K. Tappe. 1989. Predictors of adherence in the rehabilitation of athletic injuries: An application of personal investment theory. *Journal of Sport & Exercise Psychology*. 11: 367-81.

Evans, L., and L. Hardy. 1995. Sport injury and grief response: A review. *Journal of Sport & Exercise Psychology*. 17: 227-45.

Fisher, A.C., and L.L. Hoisington. 1998. Injured athletes' attitudes and judgments toward rehabilitation adherence. *Journal of Athletic Training*. 28: 43-47.

Fisher, A.C., K.C. Scriber, M.L. Matheny, M.H. Alderman, and L.A. Bitting. 1993. Enhancing athletic injury rehabilitation adherence. *Journal of Athletic Training*. 28: 312-18.

Gieck, J. 1990. Psychological considerations in rehabilitation. In W.E. Prentice (ed.), *Rehabilitation techniques in sports medicine*. St. Louis: Mosby, pp. 107-21.

Gould, D., E. Udry, D. Bridges, and L. Beck. 1997a. Stress sources encountered when rehabilitating from season-ending ski injuries. *The Sport Psychologist*. 11: 361-78.

Gould, D., E. Udry, D. Bridges, and L. Beck. 1997b. Coping with season-ending injuries. *The Sport Psychologist*. 11: 379-99.

Grove, J.R. 1993. Personality and injury rehabilitation among sport performers. In D. Pargman (ed.), *Psychological bases of sport injuries*. Morgantown, WV: Fitness Information Technology, pp. 99-120.

Gyurscik, N. 1995. *Athletes: Retrospectives on serious sports injuries*. Presentation at the meeting of the Association for the Advancement of Applied Sport Psychology, New Orleans, LA.

Haggman, S., C.G. Maher, and K.M. Refshauge. 2004. Screening for symptoms of depression by physical therapists managing low back pain. *Physical Therapy*. 84 (12): 1157-66.

Heil, J. 1993. *Psychology of sport injury*. Champaign, IL: Human Kinetics.

Ievleva, L., and T. Orlick. 1991. Mental links to enhanced healing: An exploratory study. *The Sport Psychologist*. 5: 25-40.

Kübler-Ross, E. 1969. *On death and dying*. New York: Macmillan.

Laubach, W.J., B.W. Brewer, J.L. Van Raalte, and A.J. Petitpas. 1996. Attributions for recovery and adherence to sport injury rehabilitation. *Australian Journal of Science and Medicine in Sport*. 28: 30-34.

Lazarus, R.S. 1991. *Emotion and adaptation*. London: Oxford University Press.

Leddy, M.H., M.J. Lambert, and B.M. Ogles. 1994. Psychological consequences of athletic injury among high level competition. *Research Quarterly for Exercise and Sport*. 64: 349-54.

Lipowski, Z.J. 1988. Somatization: The concept and its clinical application. *American Journal of Psychiatry*. 145: 1358–68.

Locke, E., and G.P. Latham. 1985. The application of goal setting in sports. *Journal of Sport Psychology*. 7: 205–11.

Maehr, M., and L. Braskamp (eds.). 1986. *The motivation factor: A theory of personal investment*. Lexington, MA: Lexington Books.

McDonald, S.A., and C.J. Hardy. 1990. Affective response patterns of the injured athlete: An exploratory analysis. *The Sport Psychologist*. 4: 261–74.

Messner, M.A. 1992. *Power at play: Sports and the problem of masculinity*. Boston: Beacon Press.

Miller-Keane, Marie T. O'Toole. 1992. *Miller-Keane encyclopedia & dictionary of medicine, nursing, & allied health*. 5th ed. Philadelphia: Saunders.

Miller, R.P., S. Kori, and D. Todd. 1991. The Tampa Scale: A measure of kinesiophobia. *Clin J Pain*. 7 (1): 51–52.

Murphy, G.C., P.E. Foreman, C.A. Simpson, G.N. Molloy, and E.K. Molloy. 1999. The development of a locus of control measure predictive of injured athletes' adherence to treatment. *Journal of Science and Medicine in Sport*. 2: 145–52.

Nagi, S.Z. 1965. *Some conceptual issues in disability and rehabilitation*. In M.B. Sussman (ed.), *Sociology and rehabilitation*. Washington, D.C.: American Sociological Association, pp. 100–13.

National Institute of Mental Health. 2001. *The numbers count: Mental disorders in America*. www.nimh.nih.gov/publicat/numbers.cfm. Accessed 10/20/04.

Neal, T., A. Diamond, S. Goldman, D. Klossner, E. Morse et al. 2013. Inter-association recommendations for developing a plan to recognize and refer student-athletes with psychological concerns at the collegiate level: An executive summary of a consensus statement. *Journal of Athletic Training*. 48 (5): 716–20.

Pearson, L., and G. Jones. 1992. Emotional effects of sports injuries: Implications for the physiotherapists. *Physiotherapy*. 78: 762–70.

Peppard, A., and C.R. Denegar. 1999. Depression and somatization and persistent pain in the athletic patient. *Athletic Therapy Today*: 43–47.

Peppard, A.P., and C.R. Denegar. 1994. Pain and the rehabilitation of athletic injury. *Orthopaedic Physical Therapy Clinics of North America*. 3: 439–62.

Rose, J., and R.F.J. Jevne. 1993. Psychosocial process associated with athletic injuries. *The Sport Psychologist*. 7: 309–28.

Rotella, R.J., and S.R. Heyman. 1993. Stress, injury, and the psychological rehabilitation of athletes. In J. Williams (ed.), *Applied sport psychology: Personal growth to peak performance*. 2nd ed. Mountain View, CA: Mayfield, pp. 338–55.

Smith, A.M., S.G. Scott, W.M. O'Fallon, and M.L. Young. 1990. Emotional responses of athletes to injury. *Mayo Clinic Proceedings*. 65: 38–50.

Tracey, J. 2003. The emotional response to the injury and rehabilitation process. *Journal of Applied Sport Psychology*. 15: 279–93.

Udry, E.M. 1997. Coping and social support among injured athletes following surgery. *Journal of Sport & Exercise Psychology*. 19: 71–90.

Udry, E.M., D. Gould, D. Bridges, and L. Beck. 1997. Down but not out: Athlete responses to season-ending injuries. *Journal of Sport & Exercise Psychology*. 19: 229–48.

Waddell. G., M. Newton, I. Henderson, D. Somerville, and C.J. Main. 1993. A Fear-Avoidance Beliefs Questionnaire (FABQ) and the role of fear-avoidance beliefs in chronic low back pain and disability. *Pain*. 52: 157–168.

Walker, N., J. Thatcher, and D. Lavallee. 2007. Psychological responses to injury in competitive sport: A critical review. *Journal of the Royal Society for the Promotion of Health*. 127: 174.

Wegener, S.T. 1998/1999. *Current concepts and clinical approaches in psychology of rehabilitation*. Paper presented at the National Athletic Trainers' Association 49th Annual Meeting and Clinical Symposia, Baltimore, MD, June 17, 1998, and the 50th Eastern Athletic Trainers' Association Annual Meeting, January 11, 1999.

Weiss, M.R., and R.K. Troxel. 1986. Psychology of the injured athlete. *Athletic Training*. 21: 104–9.

Wiese-Bjornstal, D.M., A.M. Smith, and E.E. LaMott. 1995. A model of psychologic responses to athletic injury and rehabilitation. *Athletic Training: Sports Health Care Perspectives*. 1: 17–30.

Wiese-Bjornstal, D.M., A.M. Smith, S.M. Shaffer, and M.A. Morrey. 1998. An integrated model of response to sport injury: Psychological and sociological dynamics. *Journal of Applied Sport Psychology*. 10: 46–69.

World Health Organization. 2002. *Towards a common language for functioning, disability, and health*. Geneva: WHO.

Worrell, T.W., and N.L. Reynolds. 1994. Integrating physiologic and psychological paradigms into orthopaedic rehabilitation. *Orthopaedic Physical Therapy Clinics of North America*. 3: 269–89.

Young, K., P. White, and W. McTeer. 1994. Body talk: Male athletes reflect on sport, injury, and pain. *Sociology of Sport Journal*. 11: 175–94.

Yukelson, D., and J. Heil. 1998. *Psychological considerations in working with injured athletes*. In P.K. Canavan (ed.), *Rehabilitation in sports medicine*. Stamford, CT: Appleton & Lange, pp. 61–70.

Chapter 3

Deyo, R.A., N.E. Walsh, D.C. Martin, L.S. Schoenfeld, and S. Ramamurthy. 1990a. A controlled trial of transcutaneous electrical nerve stimulation and exercise for chronic back pain. *New England Journal of Medicine*. 322:1627–34.

Deyo, R.A., N.E. Walsh, D.C. Martin, L.S. Schoenfeld, and S. Ramamurthy. 1990b. Can trials of physical treatments be blinded? The example of transcutaneous electrical nerve stimulation for pain. *American Journal of Physical Medicine & Rehabilitation*. 69: 6–10.

Domholdt, E. 2005. *Rehabilitation research: Principles and applications*. 3rd ed. Philadelphia: Saunders.

MacCauley, D., and T. Best. 2002. *Evidence-based sports medicine*. London: BMJ Books.

McKeon, P.O., and J. Hertel. 2008. Systematic review of postural control and lateral ankle instability, part II: Is balance training clinically effective? *Journal of Athletic Training*. 43: 305-15.

Oncel, M., S. Sencan, H. Yildiz, and N. Kurt. 2002. Transcutaneous electrical nerve stimulation for pain in patients with uncomplicated minor rib fractures. *European Journal of Cardio-Thoracic Surgery*. 22: 13-17.

Runeson, L., and E. Hacker. 2002. Iontophoresis with cortisone in the treatment of lateral epicondylalgia (tennis elbow)—a double blind study. *Scandinavian Journal of Medicine & Science in Sports*. 12: 136-42.

Vela, L.I., and C. Denegar. 2010. Transient disablement in the physically active with musculoskeletal injuries, part I: A descriptive model. *Journal of Athletic Training*. 45: 615-29.

Chapter 4

Abramson. N., and B. Melton. 2000. Leukocytosis: Basics of clinical assessment. *American Family Physician*. 62 (9): 2053-60.

Bianchetti, L., M. Barczyk, J. Cardoso, M. Schmidt, A. Bellini, and S. Mattoli. 2012. Extracellular matrix remodelling properties of human fibrocytes. *Journal of Cellular and Molecular Medicine*. 16 (3): 483-95.

Järvinen, M., L. Józsa, P. Kannus, T.L. Järvinen, M. Kvist, and W. Leadbetter. 1997. Histopathological findings in chronic tendon disorders. *Scandinavian Journal of Medicine & Science in Sports*. 7 (2): 86-95.

Kerr, M.A., C.M. Bender, and E.J. Monti. 1996. An introduction to oxygen free radicals. *Heart Lung*. 25: 200-209.

Kjaer, M. 2004. Role of extracellular matrix in adaptation of tendon and skeletal muscle to mechanical loading. *Physiological Reviews*. 84 (2): 649-98.

Kubo, K., Y. Kawakami, H. Kanehisa, and T. Fukunaga. 2002. Measurement of viscoelastic properties of tendon structures in vivo. *Scand J Med Sci Sports*. 12 (1): 3-8. PubMed PMID: 11985759.

Lech, M., and H.J. Anders. 2013. Macrophages and fibrosis: How resident and infiltrating mononuclear phagocytes orchestrate all phases of tissue injury and repair. *Biochimica et Biophysica Acta*. 1832 (7): 989-97.

Martinez-Hernandez, A., and P.S. Amenta. 1990. Basic concepts in wound healing. In W.B. Leadbetter, J.A. Buckwalter, and S.L. Gorden (eds.), *Sports induced inflammation*. Park Ridge, IL: American Academy of Orthopedic Surgeons, pp. 25-54.

Novak, M.L., and T.J. Koh. 2013. Phenotypic transitions of macrophages orchestrate tissue repair. *American Journal of Pathology*. 183 (5): 1352-63.

Sackett, D.L., S.E. Straus, W.S. Richardson, W. Rosenberg, and R.B. Haynes. 2000. *Evidence-based medicine: How to practice and teach EBM*. 2nd ed. Philadelphia: Churchill Livingstone.

Scott, R.W. 1990. *Health care malpractice*. Thorofare, NJ: Slack.

Tidball, J.G. 2005. Mechanical signal transduction in skeletal muscle growth and adaptation. *Journal of Applied Physiology*. 98 (5): 1900-8.

Ward, P.A., G.O. Till, and K.J. Johnson. 1990. Oxygen-derived free radicals and inflammation. In W.B. Leadbetter, J.A. Buckwalter, and S.L. Gorden (eds.), *Sports-induced inflammation*. Park Ridge, IL: American Academy of Orthopaedic Surgeons, pp. 315-324.

Zhang, J., C. Keenan, and J.H. Wang. 2013. The effects of dexamethasone on human patellar tendon stem cells: Implications for dexamethasone treatment of tendon injury. *Journal of Orthopaedic Research*. 31 (1): 105-10.

Zhang, X., and D.M. Mosser. 2008. Macrophage activation by endogenous danger signals. *Journal of Pathology*. 214 (2): 161-78.

Chapter 5

Asmundson, G.J.G., and K.D. Wright. 2004. Biopsychosocial approaches to pain. In T. Hadjistavropoulos and K.D. Craig (eds.), *Pain: Psychological perspectives*. Hillsdale, NJ: Erlbaum, pp. 35-57.

Berne, R.M., B.M. Koeppen, and B.A. Stanton. 2010. *Berne & Levy physiology*. Philadelphia: Mosby/Elsevier.

Bolay, H., and M.A. Moskowitz. 2002. Mechanisms of pain modulation in chronic syndromes. *Neurology*. 59: 2-7.

Bruehl, S. 2010. An update on the pathophysiology of the complex regional pain syndrome. *Anesthesiology*. 113 (3): 713-25.

Denegar, C.R., and E.F.H. Bowman. 1996. Electrotherapy in the treatment of athletic injuries. *Athletic Training and Sports Health Care*. 2 (2): 108-15.

Denegar, C.R., and A. Peppard. 1997. Evaluation and treatment of persistent pain and myofascial pain syndrome. *Athletic Therapy Today*. 2 (4): 40.

ICSI (Institute for Clinical Systems Improvement). 2009. Assessment and management of chronic pain. www.icsi.org/guidelines__more/catalog_guidelines_and_more/catalog_guidelines/catalog_neurological_guidelines/pain

International Association for the Study of Pain. 1979. Pain terms: A list with definitions and notes on usage. *Pain*. 6: 249-52.

Jessell, T.M., and D.D. Kelly. 1991. Pain and analgesia. In E.R. Kandel, J.H. Schwartz, and T.M. Jessell (eds.), *Principles of neural science*. 3rd ed. New York: Elsevier, pp. 385-99.

Knight, Kenneth L. 1995. *Cryotherapy in sport injury management*. Champaign, IL: Human Kinetics.

Ladd, A.L., K.E. DeHaven., J. Thanik., R.B. Patt, and M. Feuerstein. 1989. Reflex sympathetic imbalance. *Am J Sports Med*. 17:660-667.

Melzack, R. 2001. Pain and the neuromatrix in the brain. *Journal of Dental Education*. 65 (12): 1378-82.

Merskey, H., and N. Bogduk (eds.) 1994. *Classification of chronic pain. IASP Task Force on Taxonomy*. Seattle: IASP Press, pp. 209-14.

Millan, M.J. 2002. Descending control of pain. *Progress in Neurobiology.* 66 (6): 355-474.

Peppard, A., and C.R. Denegar. 1994. Pain and the rehabilitation of athletic injury. *Orthopaedic Physical Therapy Clinics of North America.* 3: 439-62.

Wilmore, J.H., and D.L. Costill. 1999. *Physiology of sport and exercise.* 2nd ed. Champaign, IL: Human Kinetics, pp. 67 and 72.

Chapter 6

Carley, P.J., and S.F. Wainapel. 1985. Electrotherapy for acceleration of wound healing: Low intensity direct current. *Archives of Physical Medicine and Rehabilitation.* 66: 443-46.

Cesare P., and P. McNaughton. 1997. Peripheral pain mechanisms. *Current Opinion in Neurobiology.* 7: 493-99.

Denegar, C.R., and A. Peppard. 1997. Evaluation and treatment of persistent pain and myofascial pain syndrome. *Athletic Therapy Today.* 2 (4): 40.

Denegar, C.R., and D.H. Perrin. 1992. Effect of transcutaneous electrical nerve stimulation, cold, and a combination treatment on pain, decreased range of motion, and strength loss associated with delayed onset muscle soreness. *Journal of Athletic Training.* 27 (3): 202.

Latremoliere, A., and C.J. Woolf. 2009. Central sensitization: A generator of pain hypersensitivity by central neural plasticity. *The Journal of Pain.* 10 (9): 895-926.

Machelska, H., P.J. Cabot, S.A. Mousa, Q. Zhang, and C. Stein. 1998. Pain control in inflammation governed by selectins. *Nature Medicine.* 4, 1425-28.

Mayer, D.J., and J.C. Liebeskind, J.C. 1974. Pain reduction by focal electrical stimulation of the brain: An anatomical and behavioral analysis. *Brain Research.* 68 (1): 73-93.

Melzack, R. 2001. Pain and the neuromatrix in the brain. *Journal of Dental Education.* 65 (12): 1378-82.

Melzack, R., and K.L. Casey. 1968. Sensory, motivational, and central control of determinants of pain. In D.R. Kenshalo (ed.), *The skin senses.* Springfield, IL: Thomas, p. 423.

Melzack, R., and P. Wall. 1965. Pain mechanisms: A new theory. *Science.* 150: 971-79.

Millan, M.J. 2002. Descending control of pain. *Progress in Neurobiology.* 66 (6): 355-474.

Pollard, C.A. 1984. Preliminary validity study of the Pain Disability Index. *Perceptual and Motor Skills.* 59: 974.

Shultz, S.J., P.A. Houglum, and D.H. Perrin. 2010. *Examination of musculoskeletal injuries.* 3rd ed. Champaign, IL: Human Kinetics.

Stein, C. 1995. The control of pain in peripheral tissue by opioids. *New England Journal of Medicine.* 332: 1685-90.

Chapter 7

Kahn, M.D., C. Lee, P. Neeley, and S. Portnoy. 1987. The efficacy of titrated, low-dose ECT. *Am J Psychiatry.* 1 (44): 1.

Wilmore, J.H., and D.L. Costill. 2008 *Physiology of sport and exercise.* 4th ed. Champaign, IL: Human Kinetics, p. 92.

Chapter 8

Abelson, K., G.B. Langley, H. Sheppeard, M. Vlieg, and R.D. Wigley. 1983. Transcutaneous electrical nerve stimulation in rheumatoid arthritis. *New Zealand Medical Journal.* 96: 156-58.

Akai, M., H. Oda, Y. Shirasaki, and T. Teteishi. 1988. Electrical stimulation of ligament healing: An experimental study of the patella ligament of rabbits. *Clinical Orthopaedics and Related Research.* 235: 296-301.

Ballegaard, S., S.J. Christophersen, S.G. Dawids, J. Hesse, and N.V. Olsen. 1985. Acupuncture and transcutaneous electric nerve stimulation in the treatment of pain associated with chronic pancreatitis. A randomized study. *Scandinavian Journal of Gastroenterology.* 20: 1249-54.

Barron, J.J., W.E. Jacobson, and G. Tidd. 1985. Treatment of decubitus ulcers: A new approach. *Minnesota Medicine.* 68 (2): 103-6.

Bjordal, J.M., M.I. Johnson, and A.E. Ljunggreen 2003. Transcutaneous electrical nerve stimulation (TENS) can reduce postoperative analgesic consumption. A meta-analysis with assessment of optimal treatment parameters for postoperative pain. *European Journal of Pain.* 7 (2): 181-88.

Denegar, C.R., and D.H. Perrin. 1992. Effect of transcutaneous electrical nerve stimulation, cold and a combined treatment on pain, decreased range of motor and strength loss associated with delayed onset muscle soreness. *Journal of Athletic Training.* 27 (3): 200-06.

DeSantana, J.M., D.M. Walsh, C. Vance, B.A. Rakel, and K.A. Sluka. 2008. Effectiveness of transcutaneous electrical nerve stimulation for treatment of hyperalgesia and pain. *Current Rheumatology Reports.* 10 (6): 492-99.

Dolan, M.G., A.M. Mychaskiw, and F.C. Mendel. 2003. Cool-water immersion and high-voltage electric stimulation curb edema formation in rats. *Journal of Athletic Training.* 38 (3): 225.

Feger, M., J. Goetchius, J.N. Hertel, and S. Saliba. 2015. Electrical stimulation as a treatment intervention to improve function, edema or pain following acute lateral ankle sprains: A systematic review. *Physical Therapy in Sport.*

Glaviano, N.R., N.M. Selkow, E. Saliba, J. Hertel, and S. Saliba. 2011. No difference between doses in skin anesthesia after lidocaine delivered via iontophoresis. *Journal of Sport Rehabilitation.* 20 (2): 187-97.

Goldman, R., B. Brewley, L. Zhou, and M. Golden. 2003. Electrotherapy reverses inframalleolar ischemia: A retrospective, observational study. *Advances in Skin and Wound Care.* 16 (2): 79-89.

Grimmer, K. 1992. A controlled double blind study comparing the effects of strong burst mode TENS and high rate TENS on painful osteoarthritic knees. *Australian Journal of Physiotherapy.* 48: 49-56.

Gudeman, S.D., S.A. Eisele, R.S. Heidt, A.J. Colosimo, and A.L. Stroupe. 1997. Treatment of plantar fasciitis by iontophoresis of 0.4% dexamethasone: A randomized, double-blind, placebo-controlled study. *American Journal of Sports Medicine.* 25 (3): 312-16.

Gulick, D.T., K. Bouton, K. Detering, E. Racioppi, and M. Shafferman. 2000. Effects of acetic acid iontophoresis on heel spur reabsorption. *Physical Therapy Case Reports*. 3: 64–70.

Houghton, P.E., C.B. Kincaid, M. Lovell, K.E. Campbell, D.H. Keast, M.G. Woodbury, and K.A. Harris. 2003. Effect of electrical stimulation on chronic leg ulcer size and appearance. *Physical Therapy*. 83 (1): 17–28.

Hsueh, T.C., P.T. Cheng, T.S. Kuan, and C.Z. Hong 1997. The immediate effectiveness of electrical nerve stimulation and electrical muscle stimulation on myofascial trigger points 1. *American Journal of Physical Medicine and Rehabilitation*. 76 (6): 471–76.

Jensen, H., R. Zesler, and T. Christensen. 1991. Transcutaneous electrical nerve stimulation (TNS) for painful osteoarthrosis of the knee. *International Journal of Rehabilitation Research*. 14: 356–58.

Kumar, D., and H.J. Marshall. 1997. Diabetic peripheral neuropathy: Amelioration of pain with transcutaneous electrostimulation. *Diabetes Care*. 20: 1702–5.

Lerner, F.N., and D.L. Disch. 1981. A doubleblind comparative study of microstimulation and placebo effect in short terms treatment of the chronic back pain patient. *Journal of the American Chiropractic Association*. 15 (11): 101–06.

Lewis, B., D. Lewis, and G. Cumming. 1994. The comparative analgesic efficacy of transcutaneous electrical nerve stimulation and a non-steroidal anti-inflammatory drug for painful osteoarthritis. *British Journal of Rheumatology*. 33: 455–60.

Lewis, D., B. Lewis, and R.D. Sturrock. 1984. Transcutaneous electrical nerve stimulation in osteoarthrosis: A therapeutic alternative? *Annals of Rheumatic Diseases*. 43: 47–49.

Litke, D.S., and L.E. Dahners. 1994. Effects of different levels of direct current on early ligament healing in a rat model. *Journal of Orthopaedic Research*. 12 (5): 683–88.

Mannheimer, C., and C. Carlsson. 1979. The analgesic effect of Transcutaneous electrical Nerve Stimulation (TNS) in patients with rheumatoid arthritis. A comparative study of different pulse patterns. *Pain*. 6: 329–34.

Moore, S.R., and J. Shurman. 1997. Combined neuromuscular electrical nerve stimulation and transcutaneous electrical nerve stimulation for treatment of chronic back pain: A double-blind, repeated measures comparison. *Archives of Physical Medicine and Rehabilitation*. 78: 55–60.

Møystad, A., B.S. Krogstad, and T.A. Larheim. 1990. Transcutaneous nerve stimulation in a group of patients with rheumatic disease involving the temporomandibular joint. *Journal of Prosthetic Dentistry*. 64: 596–600.

Nash, T.P., J.D. Williams, and D. Machin. 1990. TENS: Does the type of stimulus really matter? *Pain Clinic*. 3: 161–68.

Nessler, J.P., and D.P. Mass. 1987. Direct-current electrical stimulation of tendon healing in vitro. *Clinical Orthopaedics and Related Research*. 217: 303.

Owoeye, I., N.I. Spielholz, J. Fetto, and A.J. Nelson. 1987. Low-intensity pulsed galvanic current and the healing of tenotomized rat Achilles tendons: Preliminary report using load-to-breaking measurements. *Archives of Physical Medicine and Rehabilitation*. 68 (7): 415–18.

Pietrosimone, B.G., S.A. Saliba, J.M. Hart, J. Hertel, D.C. Kerrigan, and C.D. Ingersoll. 2011. Effects of transcutaneous electrical nerve stimulation and therapeutic exercise on quadriceps activation in people with tibiofemoral osteoarthritis. *Journal of Orthopaedic and Sports Physical Therapy*. 41 (1): 4–12.

Runeson, L., and E. Haker. 2002. Iontophoresis with cortisone in the treatment of lateral epicondylalgia (tennis elbow)—a double-blind study. *Scandinavian Journal of Medicine and Science in Sports*. 12 (3): 136–42.

Saliba, S.A., C.L. Teeter-Heyl, P. McKeon, C.D. Ingersoll, and E.N. Saliba. 2011. Effect of duration and amplitude of direct current when lidocaine is delivered by iontophoresis. *Pharmaceutics*. 3 (4): 923–31.

Sluka, K.A., and D. Walsh. 2003. Transcutaneous electrical nerve stimulation: Basic science mechanisms and clinical effectiveness. *Journal of Pain*. 4 (3): 109–21.

Smith, C.R., G.T. Lewith, and D. Machin. 1983. Preliminary study to establish a controlled method of assessing transcutaneous nerve stimulation as treatment for the pain caused by osteo-arthritis of the knee. *Physiotherapy*. 69: 266–68.

Smutok, M.A., M.F. Mayo, C.L. Gabaree, K.E. Ferslew, and P.C. Panus. 2002. Failure to detect dexamethasone phosphate in the local venous blood postcathodic iontophoresis in humans. *Journal of Orthopaedic and Sports Physical Therapy*. 32 (9): 461–68.

Taylor, P., M. Hallett, and L. Flaherty. 1981. Treatment of osteoarthritis of the knee with transcutaneous electrical nerve stimulation. *Pain*. 11: 233–40.

Thorsteinsson, G., H.H. Stonnington, G.K. Stillwell, and L.R. Elveback. 1978. The placebo effect of transcutaneous electrical stimulation. *Pain*. 5: 31–41.

Vinterberg, H., R. Donde, and R.B. Andersen. 1978. Transcutaneous nerve stimulation for relief of pain in patients with rheumatoid arthritis. *Ugeskr Laeger*. 140: 1149–50.

Chapter 9

Arna Risberg, M., M. Lewek, and L. Snyder-Mackler. 2004. A systematic review of evidence for anterior cruciate ligament rehabilitation: How much and what type? *Physical Therapy in Sport*. 5: 125–45.

Bernier, J.N., and D. H. Perrin. 1998. Effect of coordination training on proprioception of the functionally unstable ankle. *Journal of Orthopaedic and Sports Physical Therapy*. 27: 264–75.

Brown, J.M., and W. Gilleard. 1991. Transition from slow to ballistic movement: Development of triphasic electromyogram patterns. *European Journal of Applied Physiology*. 63: 381–86.

Burch, F.X., J.N. Tarro, J.J. Greenberg, et al. 2008. Evaluating the benefit of patterned stimulation in the treatment of osteoarthritis of the knee. *Osteoarthritis and Cartilage*. 16 (8): 865–72.

Cooke, J.D., and S.H. Brown. 1990. Movement-related phasic muscle activation II. Generation and functional role of the triphasic pattern. *Journal of Neurophysiology.* 63: 465–72.

Currier, D.P., J. Lehman, and P. Lightfoot. 1979. Electrical stimulation in exercise of the quadriceps femoris muscle. *Physical Therapy.* 59: 1508–12.

Currier, D.P., J.M. Ray, J. Nyland, J.G. Rooney, J.T. Noteboom, and R. Kellogg. 1993. Effects of electrical and electromagnetic stimulation after anterior cruciate ligament reconstruction. *Journal of Orthopaedic and Sports Physical Therapy.* 17: 177–84.

Docherty, C.L., T.C. Valovich McLeod, and S.J. Shultz. 2006. Postural control deficits in participants with functional ankle instability as measured by the balance error scoring system. *Clinical Journal of Sports Medicine.* 16: 203–8.

Draper, V., and L. Ballard. 1991. Electrical stimulation versus electromyographic biofeedback in the recovery of quadriceps femoris muscle function following anterior cruciate ligament surgery. *Physical Therapy.* 71: 455–61.

Drouin, J.M., P.A. Houglum, D.H. Perrin, and B.M. Gansneder. 2003. Weight-bearing and non-weight-bearing knee-joint reposition sense and functional performance. *Journal of Sport Rehabilitation.* 12: 54–66.

Freeman, M.A.R. 1965. Instability of the foot after injuries to the lateral ligaments of the ankle. *Journal of Bone Joint Surgery.* 47B: 669–77.

Freeman, S., A. Mascia, and S. McGill. 2013. Arthrogenic neuromusculature inhibition: A foundational investigation of existence in the hip joint. *Clinical Biomechanics.* 28: 171–77.

Gauffin, H., H. Tropp, and P. Odendrick. 1988. Effect of ankle disk training on postural control in patients with functional instability of the ankle joint. *International Journal of Sports Medicine.* 9: 141–44.

Gross, M.T. 1987. Effects of recurrent lateral ankle sprains on active and passive judgment of joint position. *Physical Therapy.* 67: 1505–9.

Gulick, D.T., J.C. Castel, F.X. Palermo, and D.O. Draper. 2011. Effect of patterned electrical neuromuscular stimulation on vertical jump in collegiate athletes. *Sports Health.* 3: 152–57.

Hale, S.A., J. Hertel, and L.C. Olmsted-Kramer. 2007. The effect of a 4-week comprehensive rehabilitation program on postural control and lower extremity function in individuals with chronic ankle instability. *Journal of Orthopaedic and Sports Physical Therapy.* 37: 303–11.

Hallett, M., B.T. Shahani, and R.R. Young. 1975. EMG analysis of stereotyped voluntary movements in man. *Journal of Neurology, Neurosurgery, and Psychiatry.* 38: 1154–62.

Hart, J.M., B. Pietrosimone, J. Hertel, and C.D. Ingersoll. 2010. Quadriceps activation following knee injuries: A systematic review. *Journal of Athletic Training.* 45: 87–97.

Holme, E., S.P. Magnusson, K. Becher, T. Bieler, P. Aagaard, and M. Kjaer. 1999. The effect of supervised rehabilitation on strength, postural sway, position sense and re-injury risk after acute ankle ligament sprain. *Scandinavian Journal of Medicine and Science in Sports.* 9: 104–9.

Hopkins, J.T., and C.D. Ingersoll. 2000. Arthrogenic muscle inhibition: A limiting factor in joint rehabilitation. *Journal of Sport Rehabilitation.* 9 (2): 135–59.

Hopkins J.T., C.D. Ingersoll, J. Edwards, and T.E. Klootwyk. 2002. Cryotherapy and transcutaneous electric neuromuscular stimulation decrease arthrogenic muscle inhibition of the vastus medialis after knee joint effusion. *Journal of Athletic Training.* 37: 25.

Janssen, K.W., W. van Mechelen, and E.A. Verhagen. 2011. Ankles back in randomized controlled trial (ABrCt): Braces versus neuromuscular exercises for the secondary prevention of ankle sprains. Design of a randomised controlled trial. *BMC Musculoskeletal Disorders.* 12: 210.

Kennedy, J.C., I.J. Alexander, and K.C. Hayes. 1982. Nerve supply to the human knee and its functional importance. *American Journal of Sports Medicine.* 10: 329–35.

Kim, K.M., T. Croy, J. Hertel, and S. Saliba. 2010. Effects of neuromuscular electrical stimulation after anterior cruciate ligament reconstruction on quadriceps strength, function, and patient-oriented outcomes: A systematic review. *Journal of Orthopaedic Sports Physical Therapy.* 40: 383–91.

Kirnap, M., M. Calis, A.O. Turgut, M. Halici, and M. Tuncel. 2005. The efficacy of EMG-biofeedback training on quadriceps muscle strength in patients after arthroscopic meniscectomy. *New Zealand Medical Journal.* 118: 1224.

Kots, Y.M. 1977. Electrostimulation. Canadian-Soviet exchange symposium on electrostimulation of skeletal muscles. Concordia University, Montreal, Quebec, Canada. December 6–15. In J. Kramer and S.W. Mendryk. 1982. Electrical stimulation as a strength improvement technique. *Journal of Orthopaedic Sports Physical Therapy.* 4: 91–98.

Lee, A.J., and W.H. Lin. 2008. Twelve-week biomechanical ankle platform system training on postural stability and ankle proprioception in subjects with unilateral functional ankle instability. *Clinical Biomechanics.* 23: 1065–72.

Lieber, R.L., P.D. Silva, and D.M. Daniel. 1996. Equal effectiveness of electrical and volitional strength training for quadriceps femoris muscles after anterior cruciate ligament surgery. *Journal of Orthopaedic Research.* 14: 131–38.

Lofvenberg, R., J. Karrholm, G. Sundelin, and O. Ahlgren. 1995. Prolonged reaction time in patients with chronic lateral instability of the ankle. *American Journal of Sports Medicine.* 23: 414–17.

Lorentzon, R., L. Elmqvist, M. Sjostrom, M. Fagerlund, and A.R. Fuglmeyer. 1993. Thigh musculature in relation to chronic anterior cruciate ligament tear: Muscle size, morphology and mechanical output before reconstruction. *American Journal of Sports Medicine.* 17: 423–29.

Mattacola, C.G., and M.K. Dwyer. 2002. Rehabilitation of the ankle after acute sprain or chronic instability. *Journal of Athletic Training.* 37 (4): 413.

Mattacola, C.G., and J.W. Lloyd. 1997. Effects of a 6-week strength and proprioception training program on measures of dynamic balance: A single-case design. *Journal of Athletic Training.* 32: 127.

McKeon, P.O., C.D. Ingersoll, D.C. Kerrigan, E. Saliba, B.C. Bennett, and J. Hertel. 2008. Balance training improves function and postural control in those with chronic ankle instability. *Medicine & Science in Sports & Exercise.* 40: 1810-19.

McMullen, J., and T.L. Uhl. 2000. A kinetic chain approach for shoulder rehabilitation. *Journal of Athletic Training.* 35: 329.

Myers, J.B., and S.M. Lephart. 2000. The role of the sensorimotor system in the athletic shoulder. *Journal of Athletic Training.* 35: 351-63.

Paine, R.M., and M. Voight. 1993. The role of the scapula. *Journal of Orthopaedic and Sports Physical Therapy.* 18: 386-91.

Palermo, F.X. 1987. Patterned electric stimulation vs. upper extremity spasticity in hemiplegia. *Archives of Physical Medicine and Rehabilitation.* 68: 651.

Palermo, F.X., K. Picone, and J. Freeburg. 1991. Patterned electrical stimulation versus torticollis—Six cases. *Physical Therapy.* 71 (6): S036.

Palmieri, R.M., C.D. Ingersoll, and M.A. Hoffman. 2004. The Hoffmann reflex: Methodologic considerations and applications for use in sports medicine and athletic training research. *Journal of Athletic Training.* 39: 268.

Palmieri-Smith, R.M., A.C. Thomas, and E.M. Wojtys. 2008. Maximizing quadriceps strength after ACL reconstruction. *Clinical Sports Medicine.* 27: 405-24.

Partner, S.L, M.A. Sutherlin, S. Acocello, S.A. Saliba., E.M. Magrum, and J.M. Hart. Changes in muscle thickness after exercise and biofeedback in people with low back pain. *J Sport Rehabilitation.* 23 (4): 307-18.

Pietrosimone, B.G., J.M. Hart, S.A. Saliba, J. Hertel, and C.D. Ingersoll. 2009. Immediate effects of transcutaneous electrical nerve stimulation and focal knee joint cooling on quadriceps activation. *Medicine & Science in Sports & Exercise.* 41: 1175-81.

Pietrosimone, B.G., J. Hertel, C.D. Ingersoll, J.M. Hart, and S.A. Saliba. 2011. Voluntary quadriceps activation deficits in patients with tibiofemoral osteoarthritis: A meta-analysis. *Physical Medicine and Rehabilitation.* 3: 153-62.

Sims, J, Cosby, N, Saliba, E.N, Hertel, J, and Saliba, S.A. 2013. Exergaming and static postural control in individuals with a history of lower limb injury. *J Athletic Training* 48 (3) 314-25.

Snyder-Mackler, L., Z. Ladin, A.A. Schepsis, and J.C. Young. 1991. Electrical stimulation of the thigh muscles after reconstruction of the anterior cruciate ligament. Effects of electrically elicited contraction of the quadriceps femoris and hamstring muscles on gait and on strength of the thigh muscles. *Journal of Bone and Joint Surgery.* 73: 1025-36.

Snyder-Mackler, L., A. Delitto, S.L. Bailey, and S.W. Stralka. 1995. Strength of the quadriceps femoris muscle and functional recovery after reconstruction of the anterior cruciate ligament. A prospective, randomized clinical trial of electrical stimulation. *J Bone Joint Surg Am.* 77 (8):1166-73.

Solomonow, M., R. Baratta, B.H. Zhou, H. Shoji, W. Bose, C. Beck, and R. D'Ambrosia. 1987. The synergistic action of the anterior cruciate ligament and thigh muscles in maintaining joint stability. *American Journal of Sports Medicine.* 15: 207-13.

Spencer, J.D., K.C. Hayes, and I.J. Alexander. 1984. Knee joint effusion and quadriceps reflex inhibition in man. *Archives of Physical Medicine and Rehabilitation.* 65: 171-77.

Tropp, H., J. Ekstrand, and J. Gillquist. 1984. Factors affecting stabilometry recordings of single limb stance. *American Journal of Sports Medicine.* 12: 185-88.

Tsang, K.K.W. 2001. *The effects of induced effusion of the ankle on neuromuscular performance.* PhD Dissertation. The Pennsylvania State University.

Ward, A.R., and V.J. Robertson. 1998. Variation in torque production with frequency using medium frequency alternating current. *Archives of Physical Medicine and Rehabilitation.* 79: 1399-1404.

Wester, J.U., S.M. Jespersen, K.D. Nielsen, and L. Neumann. 1996. Wobble board training after partial sprains of the lateral ligaments of the ankle: A prospective randomized study. *Journal of Orthopaedic Sports Physical Therapy.* 23: 332-36.

Yip, S.L., and G.Y. Ng. 2006. Biofeedback supplementation to physiotherapy exercise programme for rehabilitation of patellofemoral pain syndrome: A randomized controlled pilot study. *Clinical Rehabilitation.* 20: 1050-57.

Chapter 10

Akin, M.D., K.W. Weingand, D.A. Hengehold, M.B. Goodale, R.T. Kinkle, and R.P. Smith. 2001. Continuous low-level topical heat in the treatment of dysmenorrhea. *Obstetrics & Gynecology.* 97: 343-49.

Barber, F.A., D.A. McGuire, and S. Click. 1998. Continuous-flow cold therapy for outpatient anterior cruciate ligament reconstruction. *Arthroscopy.* 14: 130-35.

Belanger, A.Y. 2002. *Evidence-based guide to therapeutic physical agents.* Philadelphia: Lippincott Williams & Wilkins.

Bleakley. C., S. McDonough, and D. MacAuley. 2004. The use of ice in the treatment of acute soft-tissue injury: A systematic review of randomized controlled trials. *American Journal of Sports Medicine.* 32: 251-61.

Bocobo, C., A. Fast, W. Kingery, and M. Kaplan. 1991. The effect of ice on intraarticular temperature in the knee of the dog. *American Journal of Physical Medicine & Rehabilitation.* 70: 181-85.

Butterfield, T.A., T.M. Best, and M.A. Merrick. 2006. The dual roles of neutrophils and macrophages in inflammation: A critical balance between tissue damage and repair. *Journal of Athletic Training.* 41: 457-65.

Cataldi, J.K., K.A. Pritchard, J.M. Hart, and S.A. Saliba. 2013. Cryotherapy effects, part 2: Time to numbness onset and numbness duration. *International Journal of Athletic Therapy & Training.* 18 (5): 26.

Cohn, B.T., R.I. Draeger, and D.W. Jackson. 1989. The effects of cold therapy in the postoperative management of pain in patients undergoing anterior cruciate ligament reconstruction. *American Journal of Sports Medicine.* 17: 344-49.

Compton, C.J., C.N. Godwin, J.B. Brucker, T.J. Demchak, J.E. Edwards, and K.C. Huxel. 2008. Effect of walking while cooling the quadriceps intramuscular tissues following a 20-minute bout of running. *Journal of Athletic Training.* 43: S-58.

Cote, D.J., W.E. Prentice Jr., D.N. Hooker, and E.W. Shields. 1988. Comparison of three treatment procedures for minimizing ankle sprain swelling. *Physical Therapy.* 68: 1072-76.

Cross, K.M., R.W. Wilson, and D.H. Perrin. 1995. Functional performance following ice immersion to the lower extremity. *Journal of Athletic Training.* 30: 231-34.

Daniel, D.M., M.L. Stone, and D.L. Arendt. 1994. The effect of cold therapy on pain, swelling, and range of motion after anterior cruciate ligament reconstructive surgery. *Arthroscopy.* 10: 530-33.

Dervin, G.F., D.E. Taylor, and G.C. Keene. 1998. Effects of cold and compression dressings on early postoperative outcomes for the arthroscopic anterior cruciate ligament reconstruction patient. *Journal of Orthopaedic and Sports Physical Therapy.* 27: 403-6.

Dover, G., and M.E. Powers. 2004. Cryotherapy does not impair shoulder joint position sense. *Archives of Physical Medicine and Rehabilitation.* 85: 1241-46.

Draper, D.O., S.T. Harris, S. Schulthies, E. Durrant, K.L. Knight, and M. Richard. 1998. Hot-pack and 1 MHz ultrasound treatments have an additive effect on muscle temperature increase. *Journal of Athletic Training.* 33: 21-24.

Edwards, D.J., M. Rimmer, and G.C. Keene. 1996. The use of cold therapy in the postoperative management of patients undergoing arthroscopic anterior cruciate ligament reconstruction. *American Journal of Sports Medicine.* 24: 193-95.

Evans, T.A., C. Ingersoll, K.L. Knight, and T.W. Worrell. 1996. Agility following the application of cold therapy (Abstract). *Journal of Athletic Training.* 31: S-53.

French, S.D., M. Cameron, B.F. Walker, J.W. Reggars, and A.J. Esterman. *Superficial heat or cold for low back pain.* Cochrane Database of Systematic Reviews 2006, Issue 1. Art. No.: CD004750. DOI: 10.1002/14651858. CD004750.pub2

Gerig, B.K. 1990. The effects of cryotherapy on ankle proprioception (Abstract). *Journal of Athletic Training.* 24: S-119.

Grant, A. 1964. Massage with ice (cryokinetics) in the treatment of painful conditions of the musculoskeletal system. *Archives of Physical Medicine and Rehabilitation.* 45: 233-38.

Greicar, M., Z. Kendrick, I. Kimura, and M. Sitler. 1996. Immediate and delayed effects of cryotherapy on functional power and agility (Abstract). *Journal of Athletic Training.* 31: S-33.

Haimovici, N. 1982. Three years experience in direct intra-articular temperature measurement. *Progress in Clinical & Biological Research.* 107: 453-61.

Hartviksen, K. 1962. Ice therapy in spasticity. *Acta Neurologica Scandinavica.* 38 (Suppl 3): 79-84.

Higgins, D., and T.W. Kaminski. 1998. Contrast therapy does not cause fluctuations in human gastrocnemius intramuscular temperature. *Journal of Athletic Training.* 33: 336-40.

Holcomb, W.R. *2003.* The effects of superficial heating before 1 MHz ultrasound on tissue temperature. *Journal of Sport Rehabilitation.* 12: 95-103.

Hopkins, J., C.D. Ingersoll, J. Edwards, and T.E. Klootwyk. 2002. Cryotherapy and transcutaneous electric neuromuscular stimulation decrease arthrogenic muscle inhibition of the vastus medialis after knee joint effusion. *Journal of Athletic Training.* 37: 25-31.

Hopper, D., D. Whittington, and J. Davies. 1997. Does ice immersion influence ankle joint position sense? *Physiotherapy Research International.* 2: 223-36.

Hubbard, T.J., S.L. Aronson, and C.R. Denegar. 2004. Does cryotherapy improve treatment outcome? A systematic review. *Journal of Athletic Training.* 29: 88-94.

Huffman, D.H., B.G. Pietrosimone, T.L. Grindstaff, J.M. Hart, S.A. Saliba, C.D. Ingersoll. 2010. Effects of menthol-based counterirritant on quadriceps motoneuron-pool excitability. *Journal of Sport Rehabilitation.* 19 (1): 30-40.

Johnson, D.J., S. Moore, J. Moore, and R.A. Oliver. 1979. Effect of cold submersion on intramuscular temperature of the gastrocnemius muscle. *Physical Therapy.* 59 (10): 1238-42.

Knight, K.L. 1995. *Cryotherapy in sport injury management.* Champaign, IL: Human Kinetics.

Knight, K.L., J. Aquino, S.M. Johannes, and C.D. Urban. 1980. A re-examination of Lewis' cold-induced vasodilation in the finger and ankle. *Journal of Athletic Training.* 15: 238-50.

Konrath, G., T. Lock, H. Goitz, and J. Scheider. 1996. The use of cold therapy after anterior cruciate ligament reconstruction: A prospective randomized study and literature study. *American Journal of Sports Medicine.* 24: 629-33.

Kuligowski, L.A., S.M. Lephart, F.P. Giannantonio, and R.O. Blanc. 1998. Effect of whirlpool therapy on the signs and symptoms of delayed-onset muscle soreness. *Journal of Athletic Training.* 33: 222-28.

LaRiviere, J., and L.R. Osternig. 1994. The effect of ice immersion on joint position sense. *Journal of Sport Rehabilitation.* 3: 58-67.

Lessard, L.A., R.A. Scudds, A. Amendola, and M.D. Vaz. 1997. The efficacy of cryotherapy following arthroscopic knee surgery. *Journal of Orthopaedic Sports Physical Therapy.* 26: 14-22.

Leutz, D.W., and H. Harris. 1995. Continuous cold therapy in total knee arthroplasty. *American Journal of Knee Surgery.* 8: 121-23.

Levy, A.S., and E. Marmar. 1993. The role of cold compression dressings in the postoperative treatment of total knee arthroplasty. *Clinical Orthopaedics and Related Research.* 297: 174-78.

Lowdon, B.J., and R.J. Moore. 1975. Determinants and nature of intramuscular temperature changes during cold therapy. *American Journal of Physical Medicine & Rehabilitation.* 54 (5): 223-33.

Mason, L., R.A. Moore, J.E. Edwards, H.J. McQuay, S. Derry, and P.J. Wiffen. 2004. Systematic review of efficacy of topical rubefacients containing salicylates for the treatment of acute and chronic pain. *British Medical Journal.* 24: 328.

McDonough, E., K. Strauss, T. Apel, C. Ingersoll, and K.L. Knight. 1996. Cooling the ankle, lower leg and both affects dynamic postural sway (Abstract). *Journal of Athletic Training.* 31: S-10.

McMaster, W.C., S. Little, and T.R. Waugh. 1978. Laboratory evaluations of various cold therapy modalities. *American Journal of Sports Medicine.* 6: 291-94.

Merrick, M.A. 2002. Secondary injury after musculoskeletal trauma: A review and update. *Journal of Athletic Training.* 37: 209-17.

Merrick, M.A. 2003. *Inflammation and secondary injury.* Paper presented at the Penn State Athletic Training Conference, March 28.

Michlovitz, S.L. 1990. *Thermal agents in rehabilitation.* 2nd ed. Philadelphia: Davis.

Mora, S., C.G. Zalavras, L. Wang, and D.B. Thordarson. 2002. The role of pulsatile cold compression in edema resolution following ankle fractures: A randomized clinical trial. *Foot and Ankle International.* 23: 999-1002.

Myer, J.W., D.O. Draper, and E. Durrant. 1994. Contrast therapy and intramuscular temperature in the human leg. *Journal of Athletic Training.* 29: 318-22.

Myer, J.W., Measom, G., Durrant, E., and G.W. Fellingham. 1997. Cold- and hot-pack contrast therapy: Subcutaneous and intramuscular temperature change. *Journal of Athletic Training.* 32: 238-41.

Nadler, S.F., D.J. Steiner, G.N. Erasala, D.A. Hengehold, S.B. Abeln, and K.W. Weingand. 2003a. Continuous low-level heatwrap therapy for treating acute nonspecific low back pain. *Archives of Physical Medicine and Rehabilitation.* 84: 329-34.

Nadler, S.F., D.J. Steiner, G.N. Erasala, D.A. Hengehold, R.T. Hinkle, M. Beth Goodale, S.B. Abeln, and K.W. Weingand. 2002. Continuous low-level heat wrap therapy provides more efficacy than ibuprofen and acetaminophen for acute low back pain. *Spine.* 27: 1012-17.

Nadler, S.F., D.J. Steiner, S.R. Petty, G.N. Erasala, D.A. Hengehold, and K.W. Weingand. 2003b. Overnight use of continuous low-level heatwrap therapy for relief of low back pain. *Archives of Physical Medicine and Rehabilitation.* 84: 335-42.

Ohkoshi, Y., M. Ohkoshi, S. Nagasaki, A. Ono, T. Hashimoto, and S. Yamane. 1999. The effect of cryotherapy on intraarticular temperature and postoperative care after anterior cruciate ligament reconstruction. *American Journal of Sports Medicine.* 27: 357-62.

Oosterveld, F.G., and J.J. Rasker. 1994. Effects of local heat and cold treatment on surface and articular temperature of arthritic knees. *Arthritis & Rheumatology.* 37: 1578-82.

Oosterveld, F.G., J.J. Rasker, J.W. Jacobs, and H.J. Overmars. 1992. The effect of local heat and cold therapy on the intraarticular and skin surface temperature of the knee. *Arthritis & Rheumatology.* 35:146-51.

Pritchard, K.A., and S.A. Saliba. 2014. Should athletes return to activity after cryotherapy? *Journal of Athletic Training.* 49 (1): 95-96.

Provins K.A., and R. Morton. 1960. Tactile discrimination and skin temperature. *Journal of Applied Physics.* 15: 155-60.

Rice, D., P.J. McNair, and N. Dalbeth. 2009. Effects of cryotherapy on arthrogenic muscle inhibition using an experimental model of knee swelling. *Arthritis & Rheumatology.* 61: 78-83.

Rivers, D., I. Kimura, M. Sitler, and Z. Kendrick. 1995. The influence of cryotherapy and aircast bracing on total body balance and proprioception (Abstract). *Journal of Athletic Training.* 30: S-15.

Robinson, V., L. Brosseau, L. Casimiro, M. Judd, B. Shea, G. Wells, and P. Tugwell. 2002. *Thermotherapy for treating rheumatoid arthritis. Cochrane Review.* Cochrane Library. Issue 1.

Rubley, M.D., C.R. Denegar, W.E. Buckley, and K.M. Newell. 2003. Cryotherapy, sensation and isometric force variability. *Journal of Athletic Training.* 38: 113-19.

Selkow, N.M., C. Day, Z. Liu, J.M. Hart, J. Hertel, and S.A. Saliba. 2012. Microvascular perfusion and intramuscular temperature of the calf during cooling. *Medicine & Science in Sports & Exercise.* 44: 850-56.

Shuler, D.E., C. Ingersoll, K.L. Knight, and J.S. Kuhlman. 1996. Local cold application to the foot and ankle, lower leg, or both: Effects on a cutting drill (Abstract). *Journal of Athletic Training.* 31: S-35.

Sloan, J.P., R. Hain, and R. Pownall. 1989. Clinical benefits of early cold therapy in accident and emergency following ankle sprain. *Archives of Emergency Medicine.* 6: 1-6.

Steinagel, M.C., J.E. Szczerba, Z.M. Guskiwicz, and D.H. Perrin. 1996. Ankle ice immersion effect on postural sway (Abstract). *Journal of Athletic Training.* 31: S-53.

Thieme, H.A., C.D. Ingersoll, K.L. Knight, and J.C. Ozmun. 1996. Cooling does not affect knee proprioception. *Journal of Athletic Training.* 31: 8-10.

Travel, J.G., and D.G. Simons. 1983. *Myofascial pain and dysfunction: The trigger point manual.* Baltimore: Williams & Wilkins.

van den Bekerom, M.P., P.A. Struijs, L. Blankevoort, L. Welling, C.N. van Dijk, and G.M. Kerkhoffs. 2012. What is the evidence for rest, ice, compression, and elevation therapy in the treatment of ankle sprains in adults? *Journal of Athletic Training.* 47: 435-43.

Wakin, L.G., A.N. Porter, and F.H. Krusen. 1951. Influence of physical agents and certain drugs on intraarticular temperature. *Archives of Physical Medicine and Rehabilitation.* 32: 714-21.

Warner, B., K. Kyung-Min, J.M. Hart, S. Salib. 2013. Lack of effect of superficial heat to the knee on quadriceps function in individuals with quadriceps inhibition. *Journal of Sport Rehabilitation.* 22: 93-99.

Wassinger, C.A., J.B. Myers, J.M. Gatti, K.M. Conley, and S.M. Lephart. 2007. Proprioception and throwing accuracy in the dominant shoulder after cryotherapy. *Journal of Athletic Training.* 42: 84–89.

West, T.F. 1998. *The role of diminished cutaneous sensory information and cryotherapy on haptic determination of rod length.* Doctoral dissertation. Pennsylvania State University.

Chapter 11

Barber, F.A., D.A. McGuire, and S. Click. 1998. Continuous-flow cold therapy for outpatient anterior cruciate ligament reconstruction. *Arthroscopy.* 14: 130–35.

Bell, G.W., and W.E. Prentice. 1998. Infrared modalities. In W.E. Prentice (ed.), *Therapeutic modalities for allied health professionals.* New York: McGraw-Hill, 201–39.

Bleakley, C.M., S.M. McDonough, D.C. MacAuley, and J. Bjordal. 2006. Cryotherapy for acute ankle sprains: A randomised controlled study of two different icing protocols. *British Journal of Sports Medicine.* 40: 700–5.

Bleakley, C.M., P. Glasgow, and D.C. MacAuley. 2012. PRICE needs updating, should we call the POLICE? *British Journal of Sports Medicine.* 46: 220–21.

Brown, W.C., and D.B. Hahn. 2009. Frostbite of the feet after cryotherapy: A report of two cases. *Journal of Foot and Ankle Surgery.* 48: 577–80.

Denegar, C.R., D.R. Dougherty, J.E. Friedman, M.E. Schimizzi, J.E. Clark, B.A. Comstock, and W.J. Kraemer. 2010. Preferences for heat, cold, or contrast in patients with knee osteoarthritis affect treatment response. *Clinical Interventions in Aging.* 5: 199–206.

Doeringer, J., M. Hoch, and A. Krause. 2009. The effect of focal ankle cooling on spinal reflex activity in individuals with chronic ankle instability. *Athletic Training and Sports Health Care.* 1: 59–64.

Draper, D.O., and M.D. Ricard. 1995. Rate of temperature decay following 3 MHz ultrasound: The stretching window. *Journal of Athletic Training.* 30: 304–7.

Dykstra, J.H., H.M. Hill, M.G. Miller, C.C. Cheatham, T.J. Michael, and R.J. Baker. 2009. Comparisons of cubed ice, crushed ice, and wetted ice on intramuscular and surface temperature changes. *Journal of Athletic Training.* 44: 136–41.

Freeman, S., A. Mascia, and S. McGill. 2013. Arthrogenic neuromusculature inhibition: A foundational investigation of existence in the hip joint. *Clinical Biomechanics.* 28: 171–77.

Hopkins, J., C.D. Ingersoll, J. Edwards, and T.E. Klootwyk. 2002. Cryotherapy and transcutaneous electric neuromuscular stimulation decrease arthrogenic muscle inhibition of the vastus medialis after knee joint effusion. *Journal of Athletic Training.* 37: 25–31.

Knight, K.L., J. Aquino, S.M. Johannes, and C.D. Urban. 1980. A re-examination of Lewis' cold-induced vasodilation in the finger and ankle. *Journal of Athletic Training.* 15: 238–50.

Knight, K.L. 1995. *Cryotherapy in sport injury management.* Champaign, IL: Human Kinetics.

Knight, C.A., C.R. Rutledge, M.E. Cox, M. Acosta, and S.J. Hall. 2001. Effect of superficial heat, deep heat, and active exercise warm-up on extensibility of the plantar flexors. *Physical Therapy.* 81: 1206–14.

Kuenze, C., J. Hertel, and J.M. Hart. 2013. Effects of exercise on lower extremity muscle function after anterior cruciate ligament reconstruction. *Journal of Sport Rehabilitation.* 22: 33–40.

Leutz, D.W., and H. Harris. 1995. Continuous cold therapy in total knee arthroplasty. *American Journal of Knee Surgery.* 8: 121–23.

Levy, A.S., and E. Marmar. 1993. The role of cold compression dressings in the postoperative treatment of total knee arthroplasty. *Clinical Orthopaedics and Related Research.* 297: 174–78.

Lewis, T. 1930. Observations upon the reactions of the vessels of the human skin to cold. *Heart.* 15: 177–208.

Lewis, S.E., P.S. Holmes, S.R. Woby, J. Hindle, and N.E. Fowler. 2012. Short-term effect of superficial heat treatment on paraspinal muscle activity, stature recovery, and psychological factors in patients with chronic low back pain. *Archives of Physical Medicine and Rehabilitation.* 93: 367–72.

Mailler-Savage, E.A., and D.F.J. Mutasim. 2008. Cold injury of the knee and lower aspect of the leg after knee surgery and use of a cold therapy system. *Journal of the American Academy of Dermatology.* 58 (5 Suppl 1): S106–8.

Nadler, S.F., D.J. Steiner, S.R. Petty, G.N. Erasala, D.A. Hengehold, and K.W. Weingand. 2003. Overnight use of continuous low-level heatwrap therapy for relief of low back pain. *Archives of Physical Medicine and Rehabilitation.* 84: 335–42.

Ohkoshi. Y., M. Ohkoshi, S. Nagasaki, A. Ono, T. Hashimoto, and S.Yamane. 1999. The effect of cryotherapy on intraarticular temperature and postoperative care after anterior cruciate ligament reconstruction. *American Journal of Sports Medicine.* 27: 357–62.

Oosterveld, F.G., J.J. Rasker, J.W. Jacobs, and H.J. Overmars. 1992. The effect of local heat and cold therapy on the intraarticular and skin surface temperature of the knee. *Arthritis & Rheumatology.* 35: 146–51.

Oosterveld, F.G., and J.J. Rasker. 1994. Effects of local heat and cold treatment on surface and articular temperature of arthritic knees. *Arthritis & Rheumatology.* 37: 1578–82.

Palmieri, R.M., C.D. Ingersoll, M.A. Hoffman, M.L. Cordova, D.A. Porter, J.E. Edwards, J.P. Babington, B.A. Krause, and M.B. Stone. 2004. Arthrogenic muscle response to a simulated ankle joint effusion. *British Journal of Sports Medicine.* 38 (1): 26–30.

Pietrosimone, B.G., S.A. Saliba, J.M. Hart, J. Hertel, and C.D. Ingersoll. 2010. Contralateral effects of disinhibitory TENS on quadriceps function in people with knee osteoarthritis following unilateral treatment. *North American Journal of Sports Physical Therapy.* 5: 111–21.

Pritchard, K.A., and S.A. Saliba. 2014. Should athletes return to activity after cryotherapy? *Journal of Athletic Training.* 49 (1): 95–96. doi: 10.4085/1062-6050-48.3.13. Epub 2013 May 31.

Rice, D., P.J. McNair, and N. Dalbeth. 2009. Effects of cryotherapy on arthrogenic muscle inhibition using an experimental model of knee swelling. *Arthritis & Rheumatology.* 61: 78–83.

Rupp, K.A., N.M. Selkow, W.R. Parente, C.D. Ingersoll, A.L. Weltman, and S.A. Saliba. 2012. The effect of cold water immersion on 48-hour performance testing in collegiate soccer players. *Journal of Strength and Conditioning Research.* 26: 2043–50.

Sedory, E.J., E.D. McVey, K.M. Cross, C.D. Ingersoll, and J. Hertel. 2007. Arthrogenic muscle response of the quadriceps and hamstrings with chronic ankle instability. *Journal of Athletic Training.* 42: 355–60.

Stokes, M., and A. Young. 1984. The contribution of reflex inhibition to arthrogenous muscle weakness. *Clinical Science.* 67 (1): 7–14.

Tao, X.G., and E.J. Bernacki. 2005. A randomized clinical trial of continuous low-level heat therapy for acute muscular low back pain in the workplace. *Journal of Occupational and Environmental Medicine.* 47: 1298–306.

Travel, J.G., and D.G. Simons. 1983. *Myofascial pain and dysfunction: The trigger point manual.* Baltimore: Williams & Wilkins.

Tsang, K.K.W., B.P. Buxton, W.K. Guion, A.B. Joyner, and K.D. Browder. 1997. The effects of cryotherapy applied through various barriers. *Journal of Sport Rehabilitation.* 6 (4): 343–54.

Tsang, K.K.W., and S.J. Truglio. 2012. The effectiveness of two forms of cold therapy through various common barriers. National Athletic Trainers' Association Annual Meeting and Clinical Symposium, Free Communications Presentation. St. Louis, MO.

Versey, N.G., S.L. Halson, and B.T. Dawson. 2013. Water immersion recovery for athletes: Effect on exercise performance and practical recommendations. *Sports Medicine.* 43: 1101–30.

Walsh, M.T. 1996. Hydrotherapy: The use of water as a therapeutic agent. In S.L. Michlovitz (ed.), *Thermal agents in rehabilitation.* 3rd ed. Philadelphia: Davis, 139–67.

Warner, B., K. Kyung-Min, J.M. Hart, and S. Saliba. 2013. Lack of effect of superficial heat to the knee on quadriceps function in individuals with quadriceps inhibition. *Journal of Sport Rehabilitation.* 22: 93–99.

Young, A., M. Stokes, and J.F. Iles. 1987. Effects of joint pathology on muscle. *Clinical Orthopaedics and Related Research.* June: 21–27.

Chapter 12

Angle, S.R., K. Sena, D.R. Sumner, and A.S. Virdi. 2011. Osteogenic differentiation of rat bone marrow stromal cells by various intensities of low-intensity pulsed ultrasound. *Ultrasonics.* 51: 281–88.

Akyol, Y., D. Durmus, G. Alayli, B. Tander, Y. Bek, F. Canturk, and S. Tastan Sakarya. 2010. Does short-wave diathermy increase the effectiveness of isokinetic exercise on pain, function, knee muscle strength, quality of life, and depression in the patients with knee osteoarthritis? A randomized controlled clinical study. *European Journal of Physical and Rehabilitation Medicine.* 46: 325–36.

Assiotis, A., N.P. Sachinis, and B.E. Chalidis. 2012. Pulsed electromagnetic fields for the treatment of tibial delayed unions and nonunions. A prospective clinical study and review of the literature. *Journal of Orthopaedic Research.* 7: 24.

Atamaz, F.C., B. Durmaz, M. Baydar, O.Y. Demircioglu, A. Iyiyapici, B. Kuran, S. Oncel, and O.F. Sendur. 2012. Comparison of the efficacy of transcutaneous electrical nerve stimulation, interferential currents, and shortwave diathermy in knee osteoarthritis: A double-blind, randomized, controlled, multicenter study. *Archives of Physical Medicine and Rehabilitation.* 93: 748–56.

Bakhtiary, A.H., E. Fatemi, M. Emami, and M. Malek. 2013. Phonophoresis of dexamethasone sodium phosphate may manage pain and symptoms of patients with carpal tunnel syndrome. *Clinical Journal of Pain.* 29: 348–53.

Barker, A.T., P.S. Barlow, J. Porter, M.E. Smith, S. Clifton, L. Andrews, and W.J. O'Dowd. 1985. A double-blind clinical trial of low-power pulsed short wave therapy in the treatment of a soft tissue injury. *Physiotherapy* 71: 500–04.

Bashardoust Tajali, S., P. Houghton, J.C. MacDermid, and R. Grewal. 2012. Effects of low-intensity pulsed ultrasound therapy on fracture healing: A systematic review and meta-analysis. *American Journal of Physical Medicine & Rehabilitation.* 91: 349–67.

Bassett, C.A. 1984. The development and application of pulsed electromagnetic fields (PEMFs) for ununited fractures and arthrodeses. *Orthopedic Clinics of North America.* 15: 61–87.

Belanger, A.Y. 2002. *Evidence-based guide to therapeutic physical agents.* Philadelphia: Lippincott Williams & Wilkins.

Brosseau, L., L. Casimiro, V. Robinson, S. Milne, B. Shea, M. Judd, G. Wells, P. Tugwell. 2001. *Therapeutic ultrasound for treating patellofemoral pain.* Cochrane Library. 4: CD003375.

Brown, M., and R.D. Baker. 1987. Effect of pulsed shortwave diathermy on skeletal muscle injury in rabbits. *Physical Therapy.* 67: 208–14.

Cagnie, B., E. Vinck, S. Rimbaut, and G. Vanderstraeten. 2003. Phonophoresis versus topical applications of ketoprofen: Comparison between tissue and plasma levels. *Physical Therapy.* 83: 707–12.

Callam, M.J., D.R. Harper, and J.J. Dale. 1987. A controlled trial of weekly ultrasound therapy in chronic leg ulceration. *Lancet.* 2: 204–6.

Cameron, M.H., and L.G. Monroe. 1992. Relative transmission of ultrasound by media customarily used by phonophoresis. *Physical Therapy.* 72: 142–48.

Chan, A.K., J.W. Myer, G.J. Measom, and D.O. Draper. 1998. Temperature changes in human patella tendon in response to therapeutic ultrasound. *Journal of Athletic Training.* 33: 130–35.

Cicone, C.D., B.G. Leggin, and J.J. Callamaro. 1991. The effects of ultrasound on trolamine salicylate phonophoresis on delayed onset muscle soreness. *Physical Therapy.* 71: 666–75.

Clarke, G.R., L.A. Willis, L. Stenners, and P.J. Nichols. 1974. Evaluation of physiotherapy in the treatment of osteoarthritis of the knee. *Rheumatology Rehabilitation.* 13: 190-97.

Crawford, F., D. Atkins, and J. Edwards. 2000. *Interventions for treating plantar heel pain. Cochrane Library.* 3.

Da Cunha, A., N.A. Parizotto, and C. Vidal Bde. 2001. The effect of therapeutic ultrasound on repair of the Achilles tendon (tendo Achilles) of the rat. *Ultrasound in Medicine and Biology.* 27: 1691-96.

Darrow, H., S. Schulthies, D. Draper, M. Ricard, and G.J. Measom. 1999. Serum dexamethasone levels after Decadron phonophoresis. *Journal of Athletic Training.* 34: 338-41.

Demchak, T.J., S.J. Straub, and L.D. Johns. 2007. Ultrasound heating is curvilinear in nature and varies between transducers from the same manufacturer. *Journal of Sport Rehabilitation.* 16: 122-30.

Downing, D.S., and A. Weinstein. 1986. Ultrasound therapy of subacromial bursitis. A double blind trial. *Physical Therapy.* 66: 194-99.

Draper, D.O. 1996. Ten mistakes commonly made with ultrasound use: Current research sheds light on myths. *Athletic Training and Sports Health Care Perspectives* 2: 95-107.

Draper, D.O. 1999. *A breakthrough on comfortable ultrasound treatments: Beam non-uniformity ratio is only half the equation.* Paper presented at Annual Meeting and Clinical Symposium of the National Athletic Trainers' Association, June 18, Kansas City, MO.

Draper, D.O. 2002. Don't disregard ultrasound yet—the jury is still out. *Physical Therapy.* 82: 190.

Draper, D.O. 2010. Ultrasound and joint mobilizations for achieving normal wrist range of motion after injury or surgery: A case series. *Journal of Athletic Training.* 45: 486-91.

Draper, D.O. 2011. Injuries restored to ROM using PSWD and mobilizations. *International Journal of Sports Medicine.* 32: 281-86.

Draper, D.O. 2014. Pulsed shortwave diathermy and joint mobilizations for achieving normal elbow range of motion after injury or surgery with implanted metal: A case series. *Journal of Athletic Training.* 49: 851-55.

Draper, D.O., C. Anderson, S.S. Schulthies, and M.C. Richard. 1998. Immediate and residual changes in dorsiflexion range of motion using an ultrasound heat and stretch routine. *Journal of Athletic Training.* 33: 141-44.

Draper, D.O., J.C. Castel, and D. Castel. 1995. Rates of temperature increase in human muscle during 1 MHz and 3 MHz continuous ultrasound. *Journal of Orthopaedic and Sports Physical Therapy.* 22: 142-50.

Draper, D.O., J.L. Castro, B. Feland, S. Schulties, and D. Eggett. 2004. Shortwave diathermy and prolonged stretching increase hamstring flexibility more than prolonged stretching alone. *Journal of Orthopaedic & Sports Physical Therapy.* 34: 13-20.

Draper, D.O., K.K. Knight, T. Fujiwara, and J.C. Castel. 1999. Temperature change in human muscle during and after pulsed short-wave diathermy. *Journal of Orthopaedic & Sports Physical Therapy.* 29: 13-22.

Draper, D.O., and M.D. Ricard. 1995. Rate of temperature decay following 3 MHz ultrasound: The stretching window. *Journal of Athletic Training.* 30: 304-7.

Draper, D.O., S. Sunderland, D.T. Kirkendall, and M. Richard. 1993. A comparison of temperature rise in human calf muscles following applications of underwater and topical gel ultrasound. *Journal of Orthopaedic and Sports Physical Therapy.* 23: 247-51.

Dyson, M., and J.B. Pond. 1970. The effect of pulsed ultrasound on tissue regeneration. *Physiotherapy.* 64: 105-8.

Dyson, M., and J. Suckling. 1978. Stimulation of tissue repair by ultrasound: A survey of mechanisms involved. *Physiotherapy.* 64: 105-8.

Ebenbichler, G.R., C.B. Erdogmus, K.I. Resch, M.A. Funovics, F. Kainberger, G. Barisani, M. Aringer, P. Nicolakis, G.F. Weisinger, M. Baghestanian, E. Preisinger, and V. Fialka-Moser. 1999. Ultrasound therapy for calcific tendinitis of the shoulder. *New England Journal of Medicine.* 340: 1533-38.

Ebenbichler, G.R., K.L. Resch, P. Nicolakis, G.F. Weisinger, F. Uhl, A.H. Ghanem, and V. Fialka. 1998. Ultrasound treatment for treating the carpal tunnel syndrome: Randomized "sham" controlled study. *British Medical Journal.* 316: 731-35.

El-Bialy, T., A. Alhadlaq, and B. Lam. 2012. Effect of therapeutic ultrasound on human periodontal ligament cells for dental and periodontal tissue engineering. *Open Dentistry Journal.* 6: 235-59.

Erikson, S.V., T. Lundeberg, and M. Malm. 1991. A placebo controlled trial of ultrasound in chronic leg ulceration. *Scandinavian Journal of Rehabilitation Medicine.* 3: 211-13.

Enwemeka, C.S., O. Rodriquez, and S. Mendosa. 1989. The effects of therapeutic ultrasound on tendon healing. *American Journal of Physical Medicine & Rehabilitation.* 6: 283-87.

Foley-Nolan, D., C. Barry, R.J. Coughlan, P. O'Connor, and D. Rodeo. 1990. Pulsed high frequency (27 MHz) electromagnetic therapy for persistent neck pain: A double blind, placebo controlled study of 20 patients. *Orthopedics.* 13: 445-51.

Foley-Nolan, D., K. Moore, M. Codd, P. O'Connor, and R.J. Coughlan. 1992. Low energy high frequency pulsed electromagnetic therapy for acute whiplash injuries. A double blind randomized controlled study. *Scand J Rehabil Med.* 24 (1): 51-9.

Forrest, G., and K. Rosen. 1989. Ultrasound: Effectiveness of treatments given under water. *Archives of Physical Medicine and Rehabilitation.* 70: 28-29.

Forrest, G., and K. Rosen. 1992. Ultrasound treatments in degassed water. *Journal of Sport Rehabilitation.* 1: 284-89.

Friedar, S. 1988. A pilot study: The therapeutic effect of ultrasound following partial rupture of Achilles tendons in rats. *Journal of Orthopaedic & Sports Physical Therapy.* 10: 39-45.

Frye, J.L., L.D. Johns, J.A. Tom, and C.D. Ingersoll. 2007. Blisters on the anterior shin in 3 research subjects after a

1-MHz, 1.5-W/cm, continuous ultrasound treatment: A case series. *Journal of Athletic Training.* 42: 425-30.

Fukuda, T.Y., R. Alves da Cunha, V.O. Fukuda, F.A. Rienzo, C. Cazarini, Jr., A. Carvalho Nde, and A.A. Centini. 2011. Pulsed shortwave treatment in women with knee osteoarthritis: A multicenter, randomized, placebo-controlled clinical trial. *Physical Therapy.* 91: 1009-17.

Fyfe, M.C., and L.A. Chahl. 1980. The effect of ultrasound on experimental oedema in rats. *Ultrasound in Medicine and Biology.* 6: 107-11.

Fyfe, M.C., and L.A. Chahl. 1985. The effect of single or repeated applications of "therapeutic" ultrasound on plasma extravasation during silver nitrate induced inflammation of the rat hindpaw ankle joint in vivo. *Ultrasound in Medicine and Biology.* 11: 273-83.

Gam, A.N., and F. Johannsen. 1995. Ultrasound therapy in musculoskeletal disorders: A meta-analysis. *Pain.* 63: 85-91.

Gersten, J. 1958. Effect of metallic objects on temperature rises produced in tissue by ultrasound. *American Journal of Physical Medicine.* 37: 75-82.

Goldon, J.H., N.R.G. Broadbent, J.D. Nancarrow, and T. Marshall. 1981. The effects of Diapulse on the healing of wounds: A double blind randomized controlled trial in man. *British Journal of Plastic Surgery.* 34: 267-70.

Griffin, J.E., J.L. Echternach, R.E. Price, and J.C. Touchstone. 1967. Patients treated with ultrasonic driven cortisone and with ultrasound alone. *Physical Therapy.* 44: 20-27.

Griffin, J.E., and J.C. Touchstone. 1972. Effects of ultrasonic frequency on phonophoresis of cortisol in swine tissue. *American Journal of Physical Medicine & Rehabilitation.* 51: 62-78.

Hacker, E., and T. Lundeberg T. 1991. Pulsed ultrasound treatment in lateral epicondylalgia. *Scandinavian Journal of Rehabilitation Medicine.* 23: 115-18.

Hawkes, A.R., D.O. Draper, A.W. Johnson, M.T. Diede, and J.H. Rigby. 2013. Heating capacity of rebound shortwave diathermy and moist hot packs at superficial depths. *Journal of Athletic Training.* 48: 471-76.

Hayes, B.T., M.A. Merrick, M.A. Sandrey, and M.L. Cordova. 2004. Three-MHz ultrasound heats deeper into the tissues than originally theorized. *Journal of Athletic Training.* 39: 230-34.

Holcomb, W.R., and C.J. Joyce. 2003. A comparison of temperature increases produced by two commonly used ultrasound units. *Journal of Athletic Training.* 38: 24-27.

Holmes, G.B., Jr. 1994. Treatment of delayed unions and nonunions of the proximal fifth metatarsal with pulsed electromagnetic fields. *Foot and Ankle International.* 15: 552-56.

Huang, M.H., Y.S. Lin, C.L. Lee, and R.C. Yang. 2005. Use of ultrasound to increase effectiveness of isokinetic exercise for knee osteoarthritis. *Archives of Physical Medicine and Rehabilitation.* 86: 1545-51.

Itoh, M., J.S. Montemayor, Jr., E. Matsumoto, A. Eason, M.H. Lee, and F.S. Folk. 1991. Accelerated wound healing of pressure ulcers by pulsed high peak power electromagnetic energy (Diapulse). *Decubitus.* 4: 24-30.

Johns, L.D., T.J. Demchak, S.J. Straub, and S.M. Howard. 2007. The role of quantitative Schlieren assessment of physiotherapy ultrasound fields in describing variations between tissue heating rates of different transducers. *Ultrasound in Medicine and Biology.* 33: 1911-17.

Johns, L.D., S.J. Straub, and S.M. Howard. 2007. Variability in effective radiating area and output power of new ultrasound transducers at 3 MHz. *Journal of Athletic Training.* 42: 22-28.

Klucinec, B. 1996. The effectiveness of the aquaflex gel pad in the transmission of acoustic energy. *Journal of Athletic Training.* 31: 313-17.

Klucinec, B., M. Scheidler, C. Denegar, E. Domholt, and S. Burgess. 2000. Transmissivity of common coupling agents used to deliver ultrasound through indirect methods. *Journal of Orthopaedic and Sports Physical Therapy.* 30: 263-69.

Kristiansen, T.K., J.P. Ryaby, J. McCabe, J.J. Frey, and L.R. Roe. 1997. Accelerated healing of distal radial fractures with the use of specific, low-intensity ultrasound. A multicenter, prospective, randomized, double-blind, placebo-controlled study. *Journal of Bone and Joint Surgery.* 79: 961-73.

Kumagai, K., R. Takeuchi, H. Ishikawa, Y. Yamaguchi, T. Fujisawa, T. Kuniya, S. Takagawa, G.F. Muschler, and T. Saito. 2012. Low-intensity pulsed ultrasound accelerates fracture healing by stimulation of recruitment of both local and circulating osteogenic progenitors. *Journal of Orthopaedic Research.* 30: 1516-21.

Lehmann, J.F., B. Delateur, and D.R. Silverman. 1966. Selective heating effects of ultrasound in human beings. *Archives of Physical Medicine and Rehabilitation.* 47: 331-38.

Loyola-Sánchez, A., J. Richardson, K.A. Beattie, C. Otero-Fuentes, J.D. Adachi, and N.J. MacIntyre. 2012. Effect of low-intensity pulsed ultrasound on the cartilage repair in people with mild to moderate knee osteoarthritis: A double-blinded, randomized, placebo-controlled pilot study. *Archives of Physical Medicine and Rehabilitation.* 93: 35-42.

McCray, R.E., and N.J. Patton. 1984. Pain relief at trigger points: A comparison of moist heat and shortwave diathermy. *Journal of Orthopaedic and Sports Physical Therapy.* 5: 175-78.

McGill, S.N. 1998. The effect of pulsed shortwave therapy on lateral ligament sprain of the ankle. *New Zealand Journal of Physiotherapy.* 10: 21-24.

Moffett, J.A., P.H. Richardson, H. Prost, and A. Osborn. 1996. A placebo-controlled double blind trial to calculate the effectiveness of pulsed shortwave diathermy for osteoarthritic hip and knee pain. *Pain.* 67: 121-27.

Nyanzi, C.S., J. Langridge, J.R.C. Heyworth, and R. Mani. 1999. Randomized controlled study of ultrasound therapy in the management of acute lateral ligament sprains of the ankle joint. *Clinical Rehabilitation.* 31: 16-22.

Nykanen, M. 1995. Pulsed ultrasound treatment of the painful shoulder: A randomized, double blind, placebo-controlled study. *Scandinavian Journal of Rehabilitation Medicine.* 27: 105-8.

Oosterveld, F.G., J.J. Rasker, J.W. Jacobs, and H.J. Overmars. 1992. The effect of local heat and cold therapy on the intraarticular and skin surface temperature of the knee. *Arthritis & Rheumatology*. 35: 146–51.

Ozgüçlü, E., A. Cetin, M. Cetin, and E. Calp. 2010. Additional effect of pulsed electromagnetic field therapy on knee osteoarthritis treatment: A randomized, placebo-controlled study. *Clinical Rheumatology*. 29: 927–31.

Oziomek, R.S., D.H. Perrin, D.A. Harrold, and C.R. Denegar. 1991. Effect of ultrasound intensity and mode on serum salicylate levels following phonophoresis. *Medicine and Science in Sports Exercise*. 23: 397–401.

Pasila, M., T. Visuri, and A. Sundholm. 1978. Pulsating shortwave diathermy: Value in treatment of recent ankle and foot sprains. *Archives of Physical Medicine and Rehabilitation*. 59: 383–86.

Penderghest, C.E., I.F. Kimura, and D.T. Gulick. 1998. Double-blind clinical efficacy study of pulsed phonophoresis on perceived pain associated with traumatic tendinitis. *Journal of Sport Rehabilitation*. 7: 9–19.

Ryang We, S., Y.H. Koog, K.I. Jeong, and H. Wi. 2013. Effects of pulsed electromagnetic field on knee osteoarthritis: A systematic review. *Rheumatology* (Oxford). 52: 815–24.

Rattanachaiyanont, M., and V. Kuptniratsaikul. 2008. No additional benefit of shortwave diathermy over exercise program for knee osteoarthritis in peri-/post-menopausal women: An equivalence trial. *Osteoarthritis Cartilage*. 16: 823–28.

Robertson, V.J., and K.G. Baker. 2001. A review of therapeutic ultrasound: Effectiveness studies. *Physical Therapy*. 81: 1339–50.

Robinson, V.A., L. Brosseau, J. Peterson, B.J. Shea, P. Tugwell, and G. Wells. 2001. *Therapeutic ultrasound for osteoarthritis of the knee. Cochrane Database of Systematic Reviews*. Issue 3.

Rose, S., D.O. Draper, S.S. Schulthies, and E. Durant. 1996. The stretching window part two: Rate of thermal decay in deep muscles following 1 MHz ultrasound. *Journal of Athletic Training*. 31: 139–43.

Rubley, M.D., M.N. Peluaga, J. Meddoza, J. Threat, W.R. Holcolm, A.J. Tritsch, and R.D. Tandy. 2008. Ultrasound heating of the Achilles tendon: A comparison of direct and indirect applications techniques. *Journal of Athletic Training*. 43: S-58.

Saini, N.S., K.S. Roy, P.S. Bansal, B. Singh, and P.S. Simran. 2002. A preliminary study on the effect of ultrasound therapy on the healing of severed Achilles tendons in five dogs. *Journal of Veterinary Medicine. A, Physiology, Pathology, Clinical Medicine*. 49: 321–28.

Saliba, S., D.J. Mistry, D.H. Perrin, J. Gieck, and A. Weltman. 2007. Phonophoresis and the absorption of dexamethasone in the presence of an occlusive dressing. *Journal of Athletic Training*. 42: 34–54.

Seiger, C., and D.O. Draper. 2006. Use of pulsed shortwave diathermy and joint mobilization to increase ankle range of motion in the presence of surgical implanted metal: A case series. *Journal of Orthopaedic and Sports Physical Therapy*. 36: 669–77.

Sharrard, W.J.W. 1990. A double blind trial of pulsed electromagnetic fields for delayed healing of tibial fractures. *Journal of Bone and Joint Surgery*. 72B: 347–55.

Shi, H.F., J. Xiong, Y.X. Chen, J.F. Wang, X.S. Qiu, Y.H. Wang, and Y. Qiu. 2013. Early application of pulsed electromagnetic field in the treatment of postoperative delayed union of long-bone fractures: A prospective randomized controlled study. *BMC Musculoskeletal Disorders*. 14: 35.

Sicard-Rosenbaum, L., D. Lord, J.V. Danoff, A.K. Thom, and M.A. Eckhaus. 1995. Effects of continuous therapeutic ultrasound on growth and metastasis of subcutaneous murine tumors. *Physical Therapy*. 75: 3–11.

Straub, S.J., L.D. Johns, and S.M. Howard. 2008. Variability in effective radiating area at 1 MHz affects ultrasound treatment intensity. *Physical Therapy*. 88: 50–57.

Svarcova, J., K. Trnavsky, and J. Zvarova. 1987. The influence of ultrasound galvanic currents and shortwave diathermy on pain intensity in patients with osteoarthritis. *Scandinavian Journal of Rheumatology. Supplement*. 67: 83–85.

Takakura, Y., N. Matsui, S. Yoshiya, H. Fujioka, H. Muratsu, M. Tsunoda, and M. Kurosaka. 2002. Low-intensity pulsed ultrasound enhances early healing of medial collateral ligament injuries in rats. *Journal of Ultrasound in Medicine*. 21: 283–88.

Trock, D.H., A.J. Bollet, R.H. Dyer, Jr, L.P. Fielding, W.K. Miner, and R. Markoll. 1993. A double-blind trial of the clinical effects of pulsed electromagnetic fields in osteoarthritis. *Journal of Rheumatology*. 20: 456–60.

Urita, A., N. Iwasaki, M. Kondo, Y. Nishio, T. Kamishima, and A. Minami. 2013. Effect of low-intensity pulsed ultrasound on bone healing at osteotomy sites after forearm bone shortening. *Journal of Hand Surgery (American Volume)*. 38: 498–503.

Van Der Windt, D.A., G.J. Van Der Heijden, S.G. Van Den Berg, G. Ter Riet, A.F. De Winter, and L.M. Bouter. 2002. Ultrasound therapy for acute ankle sprains. *Cochrane Database of Systematic Reviews*. (1): CD001250.

Van der Windt, D.A.W.M., G.J.M.G. van der Heijden, S.G.M. van den Berg, G. ter Riet, A.F. de Winter, and L.M. Bouter. 1999. Ultrasound therapy for musculoskeletal disorders: A systematic review. *Pain*. 81: 257–71.

Walker, N.A., C.R. Denegar, and J. Preische. 2007. Low-intensity pulsed ultrasound and pulsed electromagnetic field in the treatment of tibial fractures: A systematic review. *Journal of Athletic Training*. 42: 530–35.

Warden, S.J., B.R. Metcalf, Z.S. Kiss, J.L. Cook, C.R. Purdam, K.L. Bennell, and K.M. Crossley. 2008. Low-intensity pulsed ultrasound for chronic patellar tendinopathy: A randomized, double-blind, placebo-controlled trial. *Rheumatology* (Oxford). 47: 467–71.

Welch, V., L. Brosseau, J. Peterson, B. Shea, P. Tugwell, and G. Wells. 2001. *Therapeutic ultrasound for osteoarthritis of the knee. The Cochrane Library*. 3: CD003132.

Whittaker, J.L., D.S. Teyhen, J.M. Elliot et al. 2007. Rehabilitative ultrasound imaging: Understanding the technology and its applications. *Journal of Orthopaedic and Sports Physical Therapy*. 37 (8): 434–49.

Ying, Z.M., T. Lin, and S.G. Yan. 2012. Low-intensity pulsed ultrasound therapy: A potential strategy to stimulate tendon-bone junction healing. *Journal of Zhejiang University-SCIENCE B (Biomedicine & Biotechnology)*. 13: 955–63.

Chapter 13

Bashardoust Tajali, S., P. Houghton, J.C. MacDermid, and R. Grewal. 2012. Effects of low-intensity pulsed ultrasound therapy on fracture healing: A systematic review and meta-analysis. *American Journal of Physical Medicine & Rehabilitation*. 91: 349–67.

Di Cesare, A., A. Giombini, S. Dragoni, L. Agnello, M. Ripani, V.M. Saraceni, and N. Maffulli. 2008. Calcific tendinopathy of the rotator cuff. Conservative management with 434 Mhz local microwave diathermy (hyperthermia): A case study. See comment in PubMed Commons below*Disability Rehabilitation*. 30: 1578–83.

Draper, D.O. 2010. Ultrasound and joint mobilizations for achieving normal wrist range of motion after injury or surgery: A case series. *Journal of Athletic Training*. 45: 486–91.

Draper, D.O. 2014. Pulsed shortwave diathermy and joint mobilizations for achieving normal elbow range of motion after injury or surgery with implanted metal: A case series. *Journal of Athletic Training*. 49: 851–55.

Draper, D.O., K.K. Knight, T. Fujiwara, and J.C. Castel. 1999. Temperature change in human muscle during and after pulsed short-wave diathermy. *Journal of Orthopaedic and Sports Physical Therapy*. 29: 13–22.

Draper, D.O., A.R. Hawkes, A.W. Johnson, M.T. Diede, and J.H. Rigby. 2013. Muscle heating with Megapulse II shortwave diathermy and ReBound diathermy. *Journal of Athletic Training*. 48: 477–82.

Ebenbichler, G.R., C.B. Erdogmus , K.L. Resch, M.A. Funovics, F. Kainberger, G. Barisani, M. Aringer, P. Nicolakis, G.F. Wiesinger, M. Baghestanian, E. Preisinger, and V. Fialka-Moser. 1999. Ultrasound therapy for calcific tendinitis of the shoulder. *New England Journal of Medicine*. 340: 1533–38.

Exogen (Bioventus LLC, Durham, NC, USA) www.exogen.com/us accessed 1/5/15.

Gersten, J. 1958. Effect of metallic objects on temperature rises produced in tissue by ultrasound. *American Journal of Physical Medicine*. 37: 75–82.

Hannemann, P.F., E.H. Mommers, J.P. Schots, P.R. Brink, and M. Poeze. 2014. The effects of low-intensity pulsed ultrasound and pulsed electromagnetic fields bone growth stimulation in acute fractures: A systematic review and meta-analysis of randomized controlled trials. *Archives of Orthopaedic and Trauma Surgery*. 134: 1093–106.

Incebiyik, S., A. Boyaci, and A. Tutoglu. 2014. Short-term effectiveness of short-wave diathermy treatment on pain, clinical symptoms, and hand function in patients with mild or moderate idiopathic carpal tunnel syndrome. *Journal of Back and Musculoskeletal Rehabilitation*. July 24. [Epub ahead of print].

Lehmann, J.F., B. Delateur, and D.R. Silverman. 1966. Selective heating effects of ultrasound in human beings. *Archives of Physical Medicine and Rehabilitation*. 47: 331–38.

Page, M.J., D. O'Connor, V. Pitt, N. Massy-Westropp. Therapeutic ultrasound for carpal tunnel syndrome. *Cochrane Database of Systematic Reviews* 2013, Issue 3. Art. No.: CD009601. DOI: 10.1002/14651858.CD009601.pub2.

Piravej, K., and J. Boonhong. 2004. Effect of ultrasound thermotherapy in mild to moderate carpal tunnel syndrome. *Journal of the Medical Association of Thailand*. 87 Suppl. 2: S100-6.

Punt, B.J., P.T. den Hoed, and W.P.J. Fontijne. 2008. Pulsed electromagnetic fields in the treatment of nonunion. *European Journal of Orthopaedic Surgery & Traumatology*. 18 (2): 127–33.

Seiger, C., and D.O. Draper. 2006. Use of pulsed shortwave diathermy and joint mobilization to increase ankle range of motion in the presence of surgical implanted metal: A case series. *Journal of Orthopaedic and Sports Physical Therapy*. 36:669–77.

Sicard-Rosenbaum, L., D. Lord, J.V. Danoff, A.K. Thom, and M.A. Eckhaus. 1995. Effects of continuous therapeutic ultrasound on growth and metastasis of subcutaneous murine tumors. *Physical Therapy*. 75: 3–11.

Szlosek, P.A., J. Taggart, J.M. Cavallario, and J.M. Hoch. 2014. Effectiveness of diathermy in comparison with ultrasound or corticosteroids in patients with tendinopathy: A critically appraised topic. *Journal of Sport Rehabilitation*. 23: 370–75.

Walker, N.A., C.R. Denegar, and J. Preische. 2007. Low-intensity pulsed ultrasound and pulsed electromagnetic field in the treatment of tibial fractures: A systematic review. *Journal of Athletic Training*. 42: 530–35.

Chapter 14

Abergel, R. P., C.A. Meeker, T.S. Lam,, R. M. Dwyer, M.A. Lesavoy, and J. Uitto, J. 1984. Control of connective tissue metabolism by lasers: recent developments and future prospects. *Journal of the American Academy of Dermatology*. 11 (6): 1142-50.

Alfredo, P.P., J.M. Bjordal, S.H. Dreyer, et al. 2011. Efficacy of low level laser therapy association with exercise in knee osteoarthritis: A randomized double-blinded study. *Clinical Rehabilitation*. 26 (6) 523–33.

Brown, C.G. 1999. Nitric oxide and mitochondrial respiration. *Biochimica et Biophysica Acta*. 1411: 351.

da Silva, J.P., M.A. da Silva, A.P. Almeida, et al. 2010. Laser therapy in the tissue repair process: A literature review. *Photomedicine and Laser Surgery*. 28 (1): 17–21.

Derr, V.E., and S. Fine. 1965. Free radical occurrence in some laser-irradiated biologic materials. In *Federation Proceedings*. Vol 24: SUPPL-14,

Dixit, S., A. Maiya, L. Rao, et al. 2012. Photobiomodulation by helium neon and diode lasers in an excisional wound model: A single blinded trial. *Advanced Biomedical Research*. 1: 38.

Giulivi, C., J.J. Poderoso, and A. Boveris. 1998. Production of nitric oxide by mitochondria. *Journal of Biological Chemistry*. 273 (18): 11038–43.

Hawkins, D.H. and H. Abrahamse. 2006. The role of laser fluence in cell viability, proliferation, and membrane integrity of wounded human skin fibroblasts following helium-neon laser irradiation. *Lasers in Surgery and Medicine*. 38 (1): 74–83.

Huang, Y.Y., A.C.H. Chen, J.D. Carroll, et al. 2009. Biphasic dose response in low level light therapy. *International Dose-Response*. 7 (4): 358–83.

Huang, Y.Y., K. Nagata, C.E. Tedford, et al. 2013. Low-level laser reduced oxidative stress in primary cortical neurons in vitro. *Journal of Biophotonics*. 6 (10): 829–38.

Karu, T. 1987. Photobiological fundamentals of low-power laser therapy. *IEEE Journal of Quantum Electronics*. 23 (10): 1703–17.

Karu, T. 1999. Primary and secondary mechanisms of action of visible to near-IR radiation on cells. *Journal of Photochemistry and Photobiology B: Biology*. 49: 1–17.

Karu, T.I. 1998. The science of low-power laser therapy. Amsterdam: Gordon and Breach, p. 226.

Karu, T.I., N.I. Afanasyeva, S.F. Kolyakov, et al. 2001. Changes in absorbance of monolayer living cells induced by laser radiation at 633, 670 and 820nm, IEEE J. Set. Top. *Quantum Electron*. 7: 982–88.

Kovacs, I.B., E. Mester, and P. Görög. 1974. Laser-induced stimulation of the vascularization of the healing wound. An ear chamber experiment. *Cellular and Molecular Life Sciences*. 30 (4): 341–43.

Lane, N. 2006. Cell biology: Power games. *Nature*. 443: 901–3.

Law, D. S. McDonough, C. Bleakley, G.D. Baxter, and S. Tumilty. 2015. Laser acupuncture for treating musculoskeletal pain: A systematic review with meta-analysis. *Journal of Acupuncture and Meridian Studies*. 8 (1): 2–16.

Lingard, A., L.M. Hulten, L. Svensson, et al. 2007. Irradiation at 634nm releases nitric oxide from human monocytes. *Lasers in Medical Science*. 22: 30–36.

Lubart, R., Y. Wollman, H. Friedmann, S. Rochkind, and I. Laulicht. 1992. Effects of visible and near-infrared lasers on cell cultures. *Journal of Photochemistry and Photobiology B: Biology*. 12 (3): 305–10.

Mester, E., B. Szende, and J.G. Tota. 1967. Effect of laser on hair growth of mice. *Kiserl Orvostud*. 19: 628–31.

Ozawa, Y, N. Shimizu, H. Mishima, G. Kariya, M. Yamaguchi, and Takiguchi, H. 1995. Stimulatory effects of low-power laser irradiation on bone formation in vitro. *SPIE Proceeding Series 1984*. Bellingham: 281–88.

Rodrigo, S.M., A. Cunha, D.H. Pozza, et al. 2009. Analysis of the systemic effect of red and infrared laser therapy on wound repair. *Photomedicine and Laser Surgery*. 27 (6): 929–35.

Sarti, P., M. Arese, A. Bacchi, et al. 2003. Nitric oxide and mitochondrial Complex IV. *Life*. 55 (10–11): 605–11.

Shu, B., G.X. Ni, L.Y. Zhang, et al. 2013. High-power helium-neon laser irradiation inhibits the growth of traumatic scars in vitro and vivo. *Lasers in Medical Science*. 28 (3): 693–700.

Shiva, S., and M.T. Gladwin. 2009. Shining a light on tissue NO stores: Far infrared release of NO from nitrite and nitrosylated hemes. *Journal of Molecular and Cellular Cardiology*. 46: 1–3.

Silveira, P.C., E.L. Streck, and R.A. Pinho. 2007. Evaluation of mitochondrial respiratory chain activity in wound healing by low-level laser therapy. *Journal of Photochemistry and Photobiology B: Biology*. 86 (3): 279–82.

Tumilty, S., J. Munn, S. McDonough, et al. 2010. Low level laser treatment of tendinopathy: A systematic review with meta-analysis. *Photomedicine and Laser Surgery*. 28 (1): 3–16.

Van Pelt, W.F. 1970. Laser Fundamentals and Experiments.

Xu, X., X. Zhao, T. Cheng-Yi, et al. 2008. Low-intensity laser irradiation improves the mitochondrial dysfunction of C2C12 induced by electrical stimulation. *Photomedicine and Laser Surgery*. 26 (3): 197–202.

Chapter 15

Abergel, R.P., R.F. Lyons, J.C. Castel, R.M. Dwyer, and J. Uitto. 1987. Biostimulation of wound healing by lasers: Experimental approaches in animal models and in fibroblast cultures. *Journal of Dermatologic Surgery and Oncology*. 13 (2): 127–33.

Alves, A.C., R.D. Viera, E.C. Leal-Junior, et al. 2013. Effect of low-level laser therapy on the expression of inflammatory mediators and on neutrophils and macrophages in acute joint inflammation. *Arthritis Research and Therapy*. 12; 15 (5): R116 (Epub ahead of print).

Baroni, B.M., E.C. Leal-Junior, T. DeMarchi, et al. 2010. Low level laser therapy before eccentric exercise reduces muscle damage markers in humans. *European Journal of Applied Physiology*. 110: 789–96.

Bjordal, J.M., R.A.B. Lopes-Martins, and V.V. Iversen. 2006. A randomized, placebo controlled trial of low-level laser therapy for activated Achilles tendinitis with microdialysis measurement of peritendinous prostaglandin E2 concentrations. *British Journal of Sports Medicine*. 40: 76–80.

Borsa, P.A., K.A. Larkin, and J.M. True. 2013. Does phototherapy enhance skeletal muscle contractile function and postexercise recovery? A systematic review. *Journal of Athletic Training*. 48 (1): 57–67.

Bosatra, M., A. Jucci, P. Olliaro, D. Quacci, and S. Sacchi. 1984. In vitro fibroblast and dermis fibroblast activation by laser irradiation at low energy. *Dermatology*. 168 (4): 157–62.

Choi, J.J., K. Srikantha, and W.H. Wu. 1986. A comparison of electro-acupuncture, transcutaneous electrical nerve stimulation and laser photo-biostimulation on pain relief and glucocorticoid excretion. A case report. *Acupuncture & Electro-Therapeutics Research*. 11 (1): 45–51.

de Morais, N.C., A.M. Barbosa, M.L. Vale, et al. 2010. Anti-inflammatory effect of low-level laser and light-emitting diode in zymosan-induced arthritis. *Photomedicine and Laser Surgery*. 28 (2): 227–32.

Enwemeka, C.S., J.C. Parker, D.S. Dowdy, E.E. Harkness, L.E. Harkness, and L.D. Woodruff. 2004. The efficacy of low-power lasers in tissue repair and pain control: A meta-analysis study. *Photomedicine and Laser Therapy*. 22 (4): 323–29.

Ferraresi, C., M.R. Hamblin, and N.A. Parizotto. 2012. Low-level laser (light) therapy (LLLT) on muscle tissue: Performance, fatigue and repair benefited by the power of light. *Photonics & Lasers in Medicine.* 1 (4): 267–86.

Gomez, I., N. Foundi, D. Longrois, et al. 2013. The role of prostaglandin E2 in human vascular inflammation. *Prostaglandins, Eukotrienes and Essential Fatty Acids.* 89 (2-3): 55–63.

Gum, S., G. Kesava, L. Stehno-Bittel, and C. Enwemeka. 1997. Combined ultrasound, electrical stimulation, and laser promote collagen synthesis with moderate changes in tendon biomechanics. *American Journal of Physical Medicine and Rehabilitation.* 76 (4): 288–96.

Hernandez, L.C., P. Santistaban, and M.E. del Valle Soto. 1989. Changes in mRNA of thyroglobulin, cytoskeleton of thyroid cells, and thyroid hormone levels induced by IR laser irradiation. *Laser Therapy,* 1 (4): 203–8.

Ihsan, F.R. 2005. Low-level laser therapy accelerates collateral circulation and enhances microcirculation. *Photomedicine and Laser Surgery.* 23 (3): 289–94.

Kana, J.S., and G. Hutschenreiter. 1981. Effect of low–power density laser radiation on healing of open skin wounds in rats. *Archives of Surgery.* 116 (3): 293–96.

Kelencz, C.A., I.S. Muñoz, C.F. Amorim, et al. 2010. Effect of low power gallium–aluminum–arsenium noncoherent light (640 nm) on muscle activity: A clinical study. *Photomedicine and Laser Surgery.* 28: 647–52.

Laakso, E.L., T. Cramond, C. Richardson, and J.P. Galligan. 1994. Plasma ACTH and β-endorphin levels in response to low level laser therapy (LLLT) for myofascial trigger points. *Laser Therapy.* 6: 133–42.

Larkin, K.A., J.S. Martin, E.H. Zeanah, et al. 2012. Limb blood flow after class 4 laser therapy. *Journal of Athletic Training.* 47 (2): 178–83.

Leadbetter, W.B. 2001. Soft tissue athletic injury. In F.H. Fu and D.A. Stone (eds.), *Sports injuries: Mechanisms, prevention, treatment.* Baltimore: Lippincott Williams & Wilkins, pp. 839–88.

Leal-Junior, E.C., R.A. Lopes-Martins, B.M. Baroni, et al. 2009. Effect of 830 nm low-level laser therapy applied before high-intensity exercises on skeletal muscle recovery in athletes. *Lasers in Medical Science.* 24: 857–63.

Leal-Junior, E.C., A.A. Vanin, E.F. Miranda, et al. 2013. Effect of phototherapy (low-level laser therapy and light-emitting diode therapy) on exercise performance and markers of exercise recovery: A systematic review with meta-analysis. *Lasers in Medical Science.* Nov 19 [Epub ahead of print].

Lopes-Martins, R.A.B., R. Albertini, P.S.L. Lopes-Martins, et al. 2006. Steroid receptor antagonist mifepristone inhibits the anti-inflammatory effects of photoradiation. *Photomedicine and Laser Surgery.* 24 (2): 197–201.

Maegawa, Y., T. Itoh, T. Hosokawa, K. Yaegashi, and M. Nishi. 2000. Effects of near-infrared low-level laser irradiation on microcirculation. *Lasers in Surgery and Medicine.* 27 (5): 427–37.

Meersman, P. 1999. Laser pharmacology and achilles tendinopathy. *Laser Therapy.* 11 (3): 144–50.

Mester, E., A.F. Mester, and A. Mester. 1985. The biomedical effects of laser application. *Lasers in Surgery and Medicine.* 5 (1): 31–39.

Mester, E., T. Spiry, B. Szende, and Jolan G. Tota. 1971. Effect of laser rays on wound healing. *The American Journal of Surgery.* 122 (4): 532–35

Sakurai, Y., M. Yamaguchi, and Y. Abiko. 2000. Inhibitory effect of low-level laser irradiation on LPS-stimulated prostaglandin E2 production and cyclooxygenase-2 in human gingival fibroblasts. *European Journal of Oral Sciences.* 108: 29–34.

Surinchak, J.S., M.L. Alago, R.F. Bellamy, B.E. Stuck, and M. Belkin. 1983. Effects of low-level energy lasers on the healing of full-thickness skin defects. *Lasers in Surgery and Medicine.* 2 (3): 267–74.

Tume, K., and S. Tume. 1994. *A practitioner's guide to laser therapy and musculoskeletal injuries.* Port Noarlunga South, Australia: Southern Pain Control Centre, pp. 63-77.

Tunér, J., and L. Hode. 1998. It's all in the parameters: A critical analysis of some well-known negative studies on low-level laser therapy. *Journal of Clinical Laser Medicine & Surgery.* 16 (5): 245–48.

Wohlgemuth, W.A., G. Wamser, T. Reiss, T. Wagner, and K. Bohndorf. 2001. In vivo laser-induced interstitial thermotherapy of pig liver with a temperature-controlled diode laser and MRI correlation. *Lasers in Surgery and Medicine.* 29 (4): 374–78.

Woodruff, L.D., J.M. Bounkeo, W.M. Brannon, K.S. Dawes, C.D. Barham, D.L. Waddell, and C.S. Enwemeka. 2004. The efficacy of laser therapy in wound repair: A meta-analysis of the literature. *Photomedicine and Laser Surgery.* 22 (3): 241–47.

Chapter 16

Gillespie, P.G., and R.G. Walker. 2001. Molecular basis of mechanosensory transduction. *Nature.* 413 (6852): 194–202.

Hannigan, G.E., C. Leung-Hagesteijn, L. Fitz-Gibbon, M.G. Coppolino, G. Radeva, J. Filmus, J.C. Bell, and S. Dedhar. 1996. Regulation of cell adhesion and anchorage-dependent growth by a new beta 1-integrin-linked protein kinase. *Nature.* 4; 379 (6560): 91–96.

Ingber, D.E. 1997. Tensegrity: The architectural basis of cellular mechanotransduction. *Annual Review of Physiology.* 59: 575–99.

Kjaer, M. 2004. Role of extracellular matrix in adaptation of tendon and skeletal muscle to mechanical loading. *Physiological Reviews.* 84 (2): 649–98.

Kuhn, K. 1969. The structure of collagen. *Essays in Biochemistry.* 5: 59–87.

Legate, K.R., E. Montañez, O. Kudlacek, and R. Fässler. 2006. ILK, PINCH and parvin: The tIPP of integrin signalling. *Nature Reviews Molecular Cell Biology.* 7 (1): 20–31.

Leong, D.J., Y.H. Li, X.I. Gu, L. Sun, Z. Zhou, P. Nasser, D.M. Laudier, J. Iqbal, R.J. Majeska, M.B. Schaffler, M.B. Goldring, L. Cardoso, M. Zaidi, and H.B. Sun. 2011. Physiological loading of joints prevents cartilage degradation through CITED2. *FASEB Journal.* 25 (1): 182–91.

Maffulli, N., P. Sharma, and K.L. Luscombe. 2004. Achilles tendinopathy: Aetiology and management. *Journal of the Royal Society of Medicine.* 97 (10): 472-76.

Matthews, B.D., D.R. Overby, R. Mannix, and D.E. Ingber. 2006. Cellular adaptation to mechanical stress: Role of integrins, rho, cytoskeletal tension and mechanosensitive ion channels. *Journal of Cell Science.* 119 (Pt 3): 508-18.

Ragsdale, G.K., J. Phelps, and K. Luby-Phelps. 1997. Viscoelastic response of fibroblasts to tension transmitted through adherens junctions. *Biophysical Journal.* 73 (5): 2798-808.

Raizman, I., J.N. De Croos, R. Pilliar, and R.A. Kandel. 2010. Calcium regulates cyclic compression-induced early changes in chondrocytes during in vitro cartilage tissue formation. *Cell Calcium.* 48: 232-42.

Salter, D.M., J.E. Robb, and M.O. Wright. 1997. Electrophysiological responses of human bone cells to mechanical stimulation: Evidence for specific integrin function in mechanotransduction. *Journal of Bone and Mineral Research.* 12: 1133-41.

Scott, A., H. Alfredson, and S. Forsgren. 2008. VGluT2 expression in painful Achilles and patellar tendinosis: Evidence of local glutamate release by tenocytes. *Journal of Orthopaedic Research.* 26 (5): 685-92.

Tidball, J.G. 2005. Mechanical signal transduction in skeletal muscle growth and adaptation. *Journal of Applied Physiology.* 98 (5): 1900-8.

Wang, J.H. 2006. Mechanobiology of tendon. *Journal of Biomechanics.* 39 (9): 1563-82.

Wang, J.H., and B.P. Thampatty. 2006. An introductory review of cell mechanobiology. *Biomechanics and Modeling in Mechanobiology.* 5 (1): 1-16.

Wang, J.H., B.P. Thampatty, J.S. Lin, and H.J. Im. 2007. Mechanoregulation of gene expression in fibroblasts. *Gene.* 391 (1-2): 1-15.

White, C.R., and J.A. Frangos. 2007. The shear stress of it all: The cell membrane and mechanochemical transduction. *Philosophical Transactions of the Royal Society B: Biological Sciences.* 362 (1484): 1459-67.

Wolff, J. 1892. Das Gesetz der Transformation der Knochen. Kirschwald.

Zhang, Y., K. Chen, Y. Tu, A. Velyvis, Y. Yang, J. Qin, and C. Wu. 2002. Assembly of the PINCH-ILK-CH-ILKBP complex precedes and is essential for localization of each component to cell-matrix adhesion sites. *Journal of Cell Science.* 115 (Pt 24): 4777-86.

Chapter 17

Alfredson, H., and J. Cook. 2007. A treatment algorithm for managing Achilles tendinopathy: New treatment options. *British Journal of Sports Medicine.* 41: 211-16.

Alfredson, H., and R. Lorentzon. 2000. Chronic Achilles tendinosis: Recommendations for treatment and prevention. *Sports Medicine.* 29: 135-46.

Biernat, R., Z. Trzaskoma, L. Trzaskoma, and D. Czaprowski. 2014. Rehabilitation protocol for patellar tendinopathy applied among 16- to 19-year old volleyball players. *Journal of Strength and Conditioning Research.* 28 (1): 43-52.

Crane, J.D., D.I. Ogborn, C. Cupido, S. Melov, A. Hubbard, J.M. Bourgeois, and M.A. Tarnopolsky. 2012. Massage therapy attenuates inflammatory signaling after exercise-induced muscle damage. *Science Translational Medicine.* 1 (4): 119.

Cullinane, F.L., M.G. Boocock, and F.C. Trevelyan. 2014. Is eccentric exercise an effective treatment for lateral epicondylitis? A systematic review. *Clinical Rehabilitation.* 28: 3-19.

Cyriax, J. 1984. *Textbook of orthopaedic medicine. Vol 2: Treatment by manipulation, massage and injection.* Philadelphia: Baillière Tindall.

Frost, H.M. 2001. From Wolff's law to the Utah paradigm: Insights about bone physiology and its clinical applications. *Anatomical Record.* 262: 398-419.

Joseph, M.F., K. Taft, M. Moskwa, and C.R. Denegar. 2012. Deep friction massage to treat tendinopathy: A systematic review of a classic treatment in the face of a new paradigm of understanding. *Journal of Sport Rehabilitation.* 21: 343-53.

Kongsgaard, M., K. Qvortrup, J. Larsen, P. Aagaard, S. Doessing, P. Hansen, M. Kjaer, and S.P. Magnusson. 2010. Fibril morphology and tendon mechanical properties in patellar tendinopathy: Effects of heavy slow resistance training. *American Journal of Sports Medicine.* 38 (4): 749-56.

Kraemer, W.J., J.A. Bush, R.B. Wickham, C.R. Denegar, A.L. Gómez, L.A. Gotshalk, N.D. Duncan, J.S. Volek, M. Putukian, and W.J. Sebastianelli. 2001. Influence of compression therapy on symptoms following soft tissue injury from maximal eccentric exercise. *Journal of Orthopaedic and Sports Physical Therapy.* 31: 282-90.

Kraemer, W.J., and N.A. Ratamess. 2004. Fundamentals of resistance training: Progression and exercise prescription. *Medicine & Science in Sports & Exercise.* 36 (4): 674-88.

Macdonald, G.Z., D.C. Button, E.J. Drinkwater, and D.G. Behm. 2014. Foam rolling as a recovery tool after an intense bout of physical activity. *Medicine & Science in Sports & Exercise.* 46 (1): 131-42.

Malliaras, P., C.J. Barton, N.D. Reeves, and H. Langberg. 2013. Achilles and patellar tendinopathy loading programmes: A systematic review comparing clinical outcomes and identifying potential mechanisms for effectiveness. *Sports Medicine.* 43: 267-86.

Silbernagel, K.G., R. Thomeé, P. Thomeé, et al. 2001. Eccentric overload training for patients with chronic Achilles tendon pain—A randomised controlled study with reliability testing of the evaluation methods. *Scandinavian Journal of Medicine and Science in Sports.* 11: 197-206.

Stevens, M., and C.W. Tan. 2014. Effectiveness of the Alfredson protocol compared with a lower repetition-volume protocol for midportion Achilles tendinopathy: A randomized controlled trial. *Journal of Orthopaedic and Sports Physical Therapy.* 44: 59-67.

Stanish, W.D., R.M. Rubinovich, and S. Curwin. 1986. Eccentric exercise in chronic tendinitis. *Clinical Orthopaedics and Related Research*. 208: 65-68.

Tenforde, A.S., L.M. Watanabe, T.J. Moreno, and M. Fredericson. 2012. Use of an antigravity treadmill for rehabilitation of a pelvic stress injury. *PM&R Journal of Injury, Function and Rehabilitation*. 4: 629-31.

Zainuddin, Z., M. Newton, P. Sacco, and K. Nosaka. 2005. Effects of massage on delayed-onset muscle soreness, swelling, and recovery of muscle function. *Journal of Athletic Training*. 40 (3): 174-80.

Chapter 18

Airaksinen, O., K. Partanen, P.J. Kolari, and S. Soimakallio. 1991. Intermittent pneumatic compression therapy in posttraumatic lower limb edema: Computed tomography and clinical measurements. *Archives of Physical Medicine and Rehabilitation*. 72: 667-70.

Assendelft, W.J., S.C. Morton, E.I. Yu, M.J. Suttorp, and P.G. Shekelle. 2003. Spinal manipulative therapy for low back pain. A meta-analysis of effectiveness relative to other therapies. *Annals of Internal Medicine*. 138: 871-81.

Aure, O.F., J. Hoel Nilsen, and O. Vasseljen. 2003. Manual therapy and exercise therapy in patients with chronic low back pain. A randomized, controlled trial with 1-year follow-up. *Spine*. 28: 525-31.

Beurskens, A.J., H.C. de Vet, A.J. Koke, E. Lindeman, W. Regtop, G.J. van der Heijden, and P.G. Knipschild. 1995. Efficacy of traction for non-specific low-back pain: A randomized clinical trial. *Lancet*. 346: 1596-1600.

Beurskens, A.J., H.C. de Vet, A.J. Koke, W. Regtop, G.J. van der Heijden, E. Linderman, and P.G. Knipschild. 1997. Efficacy of traction for non-specific low back pain. 12 week and 6 month results of a randomized clinical trial. *Spine*. 22: 2756-62.

Blackburn, P.G., L.R. Simons, and K.M. Crossley. 1998. Treatment of chronic exertional anterior compartment syndrome with massage: A pilot study. *Clinical Journal of Sports Medicine*. 8: 14-17.

Bronfort, G., W.J. Assendelft, R. Evans, M. Haas, and L. Bouter. 2001. Efficacy of spinal manipulation for chronic headache: A systematic review. *Journal of Manipulative & Physiological Therapeutics*. 24: 457-66.

Castien, R.F., D.A van der Windt, A. Grooten, and J. Dekker. 2011. Effectiveness of manual therapy for chronic tension-type headache: A pragmatic, randomised, clinical trial. *Cephalalgia*. 31: 133-43.

Clarke, J.A., N.W. van Tulder, S.E. Blomberg, H.C. de Vet, G.J. van der Heijden, and G. Bronfort. Traction for low-back pain with or without sciatica. *Cochrane Database Systematic Reviews*. 2005, Oct 19; (4): CD003010. Review. Update in: *Cochrane Database Systematic Reviews*. 2007; (2): CD003010.

Colachis, S.C., and B.R. Strohan. 1965. Cervical traction relationship of time to varied tractive force with constant angle of pull. *Arch Phys Med Rehabil*. 46: 815-819.

Colachis, S.C., and B.R. Strohan. 1969. Effects of intermittent traction on separation of lumbar vertebrae. *Archives of Physical Medicine and Rehabilitation*. 50: 251-58.

Conroy, D.E. and K.W. Hayes. 1998. The effect of joint mobilization as a component of comprehensive treatment for primary shoulder impingement syndrome. *Journal of Orthopaedic and Sports Physical Therapy*. 28: 3-14.

Constantoyannis, C., D. Konstantinou, H. Kourtopoulos, and N. Papadakis. 2002. Intermittent cervical traction for cervical radiculopathy caused by large-volume herniated disks. *Journal of Manipulative & Physiological Therapeutics* 25: 188-92.

Cyriax, J. 1984. *Textbook of orthopaedic medicine*. Vol. 2: *Treatment by manipulation, massage and injection*. Philadelphia: Baillie Tindal, p. l.

Denegar, C.R., J. Hertel, and J. Fonseca. 2002. The effect of lateral ankle sprain on dorsiflexion range of motion, posterior talar glide, and joint laxity. *Journal of Orthopaedic and Sports Physical Therapy*. 32: 16-73.

Escortell-Mayor, E., R. Riesgo-Fuertes, S. Garrido-Elustondo, A. Asunsolo-del Barco, B. Diaz-Pulido, M. Blanco-Diaz, and E. Bejerano-Alvarez. 2011. Primary care randomized clinical trial: Manual therapy effectiveness in comparison with TENS in patients with neck pain. *Manual Therapy*. 16 (1): 66-73.

Ferreira, M., P. Ferreira, J. Latimer, R. Herbert, and C.G. Maher. 2002. Does spinal manipulative therapy help people with chronic low back pain? *Australian Journal of Physiotherapy*. 48: 277-84.

Fond, D. and B. Hecox. 1994. Intermittent pneumatic compression. In B. Hecox, T.A. Mehreteab, and J. Weisberg (eds.), *Physical agents*. Norwalk, CT: Appleton & Lange, pp. 419-428.

Fritz, J.M., W. Lindsay, J.W. Matheson, G.P. Brennan, S.J. Hunter, S.D. Moffit, A. Swalberg, and B. Rodriquez. 2007. Is there a subgroup of patients with low back pain likely to benefit from mechanical traction? Results of a randomized clinical trial and subgrouping analysis. *Spine*. 32 (26): E793-800.

Furlan, A.D., L. Brosseau, M. Imamura, and E. Irvin. 2002. *Massage for low back pain*. Cochrane Library. 2.

Furlan, A.D., L. Brosseau, M. Imamura, and E. Irvin. *Massage for low back pain*. Abstract www.cochrane.org/reviews/en/ab001929.html. Accessed Aug. 4, 2009.

Gonzales-Iglesias, J., C. Fernandez-de-las-Penas, J.A. Cleland, F. Alburquerque-Sendin, L. Palomeque-del-Cerro, and R. Mendez-Sanchez. 2009. Inclusion of thoracic spine thrust manipulation into an electrotherapy/thermal program for the management of patients with acute mechanical neck pain: A randomized clinical trial. *Manual Therapy*. 14 (3): 306-13.

Green, T., K. Refshauge, J. Crosbie, and R. Adams. 2002. A randomized controlled trial of passive accessory joint mobilization on acute ankle inversion sprains. *Physical Therapy*. 81: 984-94.

Griffin, J.W., L.S. Newsome, S.W. Stralka, and P.E. Wright. 1990. Reduction of chronic posttraumatic hand edema: A comparison of high voltage pulsed current, intermittent pneumatic compression, and placebo treatments. *Physical Therapy* 70: 279–86.

Hernandez-Reif, M., T. Field, J. Krasnegor, and H. Theakston. 2001. Lower back pain is reduced and range of motion increased after massage therapy. *International Journal of Neuroscience.* 106: 131–45.

Hooker, D. 1998. Intermittent compression devices. In W.E. Prentice (ed.), *Therapeutic modalities for allied health professionals.* New York: Mcgraw-Hill, pp. 392–403.

Houglum, P.A. 2010. *Therapeutic exercise for musculoskeletal injuries.* 3rd ed. Champaign, IL: Human Kinetics.

Hsieh, C.Y., A.H. Adams, J. Tobis, C.Z. Hong, C. Danielson, K. Platt, F. Hoehler, S. Reinsch, and A. Rubel. 2002. Effectiveness of four conservative treatments for subacute low back pain. A randomized clinical trial. *Spine.* 27: 1142–48.

Hurwitz, E.L., H. Morgenstern, P. Harber, G.F. Kominski, T.R. Belin, F. Yu, and A.H. Adams. 2002. A randomized trial of medical care with and without physical therapy and chiropractic care with and without physical modalities for patients with low back pain: 6 month follow-up outcomes from the UCLA Low Back Pain Study. *Spine.* 27: 2193–2204.

Hurwitz E.L., E.J. Carragee, G. van der Velde, L.J. Carroll, M. Nordin, J. Guzman, P.M. Peloso, L.W. Holm, P. Côté, S. Hogg-Johnson, J.D. Cassidy, and S. Haldeman. 2009. Treatment of neck pain: Noninvasive interventions: Results of the Bone and Joint Decade 2000–2010 Task Force on Neck Pain and Its Associated Disorders. *Journal of Manipulative & Physiological Therapeutics.* 32 (2 Suppl): S141–75.

Jones, L.H., R. Kusunose, and E. Goering. 1995. *Jones Strain-Counterstrain.* Boise, ID: Jones Strain-Counterstrain.

Joseph, M.J., K. Costanzo, M. Moskwa, and C.R. Denegar. 2012. Deep friction massage for the treatment of tendinopathy: A systematic review of a classic treatment in the face of a new paradigm of understanding. *Journal of Sport Rehabilitation.* 21: 343–53.

Klaber-Moffett, J.A., G.I. Hughes, and P. Griffiths. 1990. An investigation of the effects of cervical traction. Part 1: Clinical effectiveness. *Clinical Rehabilitation.* 4: 205–11.

Kumar, S., K. Beaton, and T. Hughes. 2013. The effectiveness of massage therapy for the treatment of nonspecific low back pain: A systematic review of systematic reviews. *International Journal of General Medicine.* 4 (6): 733–41.

Lin, C.W., A.M. Moseley, M. Haas, K.M. Refshauge, and R.D. Herbert. 2008. Manual therapy in addition to physiotherapy does not improve clinical or economic outcomes after ankle fracture. *Journal of Rehabilitation Medicine.* 40: 433–39.

Meszaros, T.F., R. Olson, K. Kulig, D. Creighton, and E. Czarnecki. 2000. Effect of 10%, 30% and 60% body weight traction on straight leg raise test of symptomatic patients with low back pain. *Journal of Orthopaedic and Sports Physical Therapy.* 30: 595–601.

Mitchinson, A.R., H.M. Kim, J.M. Rosenberg, M. Geisser, M. Kirsh, D. Cikrit, and D.B. Hinshaw. 2007. Acute postoperative pain management using massage as an adjuvant therapy: A randomized trial. *Archives of Surgery.* 142: 1158–67.

Moeti, P., and G. Marchetti. 2001. Clinical outcome from mechanical intermittant cervical traction for the treatment of cervical radiculopathy: A case series. *Journal of Orthopaedic and Sports Physical Therapy.* 31: 527–38.

Moraska, A., C. Chandler, A. Edmiston-Schaetzel, G. Franklin, E.L. Calenda, and B. Enebo. 2008. Comparison of a targeted and general massage protocol on strength, function, and symptoms associated with carpal tunnel syndrome: A randomized pilot study. *Journal of Alternative and Complementary Medicine.* 14: 259–67.

Pal, B., P. Mangion, M.A. Hossain, and B.L. Diffey. 1986. A controlled trial of continuous lumbar traction in treatment of back pain and sciatica. *British Journal of Rheumatology.* 25:181–83.

Perlman, A.I., A. Sabina, A.L. Williams, V.Y. Njike, and D.L. Katz. 2006. Massage therapy for osteoarthritis of the knee: A randomized controlled trial. *Archives of Internal Medicine.* 166: 2533–38.

Preyde, M. 2000. Effectiveness of massage therapy for subacute low-back pain: A randomized controlled trial. *Canadian Medical Association Journal.* 162: 1815–20.

Quinn, C., C. Chandler, and A. Moraska. 2002. Massage therapy and frequency of chronic tension headaches. *American Journal of Public Health.* 92: 1657–61.

Rucinski, T.J., D.N. Hooker, W.E. Prentice, Jr., E.X. Shields, Jr., and D.J. Cote-Murray. 1991. The effects of intermittent compression on edema in postacute ankle sprains. *Journal of Orthopaedic and Sports Physical Therapy.* 14: 65–69.

Schiller, L. 2001. Effectiveness of spinal manipulative therapy in the treatment of mechanical thoracic spine pain. A pilot randomized clinical trial. *Journal of Manipulative & Physiological Therapeutics.* 24: 394–401.

Stockle, U., R. Hoffmann, M. Schultz, C. von Fournier, N.P. Sudkamp, and N. Haas. 1997. Fastest reduction of posttraumatic edema: Continuous cryotherapy or intermittent impulse compression? *Foot and Ankle International.* 18: 432–38.

Sucher, B.M. 1993. Myofascial manipulative release of carpal tunnel syndrome: Documentation with magnetic resonance imaging. *Journal of the American Osteopathic Association.* 93: 1273–78.

Swezey, R.L., A.M. Swezey, and K. Warner. 1999. Efficacy of home traction therapy. *American Journal of Physical Medicine & Rehabilitation.* 78: 30–32.

Tsang, K.K., J. Hertel, and C.R. Denegar. 2003. Volume decreases after elevation and intermittent compression of postacute ankle sprains are negated by gravity-dependent positioning. *Journal of Athletic Training.* 38 (4): 320–24.

Tsang, K.K.W., J.H. Hertel, C.R. Denegar, and W.E. Buckley. 2001. The effects of elevation and intermittent compression on the volume of injured ankles (Abstract). *Journal of Athletic Training.* 36: S-50.

Van der Heijden, G.J.M., A.J.H. Beurskens, M.J.M. Dirx, L.M. Bouter, and E. Lindeman. 1995. Efficacy of lumbar traction. A randomized clinical trial. *Physiotherapy.* 81: 29–35.

Vincent, K., J.Y. Maigne, C. Fischhoff, O. Lanlo, and S. Dagenais. 2013. Systematic review of manual therapies for nonspecific neck pain. *Joint Bone Spine.* 80: 508–15.

Zylbergold, R.S., and M.C. Piper. 1985. Cervical spine disorders. A comparison of three types of traction. *Spine.* 10: 867-71.

Chapter 19

Abate M. 2014. How obesity modifies tendons (implications for athletic activities). *Muscles, Ligaments, and Tendons Journal.* 4 (3): 298-302.

Alfredson H., T. Pietila, P. Jonsson, and R. Lorentzon. 1998. Heavy-load eccentric calf muscle training for the treatment of chronic Achilles tendinosis. *American Journal of Sports Medicine.* 26: 360-66.

Bjordal, J.M., R.A.B. Lopes-Martins, and V.V. Iversen. 2006. A randomised, placebo controlled trial of low level laser therapy for activated Achilles tendinitis with microdialysis measurement of peritendinous prostaglandin E$_2$ concentrations. *British Journal of Sports Medicine.* 40 (1): 76-80.

Cakir, S., S. Hepguler, C. Ozturk, M. Korkmaz, B. Isleten, and F.C. Atamaz. 2014. Efficacy of therapeutic ultrasound for the management of knee osteoarthritis: A randomized, controlled, and double-blind study. *American Journal of Physical Medicine & Rehabilitation.* 93: 405-12.

Cetin, N., A. Aytar, A. Atalay, and M.N. Akman. 2008. Comparing hot pack, short-wave diathermy, ultrasound, and TENS on isokinetic strength, pain, and functional status of women with osteoarthritic knees: A single-blind, randomized, controlled trial. *American Journal of Physical Medicine & Rehabilitation.* 87: 443-51.

Cook, J.L., and C.R. Purdam. 2009. Is tendon pathology a continuum? A pathology model to explain the clinical presentation of load-induced tendinopathy. *British Journal of Sports Medicine.* 43: 409-16.

Denegar, C.R., D.R. Dougherty, J.E. Friedman, M.E. Schmizzi, J.E. Clark, B.A. Comstock, and W.J. Kraemer. 2010. Preferences for heat, cold or contrast in patients with knee osteoarthritis affect treatment response. *Journal of Clinical Interventions in Aging.* 5: 199-206.

Draper, D.O. 2010. Ultrasound and joint mobilizations for achieving normal wrist range of motion after injury or surgery: A case series. *Journal of Athletic Training.* 45: 486-91.

Draper, D.O. 2014. Pulsed shortwave diathermy and joint mobilizations for achieving normal elbow range of motion after injury or surgery with implanted metal: A case series. *Journal of Athletic Training.* 49: 851-55.

Fitzgerald, G.K., S.R. Piva, and J.J. Irrgang. 2003. A modified neuromuscular electrical stimulation protocol for quadriceps strength training following anterior cruciate ligament reconstruction. *Journal of Orthopaedic & Sports Physical Therapy.* 33.9: 492-501.

Kearney, R., and M.L. Costa. 2010. Insertional Achilles tendinopathy management: A systematic review. *Foot & Ankle International.* 31: 689-94.

Mafi, N., R. Lorentzon, and H. Alfredson. 2001. Superior short-term results with eccentric calf muscle training compared to concentric training in a randomized prospective multicenter study on patients with chronic Achilles tendinosis. *Knee Surgery, Sports Traumatology, Arthroscopy.* 9: 42-47.

McCreesh, K., and J. Lewis. 2013. Continuum model of tendon pathology—where are we now? *International Journal of Experimental Pathology.* 94: 242-47.

Oncel, M., S. Sencan, H. Yildiz, and N. Kurt. Transcutaneous electrical nerve stimulation for pain management in patients with uncomplicated minor rib fractures. *European Journal of Cardio-Thoracic Surgery.* 22.1: 13-17.

Porcheret, M., K. Jordan, C. Jinks, and P. Croft. 2007. Primary care treatment of knee pain: A survey in older adults. *Rheumatology.* 46: 1694-1700.

Rompe, J.D., B. Nafe, J.P. Furia. 2007. Eccentric loading, shockwave treatment, or a wait-and-see policy for tendinopathy of the main body of tendo Achillis: A randomized controlled trial. *American Journal of Sports Medicine.* 35: 374-83.

Ulus, Y., B. Tander, Y. Akyol, D. Durmus, O. Buyukakıncak, U. Gul, F. Canturk, A. Bilgici, and O. Kuru. 2012. Therapeutic ultrasound versus sham ultrasound for the management of patients with knee osteoarthritis: A randomized double-blind controlled clinical study. *International Journal of Rheumatic Diseases.* 15: 197-206.

van der Worp, H., I. van den Akker-Scheek, H. van Schie, and J. Zwerver. 2013. ESWT for tendinopathy: Technology and clinical implications. *Knee Surgery, Sports Traumatology, Arthroscopy.* 21: 1451-58.

Index

About the Authors

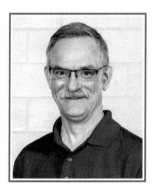

Craig R. Denegar, PhD, PT, ATC, FNATA, is a professor in the department of kinesiology and director of the doctor of physical therapy program at the University of Connecticut. He has more than 30 years of experience as an athletic trainer and physical therapist and has extensive clinical practice experience related to persistent orthopedic pain.

Denegar is a member of the National Athletic Trainers' Association (NATA) and the American Physical Therapy Association. He is editor in chief of the *Journal of Athletic Training* and serves on the editorial boards of the *Journal of Sport Rehabilitation*, *Journal of Strength and Conditioning Research*, and *Open Access Journal of Sport Medicine*. He is the former vice chair of free communications on the NATA Research and Education Foundation's Research Committee and was the 2003 recipient of the William G. Clancy Medal for Distinguished Athletic Training Research and the 2004 Distinguished Merit Award from the Pennsylvania Athletic Trainers' Society. Denegar was elected a fellow of the NATA in 2011 and recognized as a Most Distinguished Athletic Trainer by the NATA in 2014.

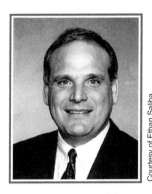

Courtesy of Ethan Saliba

Ethan Saliba, PhD, ATC, PT, has been teaching therapeutic modalities at the University of Virginia at Charlottesville for over 25 years. He is the head athletic trainer and associate athletics director for sports medicine, and he oversees 25 varsity sports. Saliba is a certified athletic trainer, licensed physical therapist, and sport-certified specialist who has written extensively on various aspects of athletic injuries and rehabilitation. Saliba was honored as the NATA Head Athletic Trainer of the Year in 2007.

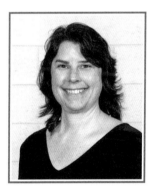

Susan Foreman Saliba, PhD, ATC, PT, is an associate professor in the Curry School of Education at the University of Virginia at Charlottesville. She has over 20 years of clinical experience and taught therapeutic modalities during that time. Susan is a member of both the NATA and the American Physical Therapy Association (APTA) and has served on the NATA Educational Executive Committee and the Free Communications Committee of the NATA Research and Education Foundation. She is conducting research on the clinical application of therapeutic modalities.

About the Contributors

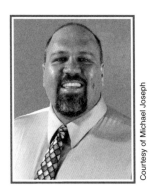

Courtesy of Michael Joseph

Michael Joseph, PhD, PT, is an assistant professor in the department of kinesiology physical therapy program at the University of Connecticut. Joseph has more than 15 years of clinical experience as a physical therapist specializing in sports medicine and is a consultant for many professional and collegiate teams. He is a member of the American Physical Therapy Association and is on the editorial board of the *Journal of Strength and Conditioning Research* and the *World Journal of Orthopedics*. Joseph teaches clinical and musculoskeletal pathology, mechanobiology, and musculoskeletal evaluation and treatment. His focus of research is the adaptation of connective tissue to physiological loading.

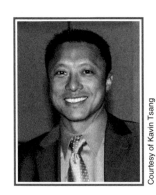

Courtesy of Kavin Tsang

Kavin Tsang, PhD, ATC, is an associate professor in the department of kinesiology at California State University at Fullerton. He is an active member of the National Athletic Trainers' Association (NATA) and an athletic trainer certified by the Board of Certification. His clinical experiences encompass physical therapy clinics, high school athletics, collegiate intramural programs, and intercollegiate athletics. He has been teaching therapeutic modalities in various athletic training education curricula for over 14 years. Tsang serves on the NATA Research and Education Foundation (NATA REF) Board of Directors, NATA REF Free Communications Committee, NATA Convention Program Committee, and Far West Athletic Trainers' Association (FWATA) Education Program Committee. He is also chair of the FWATA Research and Grants Committee.